Nanoparticle Enhanced Radiation Therapy

Principles, methods and applications

IOP Series in Global Health and Radiation Oncology

Series editor
Wilfred Ngwa
Dana Farber/Harvard Cancer Center and University of Massachusetts, Lowell, MA, USA

Editor biography
Wilfred Ngwa is the Director of the Global Health Catalyst program at Dana Farber/Harvard Cancer Center and a professor of radiation oncology and faculty medical physicist at Harvard Medical School and the University of Massachusetts. He also currently holds an international guest professorship at the University of Heidelberg, Germany. He has published two books and won several awards and prizes, including the 2015 BRIght Futures Prize for innovative new technology designed for use during radiotherapy to kill cancer cells that have spread to other parts of the body.

Aims and scope
This series will include books in the emerging area of global radiation oncology and its applications in global health. Stemming from the published book by the series editor entitled *Emerging Models for Global Health in Radiation Oncology*, it will further detail the work being done globally to promote cancer research and awareness, particularly in lower income countries.

Nanoparticle Enhanced Radiation Therapy

Principles, methods and applications

Edited by

Erno Sajo
University of Massachusetts, Lowell, MA, USA

Piotr Zygmanski
Brigham and Women's Hospital, Boston, MA, USA

IOP Publishing, Bristol, UK

ISBN 978-0-7503-2396-3 (ebook)
ISBN 978-0-7503-2394-9 (print)
ISBN 978-0-7503-2397-0 (myPrint)
ISBN 978-0-7503-2395-6 (mobi)

DOI 10.1088/978-0-7503-2396-3

Version: 20201101

IOP ebooks

British Library Cataloguing-in-Publication Data: A catalogue record for this book is available from the British Library.

Published by IOP Publishing, wholly owned by The Institute of Physics, London

IOP Publishing, Temple Circus, Temple Way, Bristol, BS1 6HG, UK

US Office: IOP Publishing, Inc., 190 North Independence Mall West, Suite 601, Philadelphia, PA 19106, USA

Contents

Editor biographies xii

Contributors xiii

Introduction xvi

Part I Radiosensitization and fundamentals

1 The role of Auger electrons versus photoelectrons in nanoparticle dose enhancement 1-1

Erno Sajo and Piotr Zygmanski

1.1 Fundamentals of the Auger process 1-1
1.2 The role of fluorescent photons 1-4
1.3 The contribution of Auger electrons and photoelectrons to dose 1-5
1.4 Angular anisotropy of electron emission from the GNP 1-9
1.5 Conclusions 1-12
References 1-13

2 Deterministic computation benchmarks of nanoparticle dose enhancement—part I. Nanometer scales 2-1

Erno Sajo, Fulya Cifter and Piotr Zygmanski

2.1 Perspectives 2-1
2.2 The radiation transport basis of high-*Z* nanoparticle dose enhancement by x-rays 2-1
2.3 Deterministic radiation transport computations 2-4
2.4 The Green's function of dose enhancement 2-6
2.5 Maximum and spatially averaged dose enhancement ratios 2-7
2.6 The optimal incident photon energy 2-10
2.7 Discussion 2-14
2.8 Conclusions 2-19
2.9 Appendix 2-20
References 2-22

3 Deterministic computation benchmarks of nanoparticle dose enhancement—part II. Microscopic to macroscopic scales 3-1

Erno Sajo, Fulya Cifter and Piotr Zygmanski

3.1 The effect of concentration distributions 3-1

3.2 Radiation transport computations 3-2
3.2.1 Case-1 geometries 3-2
3.2.2 Case-2 geometries 3-4
3.3 Macroscopic DER effects in case-1 geometries 3-5
3.3.1 Dependence on concentration in a fixed tumor volume 3-5
3.3.2 Depth and volume dependence for diffusion in one direction 3-6
3.3.3 Depth and volume dependence for diffusion in two directions 3-7
3.3.4 Kerma approximation of dose 3-8
3.3.5 The effective distance of dose enhancement 3-9
3.4 Microscopic effects in case-2 geometries—the inadequacy of spatial homogenization 3-11
3.5 Discussion 3-12
3.6 Conclusions 3-14
References 3-15

4 Mechanisms of low energy electron interactions with biomolecules: relationship to gold nanoparticle radiosensitization 4-1

Yi Zheng and Léon Sanche

4.1 Introduction 4-1
4.1.1 Gold nanoparticle (GNP) radiosensitization 4-1
4.1.2 Primary mechanisms 4-2
4.1.3 Biological damage induced by low energy electrons (LEEs) 4-4
4.2 Interaction of LEEs with condensed-phase biomolecules 4-6
4.2.1 Basic principles of interaction of LEEs with molecules 4-6
4.2.2 Transient molecular anions (TMAs) and their decay channels 4-8
4.2.3 Modification of electron capture and decay of transient anions in biological media 4-8
4.2.4 Short range and high damage efficiency of LEEs 4-10
4.3 Interaction of LEEs with water and DNA 4-11
4.3.1 LEE interaction with water and the indirect effect of radiation 4-11
4.3.2 Mechanisms of LEE-induced DNA and cellular damage 4-14
4.3.3 DNA damage from GNP-generated LEEs and LEE-bombarded GNP–DNA complexes 4-17
4.4 Conclusions and future trends 4-19
4.5 Abbreviations 4-20
Acknowledgments 4-20
References 4-20

5 Monte Carlo models of electron transport for dose-enhancement calculations in nanoparticle-aided radiotherapy **5-1**
Dimitris Emfietzoglou and Sebastien Incerti

5.1 Introduction 5-1
5.2 The challenge 5-4
5.3 Monte Carlo simulation of electron transport 5-5
5.4 Condensed-history models (class I code) 5-6
5.5 Mixed condensed-history models (class II codes) 5-10
5.6 The case of PENELOPE and Geant4 5-11
5.7 Role of condensed-history simulation in NRT 5-14
5.8 Track-structure models 5-15
5.9 Track-structure models for water 5-16
5.10 Track-structure codes for non-aqueous media 5-22
5.11 The case of TRAX and Geant4-DNA 5-24
5.12 Surface effects 5-25
5.13 Role of TS models in NRT 5-26
5.14 Monte Carlo codes in NRT 5-26
References 5-30

6 Nanoparticle-aided radiation therapy: challenges of treatment planning **6-1**
C Kirkby and B Koger

6.1 Introduction 6-1
6.2 Nature of energy absorption near high-*Z* NPs 6-3
6.3 Uptake and dispersion prediction of NPs 6-10
6.4 Nanoparticle distribution within tissues and organs 6-10
6.5 Determination of NP concentrations on the macroscopic scale 6-11
6.6 Cellular internalization 6-13
6.7 Dosimetry in the presence of NPs 6-13
6.8 NPRT dosimetry on the macroscopic scale 6-15
6.9 NPRT dosimetry on the microscopic scale 6-19
6.10 Challenges to modelling biological response 6-22
6.11 Further evidence for an NP-induced biological effect 6-23
6.12 Conclusions and a look forward 6-24
References 6-25

7 Nanoparticle enhanced radiotherapy: quality assurance perspective **7-1**
Piotr Zygmanski, Davide Brivio and Erno Sajo

7.1 General 7-1
7.2 Imaging and verification of NP distribution 7-2
7.3 Macroscopic dose calculation 7-5
7.4 Radiobiological effect from macroscopic dose enhancement 7-6
7.5 Microscopic dose calculation 7-7
7.6 Radiobiological effect from microscopic dose enhancement 7-7
7.7 Summary 7-8
7.8 Experimental/computation setup 7-8
7.9 Benchmark and validation tests and data 7-9
References 7-11

8 Optimal nanoparticle concentrations, toxicity and safety and gold nanoparticle design for radiation therapy applications **8-1**
Rajiv Kumar and Wilfred Ngwa

8.1 Introduction 8-1
8.2 Biomedical applications of gold nanoparticles 8-2
8.3 Gold nanoparticles are effective, biocompatible tumor-targeting nanocarriers 8-2
8.4 Gold nanoparticles in radiation therapy 8-3
8.5 Challenges of GNP radiotherapy 8-3
8.6 Design considerations for optimal radiosensitization using GNPs 8-4
8.7 Size and concentration/dose of GNPs 8-4
8.8 Surface charge and multi-functionalities of GNPs 8-5
8.9 Toxicity and safety associated with GNP-based radiotherapy 8-7
8.10 AuRad platform 8-7
8.11 AuRad Platform targeting tumor vasculature 8-9
8.12 AuRad platform tumor vasculature disruption 8-9
8.13 Summary 8-11
References 8-11

9 Translational nanomaterials for cancer radiation therapy **9-1**
Shady Kotb and Sijumon Kunjachan

9.1 Introduction 9-1
9.1.1 Silica-based nanoparticles 9-1
9.1.2 Superparamagnetic iron oxide nanoparticles (SPIONs) 9-2
9.1.3 Quantum dots (QDs) 9-2

9.2 High-Z metals and radiosensitization 9-2
9.2.1 Platinum nanoparticles 9-3
9.2.2 Gold nanoparticles 9-3
9.2.3 Hafnium oxide nanoparticles 9-4
9.3 Theranostics nanoparticles 9-5
9.3.1 Gadolinium nanoparticles 9-5
9.3.2 Bismuth complexes and nanoparticles 9-6
9.4 Mechanism of action 9-7
9.5 Bystander effect 9-7
References 9-8

10 Gold nanoparticle enhanced radiosensitivity of cells: considerations and contradictions from model systems and basic investigations of cell damaging for radiation therapy 10-1
Martin Falk, Michael Wolinsky, Marlon R Veldwijk, Georg Hildenbrand and Michael Hausmann

10.1 Cell viability upon cell irradiation in the presence of nanoparticles—colony formation assay (CFA) 10-5
10.2 DNA damage upon cell irradiation in the presence of nanoparticles—super-resolution microscopic analysis of γH2AX foci 10-7
10.3 Nanoparticle-mediated radio-sensitization of tumor cells independent of nuclear DNA damage 10-11
10.4 Conclusions 10-13
10.5 Materials and methods 10-15
10.5.1 Cell culture, gold nanoparticle incorporation, and specimen irradiation 10-15
10.5.2 Clonogenic assay (colony forming assay) 10-16
10.5.3 γH2AX immunostaining 10-17
10.5.4 Single molecule localization microscopy 10-17
Acknowledgement 10-18
References 10-18

Part II Imaging

11 Super-resolution microscopy of nanogold-labelling 11-1
Michael Hausmann, Götz Pilarczyk, Emanuel Maus, Jürgen Hesser and Georg Hildenbrand

11.1 Electron microscopy 11-1

11.2 Light microscopy and localization microscopy 11-3
Acknowledgments 11-7
References 11-7

12 X-ray based nanoparticle imaging **12-1**
Juergen Hesser and Davide Brivio

12.1 Computed tomography (CT) 12-1
12.2 Dual- and multi-energy CT (DECT, MECT) 12-8
12.3 X-ray fluorescence computed tomography (XFCT) 12-12
12.4 SPECT/PET 12-14
References 12-15

13 MRI based nanoparticle imaging **13-1**
Frank G Zöllner

References 13-9

14 Nanoparticle detection using photoacoustic imaging (PAI) **14-1**
Romy Mueller, Wilfred Ngwa and Juergen Hesser

References 14-5

Part III Applications

15 Radiotherapy application with *in situ* dose-painting (RAiD) via inhalation delivery **15-1**
Yao Hao

15.1 Introduction 15-1
15.2 Materials and methods 15-2
15.3 Results 15-4
15.4 Discussion 15-6
15.5 Conclusion 15-7
Acknowledgments 15-7
References 15-7

16 High-*Z* ORAYA therapy for wet AMD and ocular cancers **16-1**
Yucel Altundal and Wilfred Ngwa

16.1 Introduction 16-1
16.2 Materials and methods 16-2

16.3 Results 16-5
16.4 Discussion 16-6
References 16-7

17 Cerium oxide and titanium dioxide 17-1
Zi Ouyang and Wilfred Ngwa

17.1 Introduction 17-1
17.2 CONP mediated ROS scavenging 17-2
17.3 TONP aided radiation sensitization 17-3
17.4 Discussion 17-4
References 17-5

18 Accelerated Partial Breast Irradiation (APBI) 18-1
Gizem Cifter and Wilfred Ngwa

18.1 Methods 18-2
18.2 Results 18-5
18.3 Discussion 18-8
18.4 Conclusion 18-10
References 18-10

Editor biographies

Erno Sajo

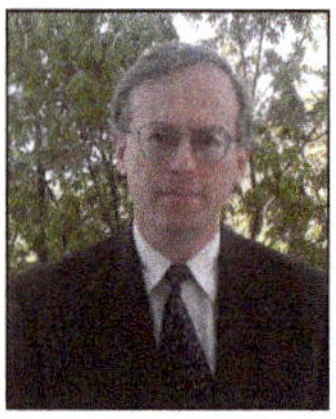

Erno Sajo, PhD, is a Professor and Director of Medical Physics at the University of Massachusetts Lowell where he also serves as the Director of Biomedical Engineering and Biotechnology. He has an MS degree in Mechanical and Nuclear Engineering from the Technical University of Budapest, and a PhD in Physics from Lowell. Prior to this position, he was a faculty member at Louisiana State University, Baton Rouge. His research areas are radiation transport computations at the nanoscale with emphasis on interfacial effects, including nanoparticle transport, the physiological translocation of nanoparticles, and nanoparticle-enhanced radiation therapy. Dr Sajo has nearly two hundred scientific publications in physics, biophysics and nuclear sciences. He is an associate editor of the *Health Physics Journal* and has also served as ad-hoc editor of *Medical Physics*.

Piotr Zygmanski

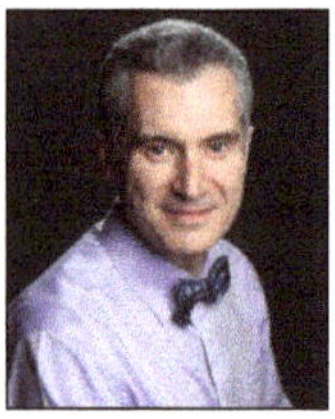

Piotr Zygmanski, PhD, is Associate Professor of Radiation Oncology at the Harvard Medical School and Medical Physicist at the Brigham and Women's Hospital/Dana Farber Cancer Institute, Boston, Massachusetts. He has an MSc degree in Applied Physics and Mathematics and a PhD in Physics. Prior to his present position he acquired his clinical training at the Massachusetts General Hospital, Boston, and the Harvard Cyclotron Laboratory, Cambridge, Massachusetts. His research interests include multiscale radiation transport computations, detection of radiation and mathematical modeling for the standard and nanoparticle-enhanced radiotherapy.

Contributors

Yücel Altundal
Flushing Radiation Oncology Services,
Flushing, USA

Davide Brivio
Brigham and Women's Hospital,
Dana Farber Cancer Institute,
Harvard Medical School, Boston, Massachussetts, USA

Fulya Cifter
Precess Medical Derivatives, Inc., Short Hills, NJ, USA

Gizem Cifter
Rush University Medical Center,
Chicago, Illinois, USA

Dimitris Emfietzoglou
University of Ioannina Medical Physics Laboratory, University of Ioannina Medical School, Ioannina, Greece

Martin Falk
Institute of Biophysics of the CAS,
Brno, Czech Republic

Yao Hao
Washington University in St. Louis
St Louis, Missouri, USA

Michael Hausmann
Kirchhoff-Institute for Physics,
Heidelberg University, Heidelberg, Germany

Jürgen Hesser
Department of Radiation Oncology,
Universitätsmedizin Mannheim, Mannheim, Germany

Georg Hildenbrand
Kirchhoff-Institute for Physics,
Heidelberg University, Heidelberg, Germany

Sebastien Incerti
Université de Bordeaux,
Centre d'Études Nucléaires de Bordeaux, Gradignan, France

Charles Kirkby
University of Calgary, Department of Medical Physics, Jack Ady Cancer Centre,
Lethbridge, Alberta, Canada

Brandon Koger
University of Pennsylvania,
Department of Radiation Oncology,
Philadelphia, USA

Shady Kotb
Department of Radiation Oncology, Brigham and Women's Hospital,
Dana Farber Cancer Institute, Harvard Medical School,
Boston, Massachussetts, USA

Rajiv Kumar
Nanomedicine Science and Technology Center,
Northeastern University, Boston, Massachusetts, USA

Sijumon Kunjachan
Department of Radiation Oncology,
Brigham and Women's Hospital,
Dana-Farber Cancer Institute and Harvard Medical School,
Boston, Massachussetts, USA

Emanuel Maus
Kirchhoff-Institute for Physics,
Heidelberg University, Heidelberg, Germany

Romy Mueller
Brigham and Women's Hospital, Dana Farber Cancer Institute, Harvard Medical School, Boston, Massachussetts, USA

Wilfred Ngwa
Brigham and Women's Hospital, Dana Farber Cancer Institute,
Harvard Medical School, Boston, Massachussetts, USA

Zi Ouyang
Department of Radiation Oncology,
University Hospitals Seidman Cancer Center,
Cleveland, Ohio, USA

Götz Pilarczyk
Kirchhoff-Institute for Physics,
Heidelberg University, Heidelberg, Germany

Erno Sajo
University of Massachusetts Lowell,
Lowell, Massachusetts, USA

Leon Sanche
Université de Sherbrooke, Département de Médecine Nucléaire et Radiobiologie,
Faculté de médecine et des sciences de la santé, Sherbrooke, QC, Canada

Marlon R Veldwijk
Department of Radiation Oncology, Universitätsmedizin Mannheim, Mannheim, Germany

Michael Wolinsky
Department of Radiation Oncology,
Universitätsmedizin Mannheim, Mannheim, Germany

Yi Zheng
Fuzhou University Shangjie Town, Minhou County, Fuzhou, China

Frank G Zöllner
Computer Assisted Clinical Medicine, Mannheim Institute for Artificial Intelligence in Medicine
Medical Faculty Mannheim, Heidelberg University, Mannheim, Germany

Piotr Zygmanski
Brigham and Women's Hospital,
Dana Farber Cancer Institute,
Harvard Medical School, Boston,
Massachusetts, USA

Introduction

Rationale of nanoparticle-enhanced radiotherapy

Improved targeting of abnormal cells and tissue in the radiotherapy of cancer has been a long-standing goal of researchers. The central purpose in nanoparticle-enhanced radiotherapy (NPRT) is to more precisely control where the radiation dose is delivered, desirably with sub-cellular precision, provided we can find a method to bring the nanoparticles to target and control their concentration and size distribution. Thus, even though the macroscopic dose delivered to the tumor may be unchanged, the radiation-induced damage is concentrated to specific cellular foci, such as the DNA, cell membrane, or endothelial cells of the microvasculature supplying the neoplastic tissue. In this way, radiation effects may be confined to cancer cells while sparing normal cells and organs and avoiding or lessening unnecessary morbidity.

Interaction of therapeutic radiation with high atomic number (high-Z) nanoparticles enhances and localizes the energy deposition pattern to the vicinity of the nanoparticle, ranging from nano- to microscopic distances. It converts sparsely ionizing, low linear energy transfer (LET) radiation that has a diffuse energy deposition pattern that affects a large volume of tissue to densely ionizing high-LET radiation that is concentrated to the tumor cells. This higher LET boost may be very large and may have radio-sensitizing effects beyond purely physical dose enhancement. Deposition of energy from high-Z nanoparticles in the cellular environment is extremely heterogeneous and it is complex to model or otherwise determine. The induced biological damage depends on many factors, including the energy of the primary radiation, macroscopic and microscopic nanoparticle concentration and particle size distribution, nanoscale clustering patterns and morphology, the localization within the cellular targets, as well as the biological response of cells.

Historically, the idea of using Auger electrons for radio-sensitization started with the concept of Auger therapy, from which significant understanding of radiochemistry and radiobiology was gained [1–4] and the foundations of Auger dosimetry were established [5]. In that proposed therapy, either a radioactive atom decaying via Auger emission or a stable atom that emits Auger electrons following photoelectric (PE) absorption of x-rays is placed within the DNA molecule. Low-energy electrons originating directly in the DNA deposit most of their energy within the chromosome in almost as dense ionization tracks as alpha particles. Initial inferences of nanoscale energy deposition, including local versus remote effects and optimal incident energies, resulted from these studies [6–8]. However, incorporating radionuclides or high-atomic number atoms within the DNA in sufficient atomic density to permit successful tumor control has proven to be difficult. This led to the idea of using nanoparticles that concentrate a much larger number of dose-enhancing atoms, capable of delivering much higher levels of radiosensitization without the necessity of incorporating them in the DNA.

One of the promising methods centers on locally increasing the radiation dose using a high-Z material introduced into the tumor volume by intravenous injection or interstitially [9]. Because of the dose-enhancing properties of these materials via their large photoelectric and scattering cross-sections the aim of this treatment is to substantially increase the energy deposition in the tumor cells or tumor micro-vasculature possessing high permeability, retention and cellular uptake. Locally inducing low-energy secondary electron emission best works when the incident radiation is x-rays or gamma rays. Although high-energy charged particles can cause impact ionization, which can also lead to low-energy secondary electron emission, the respective interaction cross-sections for this type of reactions are far lower than for photoelectric absorption.

Recently, the interest in gold as a possible dose-enhancing agent has increased due to its advantageous chemical and physical properties. In addition, the accelerated development of nanotechnology has led to an increase in the number of studies involving gold nanoparticles (GNP) in many applications. Besides its high proton number and bulk density compared to other elements of possible choice, gold is biologically inert with minimal inherent cytotoxicity [10]. At low concentrations of less than 50 mg g^{-1} tissue, discussed in the literature [11–14], local dose enhancement at the level of individual cells can be achieved without significantly altering the macroscopic (tissue or organ-level) distribution and magnitude of dose. This presents a potential advantage over other, e.g. iodine, contrast agents, which require large concentrations to observe appreciable changes in the dose enhancement.

The organization of this book

This book synthesizes the most important advances in nanoparticle-aided radiation therapy over the last decade. It has a three-tier organization, first focusing on the fundamental physics and radiation transport simulations with applications, then continues with imaging methods and concludes with various clinical applications.

We start with the review of basic characteristics of the photoelectric absorption process, which is the main mechanism in the dose enhancement, including the properties of photoelectrons and Auger electrons (chapter 1), and provides examples of dose enhancement from GNP in water using deterministic radiation transport computations that can also serve as benchmarks for other studies (chapters 2 and 3).

Next, the book discusses DNA damage due to very low energy electrons (chapter 4) and the corresponding clustered damages related to the particles' energy deposition patterns based on track structure Monte Carlo simulations (chapter 5).

This is followed by addressing the dose enhancement effects from the perspective of treatment planning of cancer, considering clinical aspects (chapter 6) as well as methodologies for accurate and safe quantitative imaging and implementation of radiation transport computations for NPRT (chapter 7).

The questions of optimal nanoparticle sizes for maximum uptake are discussed (chapter 8) and the types of nanoparticles for specific clinical endpoints are explored (chapter 9).

Microscopic image-based modeling of nanoparticle distribution and the resulting biological damage are presented in chapters 10 and 11. Followed by review of x-ray (chapter 12), MRI (chapter 13) and photo-acoustic (chapter 14) imaging methods for macroscopic mapping of nanoparticles in patients or animals.

The book is concluded by reviewing several state-of-the art applications of NPRT (chapters 15–18).

Erno Sajo and Piotr Zygmanski

References

[1] Kassis A I, Makrigiorgos G and Adelstein S J 1990 Implications of radiobiological and dosimetric studies of DNA-incorporated I-123: The use of the Auger effect as a biological probe at the nanometre level *Radiat. Prot. Dosim.* **31** 333–8

[2] Sastry K S 1992 Biological effects of the Auger emitter iodine-125: a review. Report No. 1 of AAPM Nuclear Medicine Task Group No. 6 *Med. Phys.* **19** 1361–70

[3] Terrissol M, Edel S and Pomplun E 2004 Computer evaluation of direct and indirect damage induced by free and DNA-bound iodine-125 in the chromatin fibre *Int. J. Radiat. Biol.* **80** 905–8

[4] Wright H A, Hamm R N, Turner J E, Howell R W, Rao D V and Sastry K S R 1990 Calculations of physical and chemical reactions with DNA in aqueous solution from Auger cascades *Radiat. Prot. Dosim.* **31** 59–62

[5] Humm J L, Howell R W and Rao D V 1994 Dosimetry of Auger-electron-emitting radionuclides: report no. 3 of AAPM Nuclear Medicine Task Group No. 6. *Med. Phys.* **21** 1901–15

[6] Feinendegen L E and Neumann R D 2004 Dosimetry and risk from low- versus high-LET radiation of Auger events and the role of nuclide carriers *Int. J. Radiat. Biol.* **80** 813–22

[7] Karnas S J, Yu E, McGarry R C and Battista J J 1999 Optimal photon energies for IUdR K-edge radiosensitization with filtered x-ray and radioisotope sources *Phys. Med. Biol.* **44** 2537–49

[8] Watanabe R, Yokoya A, Fujii K and Saito K 2004 DNA strand breaks by direct energy deposition by Auger and photo-electrons ejected from DNA constituent atoms following K-shell photoabsorption *Int. J. Radiat. Biol.* **80** 823–32

[9] Hainfeld J F, Slatkin D N, Focella T M and Smilowitz H M 2006 Gold nanoparticles: a new x-ray contrast agent *Br. J. Radiol.* **79** 248–53

[10] Weinberg R 2006 *The Biology of Cancer* (New York: Garland Science)

[11] Berbeco R I, Ngwa W and Makrigiorgos G M 2011 Localized dose enhancement to tumor blood vessel endothelial cells via megavoltage x-rays and targeted gold nanoparticles: new potential for external beam radiotherapy *Int. J. Radiat. Oncol. Biol. Phys.* **81** 270–6

[12] Cho S H 2005 Estimation of tumour dose enhancement due to gold nanoparticles during typical radiation treatments: a preliminary Monte Carlo study *Phys. Med. Biol.* **50** N163–73

[13] Cho S H, Jones B L and Krishnan S 2009 The dosimetric feasibility of gold nanoparticle-aided radiation therapy (GNRT) via brachytherapy using low-energy gamma-/x-ray sources *Phys. Med. Biol.* **54** 4889–905

[14] Hainfeld J F, Slatkin D N and Smilowitz H M 2004 The use of gold nanoparticles to enhance radiotherapy in mice *Phys. Med. Biol.* **49** N309–15

Part I

Radiosensitization and fundamentals

Chapter 1

The role of Auger electrons versus photoelectrons in nanoparticle dose enhancement

Erno Sajo and Piotr Zygmanski

1.1 Fundamentals of the Auger process

The primary radiation interaction mechanism by which dose enhancement occurs when photons are incident on high-Z nanoparticles is the photoelectric effect followed by Auger emission. The nanoparticle-aided radiation therapy research literature is not unequivocal about the role of Auger electrons versus photoelectrons, and many fine details that may become important in the development of an eventual treatment planning software are often neglected. This chapter clarifies these aspects.

In the photoelectric absorption (PE) process, a photon is incident on one of the atomic orbital electrons, which completely absorbs the photon energy and it is ejected from the atom. The kinetic energy of this electron, a.k.a. photoelectron, equals the difference between the incident photon energy and the electron's binding energy. Therefore, this reaction occurs only when the incident photon energy exceeds the threshold of the shell binding energy. For example, if the incident photon energy is below the K-shell energy but above the L-shell energy, it does not have enough energy to ionize the K-electrons, but it can react with the L and higher shells. X-rays and γ photons have sufficient energy to ionize the inner shells (K, L, M) while the outer shells (N, O...) are usually ionized by UV and visible light. The ejected electron leaves a vacancy, which is filled by an electron from a higher orbital. The difference in the energies between the orbital providing the electron and the orbital where the vacancy is filled is radiated out in the form of a characteristic x-ray. The reason this x-ray is called 'characteristic' is because its energy is characteristic to the shell energy differences, which are unique for every material. The electron that fills the initial vacancy will leave its own vacancy, which is again filled by another electron from a higher shell. In this way, a series of characteristic x-rays is emitted,

doi:10.1088/978-0-7503-2396-3ch1

often called 'fluorescent radiation', which correspond to the energy levels of the involved shells.

Sometimes instead of releasing a fluorescent photon, in a radiation-less transition the excited atom releases another electron, making the atom a doubly charged ion. This is known as Auger process, in which the released electron is called an Auger electron after its discoverer, Pierre Victor Auger (1899–1993). In this way, a series of vacancies can be created and filled, and multiple Auger electrons can be emitted, which follow a probability distribution in energy, as shown in figure 1.1.

The frequency at which characteristic photons versus Auger electrons are emitted is called 'fluorescent yield'. The total energy emitted as fluorescent x-rays and Auger electrons equals the binding energy of the photoelectron. The emission of characteristic photons and Auger electrons are complementary events. Therefore, if W denotes the fluorescent yield, the Auger yield is $(1 - W)$. The fluorescent yield is greater for high atomic number (Z) elements than for low atomic number elements (figure 1.2). For low-Z elements, Auger emission has much higher probability to occur, and the most probable transition is KLL. That is, following K-electron ionization, an L-electron fills the vacancy and another L-electron is emitted as Auger. Higher Z elements have LMM, MNN, LMN, MNO, etc transitions. Above $Z = 25$, fluorescent emission starts to dominate. Because of the atomic shell structure, the

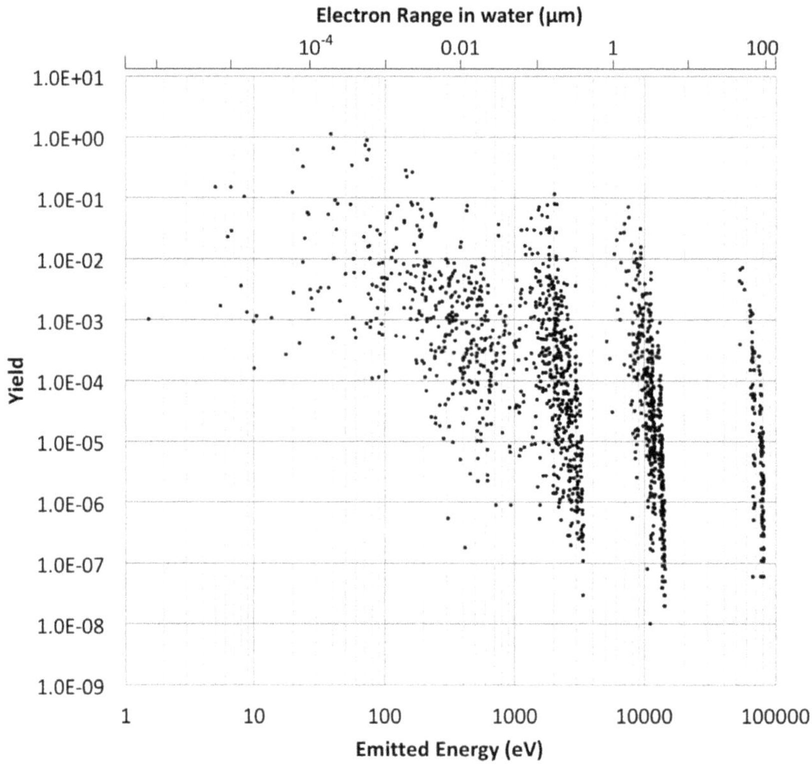

Figure 1.1. Auger emission per K-shell vacancy from gold as a function of energy and range in water [1].

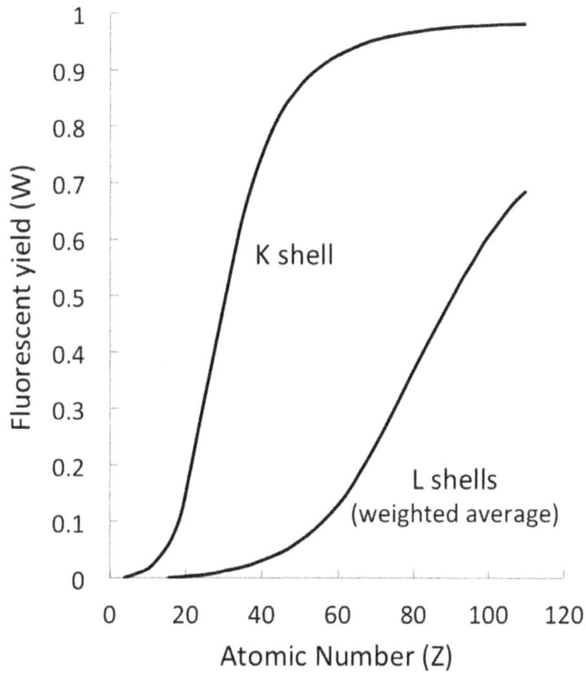

Figure 1.2. Fluorescent yield for K- and L-shell vacancies versus atomic number.

photoelectric absorption cross-section increases as the incident photon energy decreases. This is illustrated in figure 1.3. The sharp edges correspond to the atomic shell energies. For gold, the shell energies are high while for water the shell energies of the constituents H and O are below 0.001 MeV, therefore they are not shown in the plotted energy range. The photoelectric cross-section may be estimated using the following formula, in which the exponents m and n vary with the incident photon energy, as indicated:

$$\sigma_{PE}(E) \propto \frac{Z^n}{E^m} \quad \text{For } E \leqslant 0.1 \text{ MeV: } n = 4, \ m = 3.$$

The photoelectric effect is most important below about 100 keV. Above this energy, n gradually rises to 4.6 at 3 MeV and m decreases to about 1 at 5 MeV [3]. A comprehensive overview of similar approximations is given by Fornalski [4]. This formula, as well as most tabulated values and graphical representations show the total photoelectric cross-sections. That is, the combined cross-sections for interacting with all the shell electrons at ground state. Partial or shell-wise cross-sections may be obtained using quantum mechanics. When the incident photons are not polarized and when the spin of the ejected photoelectron is not resolved or observed, the partial cross-sections become a function of the emitted photoelectron direction. The angular dependencies will be explored later in this chapter.

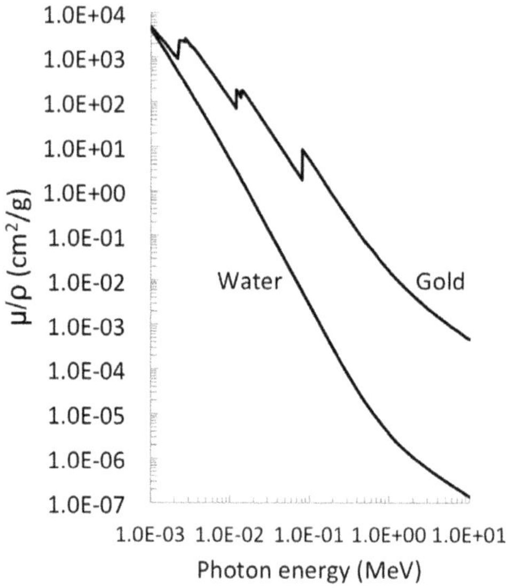

Figure 1.3. Photoelectric cross-sections for water and gold.

1.2 The role of fluorescent photons

Fluorescent photons, following initial PE absorption in the K- and L-shells have an important role, as they can be reabsorbed within the same or in other nearby nanoparticles, which can lead to further PE events in the higher shells due to the substantially (order-of-magnitude) higher cross-sections at these energies. As an example, figure 1.4(left) shows the photon spectrum in the center of the gold nanoparticle (GNP) exposed to 30 keV incident photons. The L and M fluorescent emissions as well as the Compton valley are clearly identifiable. If the GNP is too small, these photons may escape without further interaction and they will contribute to the dose farther away in the tissue, resulting in a low-gradient dose enhancement ratio (DER) curve. However, at larger GNP sizes the higher shells absorb a greater fraction of these fluorescent photons, and the subsequent PE electrons are energetic enough to escape a relatively large GNP. For example, when Lα, Lβ and Lγ fluorescent emissions ionize the M-shell the resulting PE electrons have energies between 6.2–11.2 keV (table 1.1), with respective ranges in gold of 170–440 nm. Ionization of N-shell electrons yields even more energetic photoelectrons with a minimum of 8.9 keV. When Kα and Kβ fluorescent emissions are absorbed by the L and higher shells the resulting PE electrons have a minimum of 52.6 keV with 5.5 μm range in gold.

This conclusion is valid even for very low energy fluorescent photons, at the Mα emissions. At these energies (~2 keV) larger GNPs have increasingly greater photoabsorption probabilities, resulting in N-shell ionizations, which yield photoelectrons at ~1.5 keV (not shown in table 1.1) with an escape depth of 16 nm (table 1.2). Note that ionizations of higher shell electrons (N and up) by fluorescence

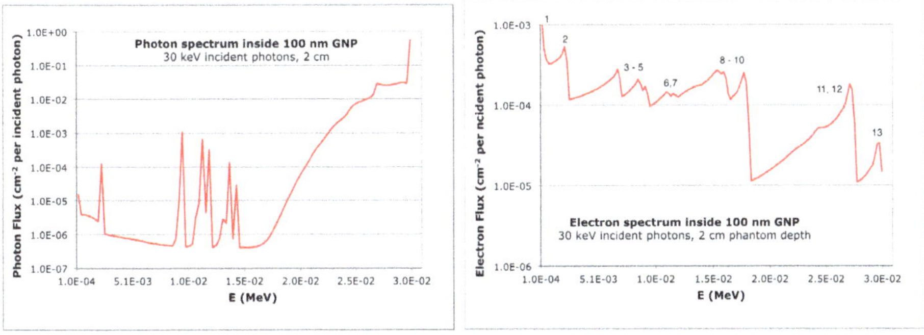

Figure 1.4. Photon (left) and electron (right) spectra in the center of a 100 nm GNP located at 2 cm phantom depth, exposed to 30 keV photons. The electron peaks are: (1) ~100–600 eV Auger following vacancy in the L-shell. (2) ~2 keV Auger following L vacancy combined with ~1.5 keV from L due to Lγ absorption and from N due to Mα. (3–5) 6–9 keV from M-shell by Lα and Lβ and from N by Lα fluorescence. (6–7) ~10–11 keV from M-shell by Lγ. (8–10), (11–12) and (13) photoelectrons from primary photon interactions with L-, M- and N-shells, respectively, with energies 15–18 keV, 24–28 keV, and 29.6 keV. Radiation transport simulations were performed using the CEPXS/ONDANT code [2].

do not contribute to the dose enhancement via Auger but they do via photoelectron emission. This is because for these events the Auger electron energies are generally below 300 eV and they are absorbed within the GNP. Figure 1.4(right) shows the electron spectrum in the center of the 100 nm GNP exposed to 30 keV photons. The numbers identify the peaks that are listed in the figure caption and can be compared to the above discussion.

Fluorescent photons, therefore, give rise to a cascade of photoelectrons originating in the higher shells with sufficient energy to escape the GNP, similar to Auger electrons above 1 keV, having similarly dense ionization tracks. Because the fluorescence yield from the K-shell is 87%–96% and from the L-shell it is ~37% [5, 6], the combined contribution of the photoelectron cascade to the dose enhancement is comparable to that of Auger electrons.

1.3 The contribution of Auger electrons and photoelectrons to dose

The relevant literature is not clear about the role of different secondary electrons in dose enhancement. McMahon and colleagues investigated the differential contribution of Auger, photo- and Compton electrons to the dose in the vicinity of 20 nm GNP exposed to 40 keV photons [7]. Their results show that Auger electrons dominate the energy deposition near the GNP surface, with relatively minor involvement of photoelectrons and a negligible role of Compton electrons. They indicate that the Auger contribution is by a factor of ~12 greater compared to all other processes combined, and it remains almost twice as high throughout the computational domain. These results appear somewhat high but tend to support the data presented here.

Figure 1.5 shows the DER for the case when the atomic relaxation cascade is turned off in the computations, which means that the Auger electrons as well as the

Table 1.1. Photoelectron energies produced by fluorescent photons in gold at the indicated emission lines. Emission energies are in parentheses. All values are in keV.

Shell	$K\alpha_1$ (68.8)	$K\alpha_2$ (67.0)	$K\beta_1$ (78.0)	$L\alpha_1$ (9.7)	$L\alpha_2$ (9.6)	$L\beta_1$ (11.4)	$L\beta_2$ (11.6)	$L\gamma_1$ (13.4)
L1	54.45	52.64	63.63	—	—	—	—	—
L2	55.07	53.26	64.25	—	—	—	—	—
L3	56.88	55.07	66.07	—	—	—	—	1.46
M1	65.38	63.56	74.56	6.29	6.20	8.02	8.16	9.96
M2	65.66	63.84	74.84	6.57	6.48	8.29	8.44	10.23
M3	66.06	64.25	75.24	6.97	6.89	8.70	8.84	10.64
M4	66.51	64.70	75.69	7.42	7.34	9.15	9.29	11.09
M5	66.60	64.78	75.78	7.51	7.42	9.24	9.38	11.18
	Generated by primary incident photons above the K-shell energy			Generated by photons above the L-shell energy				

Table 1.2. Auger electron yields per vacancy on the K- and L-shells in energy ranges of interest and corresponding escape depths or ranges in gold.

Energy range of Auger emissions (keV)	Weighted mean[a] (keV)		Combined Auger yield[b]		Corresponding escape depths from GNP (nm)
	K	L	K	L	
0.0–0.30	0.077	0.078	9.300	10.840	0–0.1
0.30–0.48	0.400	0.399	0.316	0.314	0.1–1.0
0.48–1.00	0.650	0.636	0.163	0.179	1.0–7.5
1.00–1.50	1.289	1.288	0.247	0.301	7.5–16.0
1.50–2.03[c]	1.787	1.784	0.829	1.001	16.0–27.0
2.03[c]–3.00	2.210	2.195	0.231	0.293	27.0–52.0
3.00–6.00	5.600	5.445	0.014	0.015	52.0–162.0
6.00–7.00	6.641	6.643	0.124	0.138	162.0–205.0
7.00–8.00	7.492	7.516	0.155	0.178	205.0–258.0
8.00–10.00	9.036	9.041	0.187	0.239	258.0–370.0
10.00–15.00	11.073	11.174	0.056	0.083	370.0–710.0
>15.00	58.822	–	0.041	–	710.0–

[a] Weighting by emission probability in the given energy range. Shell-dependent.
[b] Auger yield per shell-absorption event is greater than 1.
[c] The energy boundary is selected so as to include a series of emissions near 2 keV.

fluorescent photons from shells higher than K are excluded. Because in this way the effect of the Auger electrons cannot be separated from that of the fluorescence, the resultant DER underpredicts the value if only the Auger electrons were excluded. However, even with this suboptimal estimate, the computations show that the DER near the GNP is only about a factor of 3 smaller than when the cascade is enabled. Therefore, our results show a much greater contribution by photoelectrons than suggested by the literature, in accordance with the arguments provided above.

It is also seen that there are three distinctly identifiable regions of dose deposition: in the immediate vicinity of the GNP, energy deposition by low-energy Auger electrons is dominant. This region is marked by a sharp dose fall-off within a distance up to about 10–20 nm, which corresponds to electrons leaking from the GNP with energies below 1 keV. In the intermediate region, extending from about 20 nm to 150 nm, the contributions of more energetic Auger electrons along with photoelectrons influence the dose. Beyond 150 nm the combined effect of photoelectrons, Compton electrons, and fluorescent photons is observed. In addition to dose enhancement, there is an LET enhancement, as seen in figure 1.6, which has a similar drop-off with distance as that of the DER. However, farther away from the GNP its slope is somewhat less precipitous, suggesting the presence of higher energy photo- and Compton electrons.

The long-range contribution of Compton electrons is non-negligible. However, this is not due to interactions in the GNP but due to scatter of fluorescent photons in

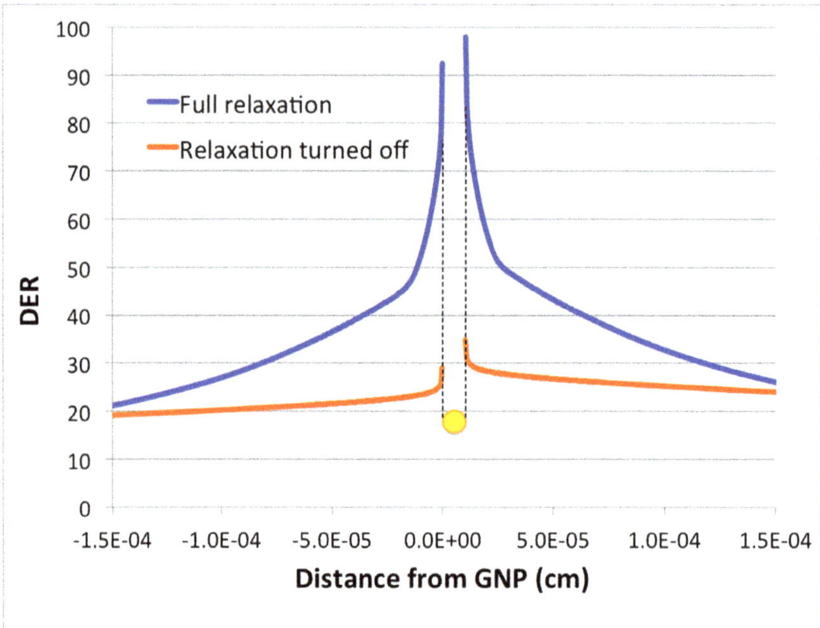

Figure 1.5. Comparison of DER with and without the effect of atomic relaxation above the K-shell. Here, a planar cluster of 100 nm GNPs at 2 cm phantom depth is exposed to 30 keV photons.

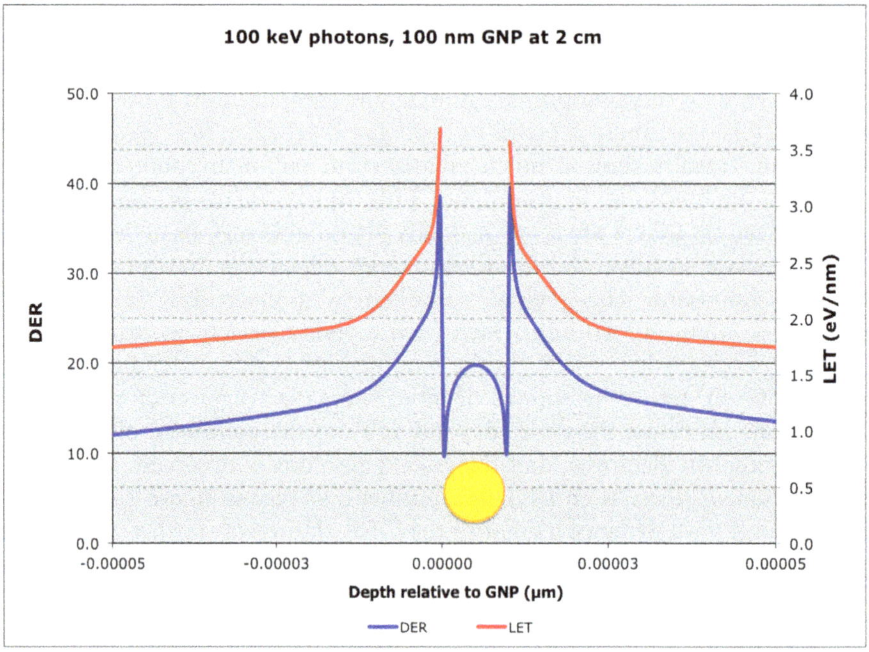

Figure 1.6. LET compared to DER generated by 100 keV photons incident on 100 nm GNP at cm water.

water where the incoherent cross-section is appreciable even at the L fluorescent emission energies (table 1.1), where it represents 3%–9% of the PE cross-section. When the K-shell fluorescent transitions are considered, the contribution of Compton electrons to dose is much greater, as incoherent scatter dominates the cross-sections. Figure 1.7(left) shows the photon flux within a 2.5-nm vicinity of a 100 nm GNP in response to 100 keV incident photons. The fluorescent photons escaping from the GNP ride on the Compton continuum in water. Figure 1.7(right) indicates that the GNP-induced increase in the electron flux and the concomitant change in its spectrum become negligible at 1 mm from the GNP surface.

1.4 Angular anisotropy of electron emission from the GNP

The literature invariably uses spherical symmetry in computing the dosimetric properties of GNP. For computational efficiency and to reduce the mounting statistical uncertainty, Monte Carlo scoring is performed in spherical shells about the GNP. Therefore, the anisotropy in the scored quantities is lost. However, depending on the GNP size and the energy of electrons generated therein, the spatial anisotropy may be non-trivial and its examination leads to important insights.

All of the main radiation interaction processes considered in nanoparticle-aided radiation therapy entail anisotropic electron scattering or emission. Compton scattering, which is the predominant photon interaction mechanism in water, produces forward-scattered electrons whose energy is usually greater than those of Auger electrons, thus they contribute to the dose far away from the nanoparticle relative to its size. The angular distribution of the photoelectrons follows the Sauter probability function, which at the limit of non-relativistic energies degenerates into the Fisher distribution [8]. In contrast to Compton scattering, in which high-energy photons have high differential cross-sections to produce low-energy laterally scattered electrons, the energy of photoelectrons increases with increasing photon energy while progressively scattering mainly in the forward direction. Because the angular distribution depends only on the energy of the photoelectron, even monoenergetic incident photons can produce many different photoelectrons via different shell interactions, resulting in different electron emission angles [9].

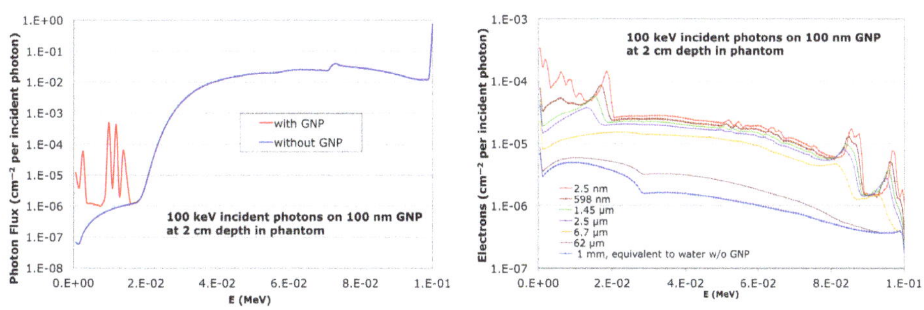

Figure 1.7. (Left) Photon flux spectrum within 2.5 nm from the proximal surface of a GNP. (Right) Electron flux spectra at various distances from the proximal surface of GNP. Computer simulations were performed using the CPEXS/ONDANT code [2].

Figure 1.8 shows three different photon energies incident on the L- and K-shells of gold with respective binding energies of 13.3 keV (weighted mean) and 80.73 keV.

The angular distribution of Auger electrons is also often neglected. This is justified in macroscopic dose computations, in which due to their short range, low-energy Auger electrons are assumed to deposit their energy locally. In the case of nanodosimetry, however, the region of computational interest extends to distances only up to a finite number of nanoparticle diameters, which is still within the range of many Auger electrons.

The emission of Auger electrons is angularly correlated with the direction of photoelectrons with respect to the incident photon. The angular correlation function depends on the ratio of shell population probabilities via an asymmetry parameter whose value is restricted to a range [−1, 2] corresponding to limiting spin polarization states. Radiation transport analysis coupled with quantum computations to determine the atomic electron shell population probabilities indicate that for the photoelectron emission angles characteristic to the proposed GNP-enhanced therapy (mainly between 25° and 90°), the Auger emission is preferentially along the direction of the photoelectron, forward and backward [9].

Energy deposition immediately adjacent to the GNP surface, within a few nanometers, is mainly due to leakage electrons from the GNP and less due to photon transmission and attenuation through the GNP or photons scattered or borne in and escaping from the GNP. Therefore, the ratio of doses proximal versus

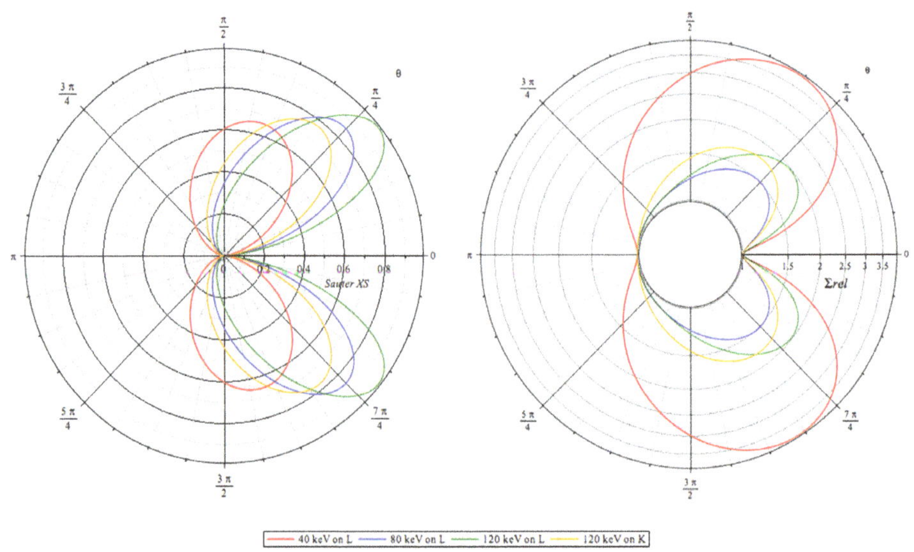

Figure 1.8. (Left) Sauter's single-differential angular probability distribution of photoelectron emission due to 40 keV, 80 keV and 120 keV photons interacting with L- and K-shell electrons in gold. (Right) the same distribution is scaled by these photons' respective PE cross-sections and plotted about a unit sphere representing the nanoparticle. The radial axis, Σ_{rel} is expressed as the cross-section relative to that at 120 keV photon energy and it is plotted in log scale. For all practical photon energies considered for GNP therapy, the photoelectron emission angle is mainly within 25° and 90°. Photons incident on left.

distal to the GNP with respect to the photon incidence is a good measure of anisotropy. Although there is a general forward scattering tendency of photo-electrons and anisotropic emission of Auger electrons, only those with the highest energy will not lose their initial direction due to multiple scattering in gold before they leak out. The angular variation in the electron leakage intensity therefore will also depend on the location within the escape depth where the photo or Auger electrons were generated, and on their initial direction. The complex combination of photo-, Auger, and Compton electron angular distributions as a function of the incident photon energy and the GNP size, which includes interaction density and self-shielding coupled with the spatial distribution of reactions within the escape depth, results in a non-trivial angular dose anisotropy. Detailed deterministic radiation transport simulations using the SCEPTRE code [10] indicate that the aggregate anisotropy effects combined with the differential attenuation of the emitted secondary electrons can result in up to about 18% relative variation in the DER as a function of nanoparticle size, incident photon energy and distance from the GNP.

The highest relative variations about the GNP are not necessarily between two diametrically opposite faces of the nanoparticle but analysis of proximal versus distal doses with respect to the incident photon direction can provide a good understanding. Figure 1.9 shows the ratio of doses proximal versus distal to the GNP. It is readily seen that at low incident photon energies the distal dose is greater than the proximal one, and that the ratio of doses is sensitive to the variation in the PE cross-section. When the incident photon is very close to one of the shell energies, the generated photoelectron may have lower energy than many of the subsequent Auger electrons and most of them will be captured locally, within the GNP. Thus, in this case the non-relativistic Fisher distribution applies to the photoelectrons, and because very few of these electrons emerge from the GNP, both the dose and the dose anisotropy near the GNP surface are dominated by the Auger electrons, and the latter are not substantially affected by the size of the GNP. This effect can be seen at the L-shell (~12–14 keV) and K-shell (~81 keV) energies where the proximal to distal dose ratios are very close for all GNP sizes considered. This also means that the optimal incident photon energy to produce the greatest dose enhancement is greater than the electron shell energy, such that the photoelectrons can escape the GNP.

An interesting feature of the anisotropy function is that for GNP sizes between 10 and 100 nm the proximal dose becomes larger than the distal dose at a threshold energy of ~125 keV (not shown in figure 1.9). Note that the exact threshold energies may depend on the depth of the GNP in tissue or in the phantom due to changes in the photon spectrum reaching the GNP. At high incident photon energies the generated photoelectron's kinetic energy becomes so high that due to its reduced linear energy transfer (LET) it deposits most of its energy farther away from the GNP. Therefore, despite their much greater extent of forward scattering, the dose near the GNP will be larger on the proximal side.

The escaping electrons' LET also exhibits an anisotropy, but due to the variations in the angular emission of Auger electrons, its peak does not always coincide with

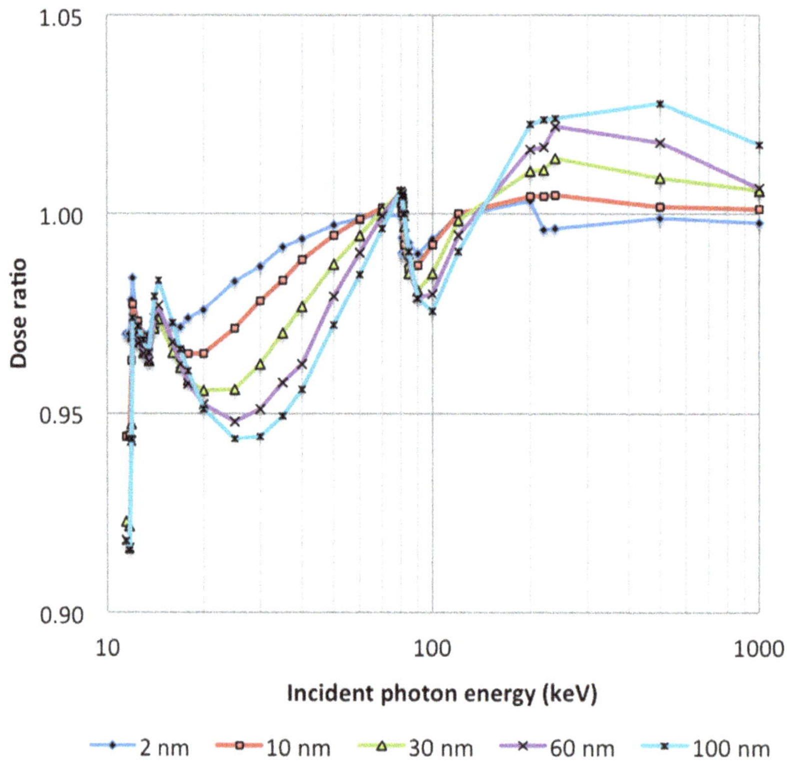

Figure 1.9. Proximal to distal anisotropy in the 2 nm voxel directly adjacent to GNPs of different sizes located at 2 cm phantom depth.

that of the DER. Figure 1.6 shows an example, in which the DER peaks on the distal side of the GNP while the LET exhibits a maximum on the proximal side.

Note that the angular anisotropy is significant for electrons only. Experimental measurements indicate that the emission of fluorescent photons following photoelectric absorption in gold is isotropic within the experimental uncertainties [11]. Compton-scattered photons possess too high energy to be a significant source of dose near the GNP. In the case of agglomerated or coagulated GNPs, the anisotropy affects the net electron current escaping from the nanoparticles, but it has diminished impact in terms of the angular distribution of the dose or dose enhancement [12].

1.5 Conclusions

The significant dose enhancement in the near vicinity of the nanoparticles is clearly dominated by the contribution of Auger electrons. This is superimposed on the effect of other low-energy electrons due to interactions of fluorescent photons within the same nanoparticle. Farther away, about 1 μm and beyond, photoelectrons originating in the initial photoelectric absorption event have prevalence. The precipitous increase or decrease of the dose enhancement as a function of distance from the nanoparticle is not only due to the increased number of leakage electrons but also due to the enhanced LET of these electrons. Dose and LET anisotropy about nanoparticles is primarily a local effect, which is nearly undetectable a few micrometers away, but it may be important to consider under special circumstances.

References

[1] Cullen D E 1992 *Program RELAX: A Code Designed to Calculate Atomic Relaxation Spectra of X-Rays and Electrons* (Oak Ridge, TN: US Department of Energy, Office of Scientific and Technical Information, UCRL-ID-110438)

[2] Lorence L J J and Morel J E 1992 *CEPXS/ONELD: A One-dimensional Coupled Electron-Photon Discrete Ordinates Code Package* (Albuquerque, NM: Sandia National Laboratories SAND-92-0261C)

[3] Attix F H 1986 *Introduction to Radiological Physics and Radiation Dosimetry* (New York: Wiley)

[4] Fornalski K W 2018 Simple empirical correction functions to cross sections of the photoelectric effect, Compton scattering, pair and triplet production for carbon radiation shields for intermediate and high photon energies *J. Phys. Commun.* **2** 035038

[5] Bambynek W, Crasemann B, Fink R W, Freund H-U, Mark H, Swift C D, Price R E and Rao P V 1972 X-ray fluorescence yields, Auger, and Coster–Kroning transitions probabilities *Rev. Mod. Phys.* **44** 716–813

[6] Perkins S T, Cullen D E, Hubbel J H and Kissel L 1997 *LLNL Libraries of Atomic Data, Electron Data, and Photon Data in Evaluated Nuclear Data Library (ENDL) Type Format* (Oak Ridge, TN: Oak Ridge National Laboratory RSICC Data Library Collection)

[7] McMahon S J *et al* 2011 Biological consequences of nanoscale energy deposition near irradiated heavy atom nanoparticles *Sci. Rep.* **1** 18

[8] Davisson C M and Evans R D 1952 Gamma-ray absorption coefficients *Rev. Mod. Phys.* **24** 79–107

[9] Gadoue S M, Toomeh D, Zygmanski P and Sajo E 2017 Angular dose anisotropy around gold nanoparticles exposed to x-rays *Nanomedicine* **13** 1653–61

[10] Bonhoff W J, Drumm C R, Fan W C, Pautz S D and Valdez G D 2016 *SCEPTRE: Sandia Computational Engine for Particle Transport for Radiation Effects, v. 1.7* (Albuquerque, NM: Sandia National Laboratories)

[11] Yamaoka H, Oura M, Takahiro K, Takeshima N, Kawatsura K, Mizumak I K M, Kleiman U, Kabachnik N M and Mukoyama T 2002 Angular distribution of Au and Pb L x-rays following photoionization by synchrotron radiation *Phys. Rev.* A **65** 062713-1–8

[12] Gadoue S M, Zygmanski P and Sajo E 2018 The dichotomous nature of dose enhancement by gold nanoparticle aggregates in radiotherapy *Nanomedicine* **13** 809–23

Chapter 2

Deterministic computation benchmarks of nanoparticle dose enhancement—part I. Nanometer scales

Erno Sajo, Fulya Cifter and Piotr Zygmanski

2.1 Perspectives

Nanoparticle dose enhancement is a multiscale computational problem, spanning seven orders of magnitude in spatial distance, from nanometers to centimeters, and six orders of magnitude in energy, from eV to MeV. The spatial scale, especially in Monte Carlo simulations, presents most of the difficulty, while in deterministic computations the spatial and energy resolutions are interdependent. At the nanoscale, increased energy deposition from a single nanoparticle or a cluster of nanoparticles has to be simulated by carefully considering the microbeam geometry (that part of the primary beam, which is incident on the nanoparticle and its cellular-scale surroundings) and phase space parameters in relation to the geometry of the nanoparticle region. However, at the macroscale the otherwise heterogeneous nanoscopic energy deposition pattern is averaged and other properties, such as attenuation and beam hardening, become important. In this chapter, we present deterministic radiation transport computer simulations in high spatial resolution at nanometer scales, but extending up to 2 mm, and provide examples of dose enhancement from gold nanoparticles (GNP) in water, which can also serve as benchmarks for other studies. In part II of the benchmark study, we extend the discussion to macroscopic scales.

2.2 The radiation transport basis of high-*Z* nanoparticle dose enhancement by x-rays

In the energy range of therapeutic interest, water is nearly a pure Compton scatterer while high-*Z* materials are almost pure photoelectric absorbers. For $Z = 64$–73 (e.g. Gd, Tb, Dy, Ho, Hf, Ta) photoelectric effect (PE) dominates the x-ray interactions

doi:10.1088/978-0-7503-2396-3ch2

below about 400 keV. In the range of $Z = 74–82$, which includes Re, Os, Ir, Pt, Au, Tl, Pb, photoabsorption is dominant below 500 keV. At higher energies, these materials are mainly Compton scatterers, but their PE cross-section remains relatively high. For example, at about 1 MeV photon energy the ratio of Compton versus PE cross-sections is between a factor of 5 and 10 in these materials, while in water this ratio is more than 10^4. Therefore, in high-Z materials secondary electron production via the PE mechanism remains significant even at megavoltage energies.

Because of gold's advantageous physical, chemical and biological properties, many researchers have focused on the computational description of various quantities related to GNP dose enhancement. All of these investigators employed Monte Carlo (MC) methods and used an effectively one-dimensional geometry in their scoring and assessment of the dose and other dose-related quantities, assuming and taking advantage of the spherical symmetry about the nanoparticles. A common conclusion is that low-energy incident photons tend to give rise to higher dose enhancement than do high-energy photons, which is related to the interaction cross-sections' energy dependence. Many authors disagree in the magnitude of dose enhancement and in the spatial range of this effect, with discrepancies often reaching more than an order of magnitude. In synthesizing the results a difficulty is presented by the fact that not all authors used the same metric for dose enhancement, several used atomic gold mixtures rather than nanoparticles, and many reported results normalized to disparate radiation transport quantities in different simulation geometries and using mutually exclusive assumptions.

The dose enhancement and the spatial properties of electron production were examined by Leung and colleagues [1] using three GNP sizes exposed mainly to spectral beams. They found that larger GNPs produced higher doses than small GNPs. This appears to be contrary to the findings of McMahon *et al* [2, 3], who studied a range of GNP sizes with monoenergetic and spectral photons. An important recognition was that the GNP sensitization is driven by dose inhomogeneity in the nanoscale, not over the entire cell. Because of the rapid changes in energy deposition in the short range, sub-cellular localization is important. This conclusion concurs with that of Lechtman and coworkers [4] who obtained normalized electron number intensities per photoelectric event as function of spatial range, from which the electron energy can be inferred. The conclusion was drawn that megavoltage photon sources may not be clinically feasible, which is comparable to the findings of Cho and colleagues [5, 6]. A large discrepancy, however, was found between their predicted electron range originating in 100 nm GNP exposed to 6 MV photons compared to the same scenario investigated by Leung [1], casting uncertainty on ruling out the application of megavoltage beams.

Contrary to many of the investigators cited above, in earlier studies Cho and colleagues [5, 6] used various concentrations of atomic gold, instead of nanoparticles, mixed with tissue or water and exposed mainly to spectral photon sources. Their dose enhancement was found to depend on the photon energy spectra, radial distance from the particle and the gold concentration, which was later verified by other investigators. In a follow-up study by Jones *et al* [7], the spatial range of the dose enhancement was found to extend to ~30 μm for low-energy sources, and to ~500 μm for megavoltage sources. In comparison to Leung [1], the results seem to agree well at low energies but in megavoltage the latter study shows almost ten times greater range. On the other hand, the ranges in both of these studies are orders of magnitude greater than what McMahon [2, 3] predicts.

These studies showed that radiation transport computations face numerous challenges due to the requirement of high spatial and energy resolution about the nanoparticle, and the approximations used at the interface between the macroscopic clinical beam and the nanoscopic environment. To resolve this issue and to find the origin of discrepancies between the results of various researchers, Zygmanski *et al* [8] investigated the impact of Monte Carlo simulation geometry, including phase space transitions from the macroscopic clinical beam at the water GNP interface to the nanoscopic transport of electrons leaking from the GNP. This as well as a separate study by the same research group also examined the spatial anisotropy of energy deposition about single and clustered nanoparticles [9, 10]. Computer simulations were performed for 50 nm and 100 nm GNPs irradiated in water phantom by various monoenergetic (11 keV–1 MeV) and spectral (50 kVp, 80 kVp and 120 kVp) sources using the CEPXS/ONEDANT [11] and SCEPTRE [12] deterministic code packages, and the GEANT4 Monte Carlo model. The authors found that the dose enhancement is very sensitive to the macro–micro–nano transition geometry, which explains some of the discrepancies reported in the literature, and cautions future studies and the interpretation of existing MC results obtained in different simulations geometries.

Apart from experimental and Monte Carlo simulation studies, Ngwa *et al* [13, 14] and Berbeco *et al* [15] performed analytical calculations for dose enhancement in a simplified model of endothelial cells due to GNPs as contrast agents. They showed that using megavoltage or brachytherapy sources leads to dose boost, which in turn may lead to an angio-disruptive radiotherapy. The advantage of this approach is that passive contrast agents that are based on e.g. iodine- or gadolinium-containing molecules are commonly used in imaging studies, however, their dose enhancement lags behind that of gold.

Despite the recent advances in understanding nanoparticle dose enhancement effects, the optimal size of the particle, the optimal incident energy as a function of nanoparticle size and location (depth) in the tissue, and the resulting dose enhancements alone or in combinations still require further explorations. Moreover, future computations of dose enhancement in the treatment planning systems must rely on practical methods, which would take into account the fact that in clinical beams the x-ray spectrum varies depending on the specific irradiation technique and region of interest with respect to the field center and depth [16, 17].

The present chapter provides deterministic benchmarks and introduces a Green's function approach, which makes these tasks easier to accomplish. The parameterization of dose enhancement ratio (DER) effects, which is part of obtaining the numerical representation of Green's function, has to isolate important features, which in turn can be used for finding the optimal combinations of particle size, incident photon energy, and tissue depth. Because of the rapid changes in energy deposition patterns within very short distances in the nanometer scale, such parameterization requires a large number of computations that explore various scenarios on a very fine spatial mesh. Monte Carlo (MC) simulations are potentially the most accurate in situations when the geometry of the problem is complex. However, in the case when the interaction density in the tally volume is small, large computational uncertainty results, which requires aggressive non-analog variance reduction and/or prohibitively large number of histories, which is not suitable for the required series of analysis we present here. While variance reduction techniques can speed up MC computations, they are not uniformly effective, and can lead to non-physical predictions, a few examples of which are scattered in the literature.

In order to characterize the radiosensitization properties of GNP, detailed energy deposition information is needed in the range of sub-cellular dimensions in nano-metric spatial resolution. In addition, the dosimetric quantities must be established for various incident energies, GNP sizes and locations. In this chapter we present data based on deterministic computations, which can be regarded as a parametric representation of the Green's function of GNP dose deposition, and can be used as benchmarks for other studies.

2.3 Deterministic radiation transport computations

In relatively simple geometries, such as spherical or parallelepiped, deterministic computations have been shown to provide as accurate results as Monte Carlo methods [18, 19]. Because deterministic methods do not suffer from statistical uncertainties, in cases when the required spatial resolution is much smaller than the mean free path of the tracked particles they can yield results that are superior to MC computations. In addition, the computational time necessary to reduce the MC uncertainty to acceptable levels is many orders of magnitude greater than what deterministic computations demand. Hence, the deterministic approach permits to gain parametric data for GNP dose enhancement in such detail that would be simply impossible to obtain using MC techniques in a reasonable time.

Coupled photon–electron radiation transport computations were performed using the CEPXS/ONEDANT computer code package [11, 20], which has been extensively validated and benchmarked, and has been used in a number of applications, including medical physics [18, 19, 21]. A comprehensive description is provided by Lorence *et al* [22]. Briefly, ONEDANT is an advanced discrete ordinates code that solves the one-dimensional multigroup Boltzmann transport equation in plane, cylindrical, spherical, and two-angle plane geometries over the energy range from 100 eV to 100 MeV. Regular and adjoint, inhomogeneous and homogeneous problems subject to vacuum, reflective, periodic, white, albedo, or inhomogeneous boundary flux conditions are solved. General anisotropic scattering is allowed and anisotropic inhomogeneous sources are permitted. CEPXS is a multigroup-Legendre cross-section generating code, which extracts electron cross-section information from the DATAPAC library of the ETRAN Monte Carlo system [23, 24] and produces photoelectric and pair absorption cross-sections using the Biggs–Lighthill formulation [22, 25, 26]. The model that is used for ionization/

relaxation in CEPXS is the same as that employed in the Integrated Tiger Series (ITS) Monte Carlo code system [27] which has been adopted by many other MC computer codes. With a few exceptions, CEPXS and ITS have identical cross-section data [22]. Once such exception is that the low-energy cutoff of the cross-sections in the latest CEPXS distribution of DATAPAC is extended down to 100 eV [20].

In the present work it is assumed that the GNPs may occur as single spherical particles as well as in a form of clusters that can be approximated as slabs. Particles suspended in colloidal and bimolecular dispersions have been shown to form chain- and slab-like aggregates [28], and studies of cell uptake of GNPs observed clustering in the cytoplasm [29, 30]. Because the photoelectric production is practically uniform across the GNP, dose computations can be performed in one-dimensional spherical geometry [8]. By way of a geometry transformation, this is equivalent to a 1D slab geometry [22, 31]. Therefore, the 1D calculation model (spherical or slab) is valid for a single GNP as well as a densely packed cluster of GNPs, which are the two extremes of nanoparticle morphologies that can occur. Note that the 1D assumption is also inherent in the current relevant literature of nanoparticle dose enhancement [1–7].

In this work, three GNP sizes, 10 nm, 30 nm and 100 nm, are considered, situated at two different depths, 2 cm and 20 cm in a water phantom to account for attenuation and hardening of the primary beam. In each computation the incident photons were monoenergetic ranging from 11.4 keV to 6.5 MeV, covering a total of 73 discrete energies, with sufficient energy resolution about the K- and L-edges of gold to resolve the variations in the photoelectric cross-section. In aggregate, this represents approximately 410 computational simulations in which doses and dose enhancement ratios were computed in nanometer resolution, which provides a detailed database suitable for assembling the parameterized Green's function of the GNP-induced dose enhancement.

In addition to the monoenergetic cases, four clinical photon spectra, 120 kVp (Varian OBI system), 220 kVp (small animal radiation platform, SARRP [32]), and 6.5 MV Linac (Varian 2100 EX) with and without flattening filter were also analyzed [33]. In each case investigated, the spatial resolution of the computed dose varied logarithmically as function of distance from the GNP surface and as function of incident photon energy. In the range where Auger contribution is dominant (<1.0 μm) the spatial resolution varied between 1.0 and 10.0 nm. Between 1.0 μm and 1.0 mm distances the resolution ranged from 10.0 to 100.0 nm. Beyond 1.0 mm, the resolution was generally set to 100 nm. Inside the gold the spatial mesh was 2 nm for GNP sizes 10 nm and 30 nm, and it was 5 nm for 100 nm GNP size.

Dose computations were performed with and without the GNP present in the water phantom. Because the GNP is situated at a defined depth in water, it is a spectrum of photons plus secondary electrons that reach the gold surface even if the incident photons on the phantom surface are monoenergetic. The DER was calculated as the ratio of the doses at a defined spatial point with GNP present and when the GNP was replaced with water. In this way, the spatial variation (x) of DER as function of incident photon energy (E), GNP size (t) and its location within

Table 2.1. Simulation parameters. Computations were performed for all combinations of photon energies, GNP sizes and water depths.

Incident photon energy (*E*):	14 keV–30 keV in 1 keV increments, monoenergetic 40 keV–120 keV in 20 keV increments, monoenergetic 80 keV–90 keV in 1 keV increments, monoenergetic 1 MeV, 6.5 MeV, monoenergetic 120 kVp, 220 kVp, 6.5 MV (STD) and 6.5 MV (FFF), spectral
GNP sizes (*t*):	10, 30, 60, 100 nm
Depth in water (*d*):	2 cm and 20 cm
Distance from GNP surface (*x*):	Up to 2 mm
Spatial resolution:	At GNP surface: 1 nm for sizes up to 60 nm, 2.5 nm for 100 nm 1 nm–1 μm from surface: 1–10 nm[a] 1 μm–1.0 mm from surface: 10–100 nm[a] 1 mm–2 mm from surface: 100 nm Inside GNP: 2 nm for sizes up to 60 nm 5 nm for 100 nm

[a] In logarithmically spaced zones as function of photon energy.

the phantom (d) was obtained, yielding the function, DER(x, E, t, d). Table 2.1 summarizes the simulation parameters.

2.4 The Green's function of dose enhancement

The total dose enhancement ratio is defined as the ratio of total dose in water with gold to that without gold:

$$DER = \frac{D_T^{(Au)}}{D_T^{(w)}}. \tag{2.1}$$

Assume that there is a spectrum of incident photons that can be described as a continuous distribution function $\nu(E)$, which may be discretized using a bin-wise series of $\nu_i(E_i)$, where ν_i is the number of incident photons in energy group or bin E_i. Note that here the function $\nu(E)$ is not normalized, therefore, $\sum \nu_i(E_i) \neq 1$. Let $D_i(E_i)$ represent the dose *per photon* due to incident photons in energy group E_i. In this way, the total dose can be written as the sum of doses due to photons in E_i, as follows:

$$D_T = \sum_i \nu(E_i) D_i(E_i) \equiv \sum_i \nu_i D_i. \tag{2.2}$$

This equation may be written for dose with gold, $D_i^{(Au)}$, and without gold, $D_i^{(w)}$. Hence, a dose enhancement ratio can be defined for each energy group E_i, which we may call dose enhancement kernel, DER_i:

$$DER_i = \frac{\nu_i D_i^{(Au)}}{\nu_i D_i^{(w)}} = \frac{D_i^{(Au)}}{D_i^{(w)}}. \tag{2.3}$$

In the appendix we show that the total dose (with and without GNP) can be expressed in terms of the Green's function of radiation transport, hence DER_i is a parameterized representation of the Green's function of the dose enhancement. Substituting equation (2.2) into equation (2.1), and then using equation (2.3), we have:

$$DER = \frac{\sum_i \nu_i D_i^{(Au)}}{\sum_i \nu_i D_i^{(w)}} \neq \sum_i DER_i, \tag{2.4}$$

$$DER = \frac{\sum_i \nu_i D_i^{(w)} DER_i}{\sum_i \nu_i D_i^{(w)}} = \frac{1}{D_T^{(w)}} \sum_i \nu_i D_i^{(w)} DER_i. \tag{2.5}$$

In continuous form equation (2.5) can be written as:

$$DER = \frac{1}{D_T^w} \int_E \nu(E)\ D^{(w)}(E)\ DER(E)\ dE. \tag{2.6}$$

The total dose due to the presence of gold is expressed as function of dose without gold using the dose enhancement kernel as:

$$D_T^{Au} = \sum_i \nu_i D_i^{(w)} DER_i = \int_E \nu(E)\ D^{(w)}(E)\ DER(E)\ dE. \tag{2.7}$$

The total dose and the dose enhancement kernel, defined in equation (2.3), may be expressed in terms of the Green's function, as shown in the appendix. Thus, DER_i may be regarded as the parametric Green's function of the DER. In this way, if the energy spectrum of the incident photons and the dose response is known in sufficiently fine energy group structure, this formalism permits the computation of the total dose response due to an arbitrary spectral beam.

2.5 Maximum and spatially averaged dose enhancement ratios

Owing to the escaping low-energy Auger electrons, the DER has a local maximum (DER_{MAX}) in the immediate vicinity of the GNP surface, which corresponds to the first spatial mesh point outside the GNP. The values of DER, including DER_{MAX}, reported in this work represent spatial averages over each mesh interval. In the case of DER_{MAX} the initial spatial step is invariably 1 nm, except for 100 nm GNP sizes, where it is 2.5 nm.

In addition, because of the many different electron ranges and photon energies involved in forming the total DER and because the location of the GNP with respect to cellular and sub-cellular targets may vary, we also examine the dose enhancement ratios averaged over various radiobiologically important ranges and target sizes corresponding to the DNA-histone structure and cell membrane dimensions (10 nm), chromatin structure (100 nm), cell nucleus (1 μm) and endothelial cell (2 μm). In this way, the spatially averaged DER is defined as

$$\langle DER(x)\rangle = \frac{1}{x}\int_{x_L}^{x_H} DER(x')dx'. \tag{2.8}$$

Here, x is the distance from the GNP surface along its surface normal, and it may encompass numerous mesh points. $[x_L, x_H]$ is the region of interest where $x_L \in [0, x_H)$. In this way, the optimal incident photon energy for GNP treatment may be defined as that which provides the highest DER_{MAX} near the surface or the highest $\langle DER\rangle$ at the appropriate averaging interval.

Figures 2.1–2.7 show various properties of the DER for 10 nm, 30 nm and 100 nm GNP sizes located at 2 cm and 20 cm depths in a water phantom. The spatial resolution in the figures are 2 nm for t = 10 nm and t = 30 nm GNP, and 5 nm for t = 100 nm size. Figure 2.1 is an example, which shows the mesh-wise variation of DER within one-diameter distance of a 10 nm GNP at 2 cm depth with various incident photon energies.

Figure 2.2 shows a surface plot of DER versus distance from the same GNP as function of incident photon energy. The two local maxima of the DER occur at ∼20 keV and ∼90 keV incident energies, which are slightly above the gold L- and K-shell energies at 13.3 (weighted average) and 80.73 keV, respectively. A similar pattern for the spatial variation of DER is observed for all incident energies and GNP sizes, with changes only in the magnitude of DER. From the aggregate data it is evident that within the limits of the investigated sizes (from 10 to 100 nm) the larger the GNP the greater DER is obtained.

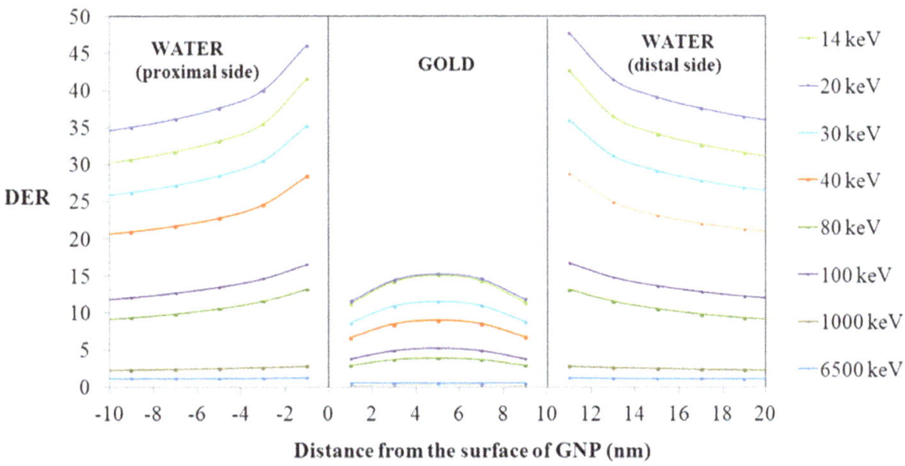

Figure 2.1. DERs across a 10 nm GNP at 2 cm depth in water with incident photon energy as parameter.

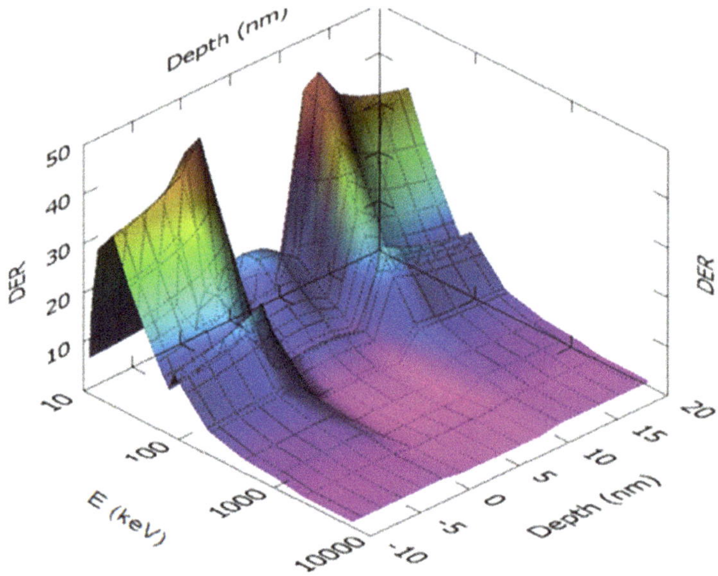

Figure 2.2. Surface plot of DER as function of incident photon energy and distance for the same GNP as in figure 2.1.

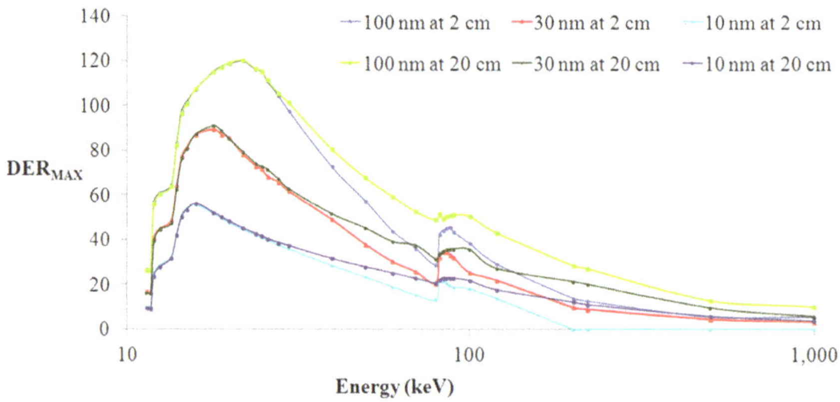

Figure 2.3. DER_{MAX} as a function of incident photon energy with GNP size and depth as parameters.

It is expected that the variation of DER with photon energy should follow the photoelectric cross section, having local maxima near the K- and L-edges of gold. The highest DER values are obtained with incident photon energies closer to the L-shell. Below the L-shell, although the potential dose enhancement for very small GNP is high, it has a decreasing practical relevance due to the very low photon energies at this range (<3 keV). This can be seen in figure 2.3, where the maximum values of the DER (which occur near the surface of the GNP) are displayed as function of incident photon energy with GNP size as parameter at two depths in the phantom, 2 cm and 20 cm.

2.6 The optimal incident photon energy

The optimal incident photon energy that produces the highest DER is determined by a complex interplay of PE reaction rates, fluorescent versus Auger yields, their energies in relation to the GNP size, and it is closely related to the energy at which electronic equilibrium is lost in the GNP. Figure 2.4 shows the DER produced by a 100 nm GNP as a function of incident photon energy together with the ratios of mass energy absorption coefficients, $(\mu_{en}/\rho)_{Au}/(\mu_{en}/\rho)_{Water}$. On the second axis, the PE cross-section (a.k.a. linear attenuation coefficient) is superimposed in a way to compare its slope with that of the DER at high energies.

At low incident photon energies, the DER closely follows the (μ_{en}/ρ) ratio, up to approximately 22 keV, at which point the two ratios are almost identical. Above this energy, the tendency of DER departs and starts to follow the slope of the PE cross-section. This indicates that charged particle equilibrium exists in this GNP up to 22 keV and disequilibrium above it. The optimal incident photon energy to produce the highest DER is at which the nanoparticle loses electronic equilibrium.

For a fixed GNP size the DER peaks near the GNP surface (DER_{MAX}), and its value is a strong function of photon energy. Figure 2.5 displays the variation of DER_{MAX} as function of GNP size (placed at 2 cm and 20 cm depths) with the incident photon energy at which the largest value of DER_{MAX} is obtained. This energy is the optimal incident photon energy for the given GNP size. Tables 2.2(a) and (b) summarize the optimal energies at which the maximum DERs occur as function of targeted shell and GNP size.

According to these results, DER_{MAX} is not very sensitive to the depth at which the GNP is located, and there is very little variation in the optimal energies between 2 cm and 20 cm depths. A much greater sensitivity is exhibited for the size of the GNP as detailed above. Note, however, that the absolute doses at 2 cm and at 20 cm

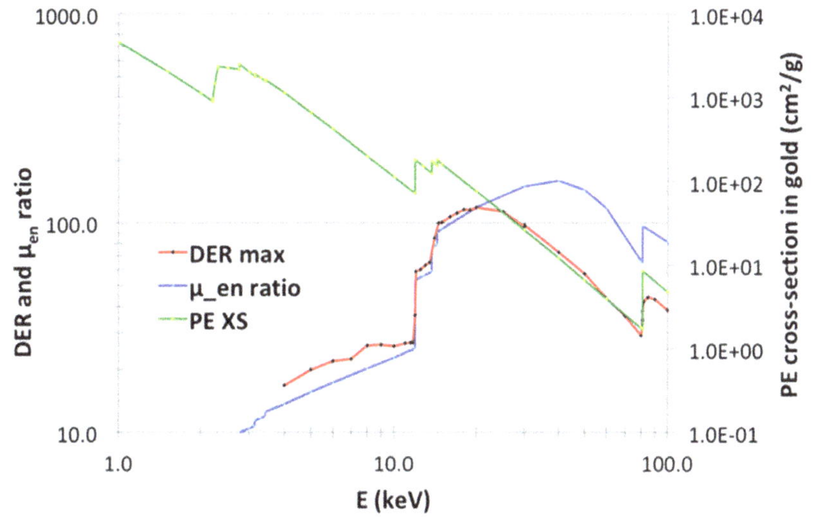

Figure 2.4. DER for 100 nm GNP at 2 cm depth in relation to the (μ_{en}/ρ) ratios and the PE XS.

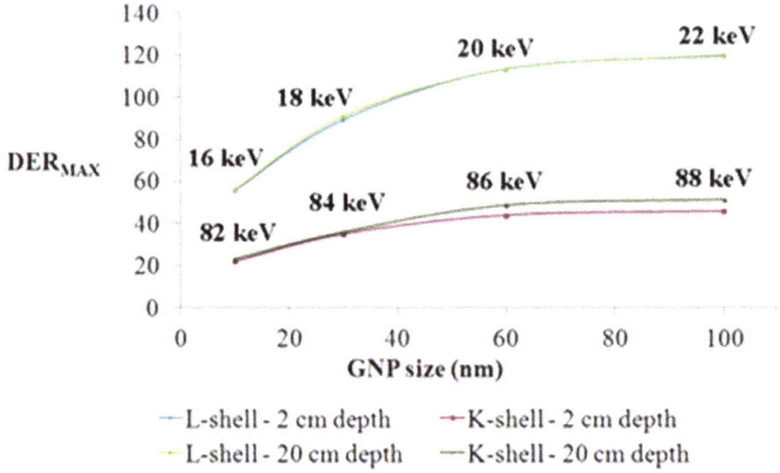

Figure 2.5. The variation of DER_{MAX} as function of GNP size. Optimal energies to achieve the highest DER_{MAX} for each size are also indicated.

Table 2.2. (a) Optimal incident photon energies targeting the L-shell as a function of GNP size.

	GNP at 2 cm depth in water phantom		GNP at 20 cm depth in water phantom	
GNP size (nm)	Optimal energy (keV)	DER_{MAX}	Optimal energy (keV)	DER_{MAX}
10	16	56	16	56
30	18	89	18	91
60	20	113	20	113
100	22	119	22	120

Table 2.2. (b) Optimal incident photon energies targeting the K-shell as function of GNP size.

	GNP at 2 cm depth in water phantom		GNP at 20 cm depth in water phantom	
GNP size (nm)	Optimal energy (keV)	DER_{MAX}	Optimal energy (keV)	DER_{MAX}
10	82–84	22	86	23
30	84–86	35	88	36
60	86–88	44	90	49
100	86–88	46	92–94	51

are obviously not identical due to differences in the photon fluence. At incident photon energies greater than 100 keV there is a non-negligible difference between the $DER(x)$ functions at 2 cm versus 20 cm GNP depths. Figure 2.6(a) illustrates that at 20 keV incident energy, for the same GNP sizes at different depths the DER as a function of distance from the surface of the gold is nearly identical. This is because at

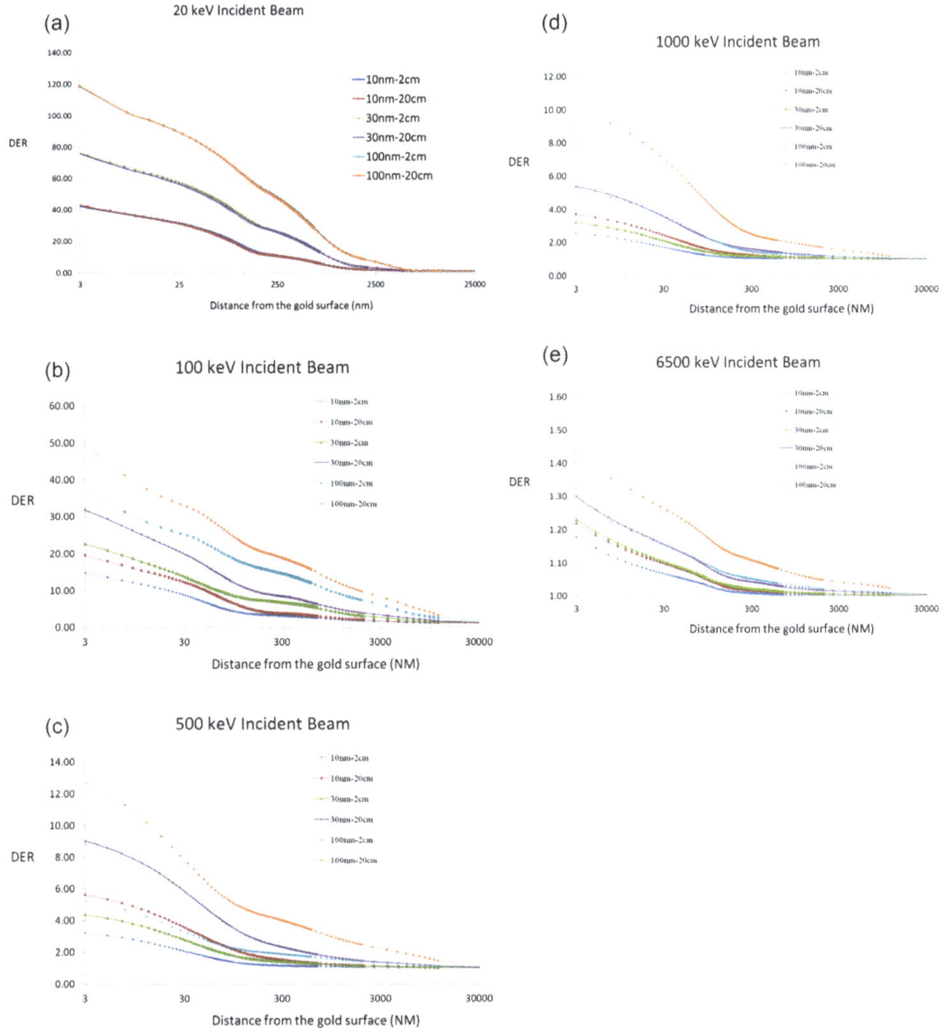

Figure 2.6. (a) (top)–(e) (bottom): Comparison of DERs as function of distance extending to 200 μm for 20 keV (a), 100 keV (b), 500 keV (c), 1000 keV (d), and 6500 keV (e) incident monoenergetic beams with GNPs located at 2 cm and 20 cm depths. DERs shown are on the distal side of the GNP (i.e. beam is incident from the left).

this low energy Compton scattering in water results in little energy loss while the mean free path is about 7.4 cm. Therefore, the photon spectrum incident on the GNP at 2 cm versus 20 cm is not substantially different. As the incident energy increases, larger fractional photon energy loss is experienced and the DER tends to be greater at 20 cm versus at 2 cm, as shown by figures 2.6(b)–(e). This effect is already present at 100 keV, which yields a nontrivial difference between $DER(x)$ at these two depths (figure 2.6(b)).

When the incident energy is 1.0 MeV or greater, the relative difference between $DER(x, d = 2\text{ cm})$ versus $DER(x, d = 20\text{ cm})$ further increases. However, at

6.5 MeV, the fractional difference between these respective $DER(x)$ values appears to be much smaller due primarily to the increased probability of forward Compton scatter with little energy loss. The range at which DER > 1 is gradually longer with increasing incident photon energy due to the increasing contribution of Compton electrons and increasing kinetic energy (and range) of photoelectrons.

Data in figure 2.6 are shown only on the distal side of the GNP, opposite from the beam incidence. At certain beam energies, a nontrivial angular variation in DER exists [10], which may be important to consider when detailed treatment planning computations are required, especially for clustered nanoparticles [9]. The impact of angular anisotropy in electron leakage from the GNP is examined in a different chapter of this book.

Because of the precipitous dose fall-off near the GNP, the *de-facto* biological target of the GNP-enhanced radiation treatment is not always obvious, and it strongly depends on the location of the GNPs with respect to the cell's organelles and structures. For example, in the case when GNPs accumulate at the cell membrane, the dose enhancement received by the chromosome may be an order of magnitude smaller than what the cell membrane receives. Therefore, we also examine the DERs averaged over various radiobiologically important ranges and target sizes corresponding to the DNA-histone structure and cell membrane dimensions (0–10 nm), chromatin structure (100 nm), cell nucleus (1 μm) and endothelial cell (2 μm). The spatially averaged $\langle DER(x) \rangle$ is defined by equation (2.8). The results are collected in figure 2.7 for various cases.

For 10 nm and 30 nm GNP sizes, the peak of the averaged DER over various regions occurs at 20 keV. However, for 100 nm size while the DER averaged over <100 nm peaks at 20 keV, for >100 nm it peaks at 30 keV. In addition, when the target size is up to 100 nm, the average DER exhibits two local maxima corresponding to the K- and L-shell energies of gold. For greater target sizes only the L-shell peak is dominant.

In addition to monoenergetic incident photons, the effects of four spectral beams are also examined using x-ray energies 120 kVp and 220 kVp, and linac-based standard 6.5 MV (STD) and 6.5 MV free of flattening filter (FFF) [33]. The highest DER values are observed using 120 kVp and 220 kVp beams (figure 2.8 and table 2.3). In the immediate vicinity of the GNPs the 120 kVp beam results in slightly larger DER than the 220 kVp beam, but it has a more rapid fall-off with distance than the DER produced by the 220 kVp beam. The two DER(x) curves cross at 17 nm from the surface of the GNP. This is related to the relative importance of the photoelectrons' contribution to the dose at these distances. The probability of photoabsorption by the 120 kVp beam is greater than that of the 220 kVp beam because in these two x-ray spectra the most probable photon energies are ~40 keV and ~70 keV, respectively. However, because of its higher mean photon energy, the 220 kVp beam produces photoelectrons with higher kinetic energies having a longer range.

As observed with the monoenergetic cases, the depth at which the GNP is located does not substantially affect the maximum values of the DER. The largest fractional difference in the DER between these depths is seen only for 100 nm size exposed to

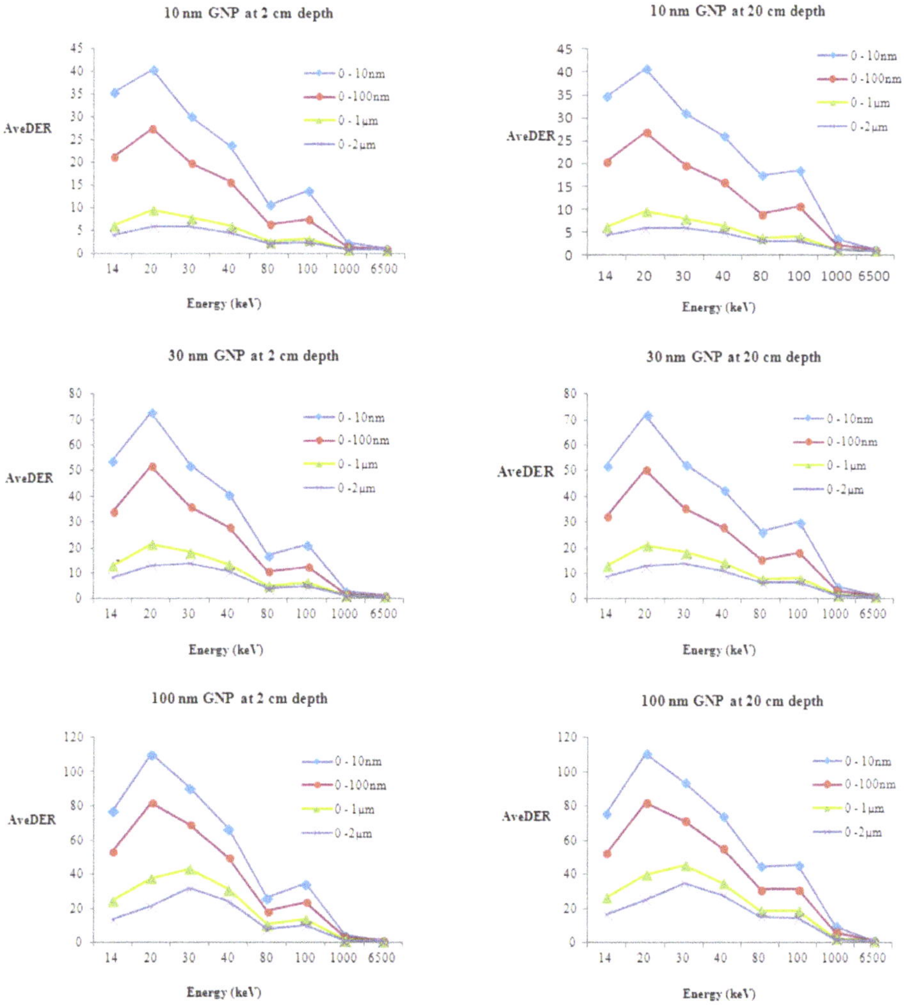

Figure 2.7. DER averaged over various target sizes as function of incident photon energy for three GNP sizes at 2 cm and 20 cm depths.

megavoltage beams. Importantly, megavoltage beams elicit a non-negligible DER when 100 nm nanoparticles are used.

2.7 Discussion

When high-*Z* nanoparticles are irradiated by photons, ionizations in K and higher shells lead to the productions of photoelectrons, Auger electrons, and fluorescent photons. Because of their small size, the photon interactions are nearly uniformly distributed across the volume of the GNPs, and the emission of fluorescent photons are isotropic [34]. Photoelectrons are emitted mostly in the forward direction, which sharply peaks only at high incident photon energies [34]. Because of this and because Auger electrons also exhibit preferential directions, there is an angular dose

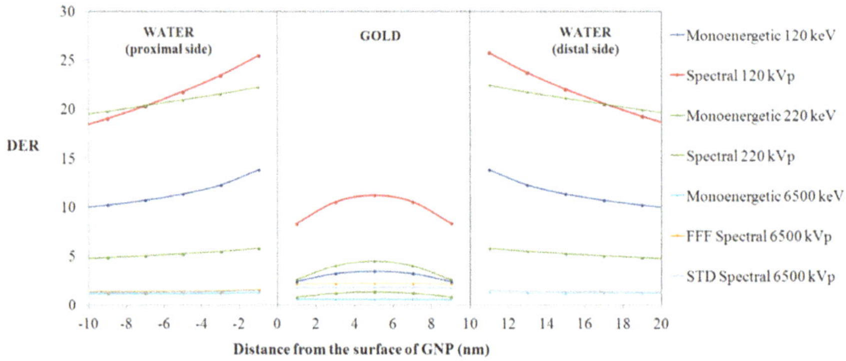

Figure 2.8. Comparison of spectral and monoenergetic cases for 10 nm GNP at 2 cm depth.

Table 2.3. Maximum DER values at 1 nm from the GNP distal surface for the spectral beams examined in this study.

Incident energy	GNP size at 2 cm depth			GNP size at 20 cm depth		
	10 nm	30 nm	100 nm	10 nm	30 nm	100 nm
120 kVp	25.7	40.1	64.5	24.6	38.1	62.7
220 kVp	22.4	42.7	60.5	21.2	40.1	56.3
6.5 MV (FFF)	2.17	2.37	3.65	2.02	2.2	5.8
6.5 MV (STD)	1.78	1.95	2.83	1.64	1.8	4.5

anisotropy about the GNP [10]. The energy deposition pattern about the nanoparticle shows various distinct regimes corresponding to the energies and ranges of escaping electrons. The sharp dose enhancement near the nanoparticle surface is not only due to the presence of low-energy leakage electrons, but also because these electrons have much higher LET. Apart from dose enhancement (DER) there is also a LET enhancement (LER) whose relations are illustrated in figure 2.9. Compared to DER, LER is more precipitously dropping near the nanoparticle surface but it rapidly tapers off to take almost a constant value within two diameters distance, which indicates the preponderance of Auger electrons and other low-energy electrons close to the nanoparticle. Because of the complex angular dependence of Auger electrons on the direction of photoelectrons, although DER shows an anisotropy in which the distal DER_{MAX} is greater than the proximal DER_{MAX}, LER_{MAX} reverses this pattern and exhibits a larger value on the proximal side of the nanoparticle.

However, this is dominant mostly in the immediate vicinity of the GNP, and farther away the dose contribution to the surrounding medium loses its angular variation, as it comes mainly from the superposition of relatively long-range photoelectrons and short-to-medium ranged Auger electrons. Escaping photons,

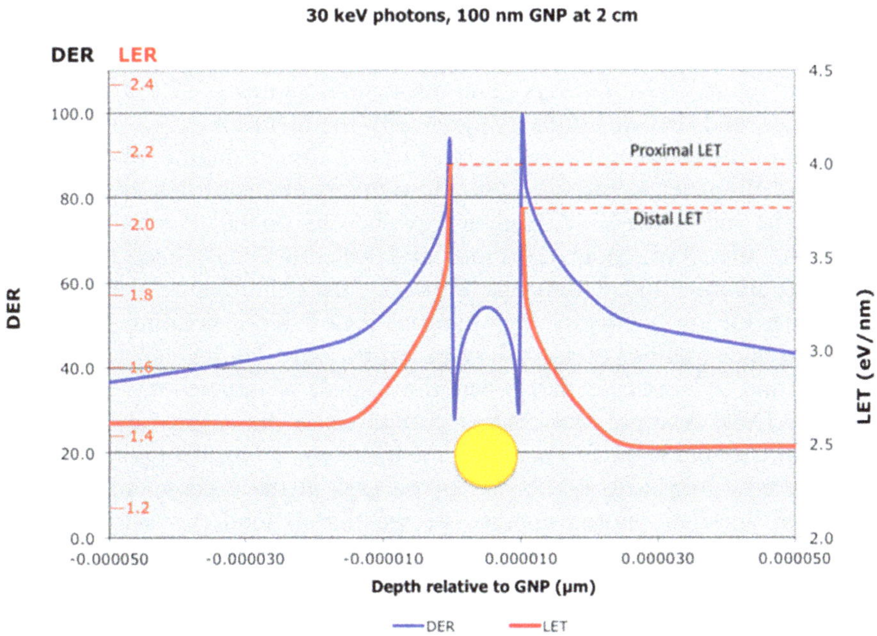

Figure 2.9. Dose enhancement versus LET enhancement about a 100 nm GNP exposed to 30 keV photons in 2 cm water depth. The behavior of DER_{MAX} and LER_{MAX} show opposite patterns in this example.

having no range and small stopping power in aqueous medium, can travel large distances, causing no significant contribution to local dose. The energy deposition in the immediate vicinity of the nanoparticle, up to about 1 µm distance, is predominantly due to low-energy and high-LET Auger electrons. In comparison, photoelectrons are energetic and they are the dominant source of dose deposition from about 1 µm from the surface of nanoparticle to distances up to hundreds of microns, as our results show. Compton electrons, which become dominant above ~500 keV of incident photons, are more energetic and also contribute to the long-range energy deposition. *Nota bene*, these effects are highly localized, and in the macroscopic scale (mm to cm) the total dose does not differ from conventional treatment doses. In the nanometer scale, however, there is a sharp local dose enhancement gradient. This feature permits localizing the dose to only tumor cells, without irradiating normal tissue if the nanoparticles are confined to the tumor volume. In this volume, the magnitude of the dose enhancement depends on the type and size of the GNP, its concentration, and on the energy spectrum of the incident radiation.

Because of the short range of electrons in gold, only those photoelectrons and Auger electrons can escape that are produced within their respective ranges from the surface of the GNP (a.k.a. escape depth). In determining the optimal size of the GNP, there are two competing processes: The most efficient size of the nanoparticle is the maximum size that permits the escape of all electrons. However, the larger the nanoparticle the greater is the volume where such electrons can be produced.

Therefore, from this perspective a large nanoparticle always generates greater total dose in its vicinity than a small nanoparticle. On the converse, the smaller the size of the nanoparticle the larger the chances of its intra-cellular uptake. These effects are clearly seen in figure 2.5 for DER_{MAX} and throughout figures 2.3, 2.6, and 2.7 for all $DER(x)$ values, and they qualitatively agree with the literature.

The effect of the incident photon energy shows a similar duality: photons below the K- or L-shells generate predominantly low-energy electrons that are unlikely to escape from the bulk of the GNP. High-energy photons, on the other hand, will have more uniform flux throughout the GNP and generate higher energy secondary electrons that are more likely to escape. However, the photoelectric absorption rate is much higher for low-energy incident photons (below K), generating more than a magnitude greater number of secondary electrons, than for high-energy photons. Figures 2.3 and 2.7 indicate that when the L-shell is targeted by the incident photons, the DER is appreciably higher compared to the case when the photon energy is near the gold K-edge. Therefore, the lower energy incident photons have a significant role even in large GNPs. When we look at the behavior of DER with respect to the incident photon energy, we see that it tends to follow the gold photoelectric cross section and exhibits local maxima at approximately 20 keV and 90 keV, somewhat above the gold L- and K-shells, respectively. The overall optimal incident photon energy varies between 16 keV and 30 keV depending on the target size over which the DER is averaged (figure 2.7) and on the GNP size (figure 2.5) but not on the depth at which the GNP is located (tables 2.1 and 2.2). The optimal incident photon energy is that at which the nanoparticle transitions from charged particle equilibrium to disequilibrium.

Owing to the escaping Auger electrons, the highest dose is obtained within 10 nm from the gold surface (figures 2.1, 2.6, and 2.8). This puts a limitation on the distance within which the largest benefit of GNPT is achieved, and as a consequence, on the biological target of GNP therapy. Therefore, if the intended target is the DNA, the GNP must penetrate the chromosome and be embedded in the chromatin structure in order to have the highest possible effect. In this case, using kilovoltage energies below the K-shell, a DER of ~40, ~73, or ~90 will be obtained for 10 nm, 30 nm and 100 nm GNP, respectively. Coating of the GNP either to functionalize it or to prevent undesired agglomeration further limits the useful range of DER. In the case when the biological target is the cell membrane, whose phospholipid bilayer is in the order of 10 nm, the DER of the GNP is likely better harvested. When the formation of various response proteins are also included the active range from the gold surface extends to more than 100 nm, where the DER values will be ~28, ~52, ~82 for the respective GNP sizes of 10, 30, and 100 nm. This behavior of the nanoparticles has important implications for the radiobiological modeling of GNPT, which was explored by Zygmanski and colleagues [35].

Various studies of GNP-aided radiotherapy suggested that combination of GNPs with low keV energy x-rays leads to higher dose enhancement [3–5, 36] by two orders magnitude or greater [1, 7]. Our results agree with this, as we obtained DER ~118 for 100 nm GNP at 2 cm depth with incident beam energy of 20 keV, whereas 6.5 MeV beam provided a DER of only ~1.3. But spectral 6.5 MV FFF and STD beams for the same case gave DER values of ~3.7 and ~2.8, respectively. The finding that low-energy incident photons generate larger dose enhancement is explained by the behavior of the photon cross-sections in this energy range. However, in some of the literature [5–7, 37] the gold used in the tissue was not in the form of nanoparticles but in terms of mean macroscopic concentrations, which inherently assumes an atomic mixture of Au with tissue constituents. These studies used a 0D (no spatial variation) or 1D formulation with respect to the gold-laden tissue in micrometer resolution, hence direct comparison to our work would be difficult and may not be appropriate.

The dose fall-off with distance is monotonously decreasing, as shown in e.g. figure 2.6, and it exhibits three regions of differing gradients corresponding to Auger electrons, photoelectrons, and Compton electrons, with respectively increasing energies. The effect of fluorescent photons superimposes on this and they mostly contribute to the dose at larger distances. These regions of energy deposition regimes are also observed by McMahon and colleagues [2]. The general trend of monotonous decrease of DER with distance agrees with all of the literature except for Jones *et al* [7] who show a widely varying behavior of their microscopic dose enhancement factor (mDEF) with distance. Leung *et al* [1] found that for 50 kVp incident photons there is a local maximum in the radial dose profile at 4 μm, which they attribute to the escaping photoelectrons. However, such a peak does not occur in other incident energies they considered. In our work we do not see such local maxima with any of the monoenergetic or spectral beams we analyzed. Also, unlike Carter *et al* [38] whose simulation shows that the energy deposition drops nearly four orders of magnitude within 100 nm from the surface of a 3 nm GNP exposed to 100 kVp, our results indicate a much more subtle gradient.

Similarly to Lechtman *et al* [4], we find that Auger electrons dominate the DER, particularly DER_{MAX}, for small GNP sizes, whereas for large sizes most of the Auger electrons are self-absorbed and it is the photoelectrons that have most of the contribution to the dose. The various regions where these electrons have their respective dominance are clearly seen in figure 2.6. A comparison can be made between our figure 2.6(a) for 20 keV incident photons with its counterpart in Lechtman [4] for a Pd-103 source. Although Lechtman computed the electron intensity as a function of range, the corresponding dose can be inferred from this information, and the spatial location of the local maxima observed by these authors correlate well with the changes in the DER gradients shown in figure 2.6(a) of this work.

The range where DER > 1 can also be compared to two previous studies by Leung *et al* [1] and Lechtman *et al* [4]. For 6.5 MV photons incident on 100 nm GNP, we find that DER ≈ 1 at a distance ~180 μm. In comparison, for 6 MV photons Lechtman concludes that the average range of electrons escaping a 100 nm GNP is ~80 μm, whereas Leung finds this distance at ~1100 μm. Note that the DER includes the effect of the fluorescent photons in addition to the electrons. Therefore, the distance at which DER = 1 is expected to be greater than the range of electrons escaping the GNP. The lack of Compton treatment and the slightly different photon spectrum used by Lechtman explain the difference between our results and their study. However, Leung's mean electron range is substantially larger than that indicated by either Lechtman or our results.

McMahon *et al* [3] computed the dose in water due to a single photoelectric ionization event in a single GNP exposed to monoenergetic and spectral photons. Energy deposition was scored in concentric shells in the water phantom about the GNP, giving rise to an effectively 1D geometry. The authors conclude that the dose deposited near the GNP is weakly connected to the incident photon energy, therefore the energy dependence of the dose enhancement would be different from that of the underlying mass-energy absorption cross sections. Our work does not support this conjecture. Figure 2.3 (with respect to DER_{MAX}), figure 2.4, and figure 2.7 (with respect to various spatial averages of DER) show a strong correlation with the photoelectric cross-section of gold. McMahon and colleagues' inference is valid only if the computational results are analyzed on a per photo-electric (PE) absorption basis, which by definition carries the assumption that the probability of PE interaction is unity. In reality, however, the dose is due to a mixture of photoelectrons, Auger electrons, and Compton electrons. The PE interaction rate is a function of incident photon energy, and it scales with the PE cross section. Therefore, the dose deposited near the GNP should and does follow the PE cross-section of gold, and the dose enhancement also follows the ratio of gold-to-water mass energy absorption coefficients in charged particle equilibrium and the PE cross-section in disequilibrium, as shown in this work.

Our study shows that the dose enhancement increases with increasing GNP size at all photon energies and phantom depths (figures 2.3 and 2.5). *Prima facie*, this is contrary to McMahon and colleagues' conclusion that smaller nanoparticles deposit larger doses in their vicinity due to their greater surface-to-volume ratio. Again, this observation is correct only when the results are normalized per PE event per nanoparticle. Because the volume of the shell (V_d) of the GNP within a fixed electron escape-depth (d) increases with the square of the GNP radius (R), $V_d(d < < R) \cong 4\pi R^2 d$, the total number of radiation interactions in this shell also commensurately increases. Therefore, there will be a proportionately larger number of secondary electrons that escape from the GNP. Hence on an absolute scale a larger nanoparticle will always deposit higher dose in its vicinity than a smaller particle.

2.8 Conclusions

In this work we have analyzed the behavior of the DER in nanometric scales for different GNP sizes, incident beam energies and GNP depths. Based on deterministic computations, a numerical representation of the Green's function of the dose enhancement was obtained. Using systematic computations of DER as a function of x-ray energy and GNP size, optimal photon energies and optimal GNP sizes were determined. We found that for all GNP sizes investigated, the highest DERs are obtained at that energy at which electronic equilibrium transitions to disequilibrium. This occurs at about ~20 keV incident beam energy, targeting the gold L-shell. With respect to the GNP size the highest dose enhancement is seen at 100 nm. Although in this work we did not investigate larger nanoparticles, figure 2.5 shows a plateau effect, indicating that it is unlikely that increased particle size would significantly benefit the maximum attainable DER. The overall highest DER_{MAX} that we found in this study was 120, which occurred using 100 nm GNP when the phantom is exposed to 22 keV photons. This value did not change significantly as function of depth in the phantom. Generally, the effect of the depth is small for the K-shell and it is negligible when the L-shell is targeted. The spatially averaged DER over radiobiologically important ranges or targets has a rapid fall-off as the target size increases (figure 2.7) with a simultaneously shifting of optimal incident photon energy from about 20 keV to 30 keV. The Green's function approach is a rigorous and convenient method suitable for future treatment-planning applications and for the radiobiological modeling of GNP treatment.

2.9 Appendix

The Green's function of radiation transport, $G(\hat{P}_S \rightarrow \hat{P}_T)$, is the angular fluence within phase space element $\hat{P}_T(\bar{r}_T, E_T, \hat{\Omega}_T)$ at the target due to a single source particle within phase space element $\hat{P}_S(\bar{r}_S, E_S, \hat{\Omega}_S)$ [39]. Here, $\bar{r}$ is the location vector, E is the energy of the particle, and $\hat{\Omega}$ is the direction of particle travel at their respective phase space coordinates. In the case of a generalized volumetric source distribution $S(\bar{r}_S, E_S, \hat{\Omega}_S)$, the angular fluence of radiation type j at the target may be written as

$$\Psi_j(\hat{P}_T) = \iiint G_j(\hat{P}_S \rightarrow \hat{P}_T)\ S(\hat{P}_S)\ dE_S\ d\hat{\Omega}_S\ dV_S. \tag{2.9}$$

Following the development presented by Shultis and Faw [39], the total dose in the target region V_T, which has mass m_T, may be expressed as the integral of the particle fluence therein folded with its respective dose response function and summed over all primary and secondary radiation types:

$$D(S \rightarrow T) = \frac{1}{m_T}\sum_j \iiint \rho(\bar{r}_T)\Psi_j(\hat{P}_T)R_j(\hat{P}_T)dE_T\ d\hat{\Omega}_T\ dV_T. \tag{2.10}$$

Here, $\rho(\bar{r}_T)$ is the material density at the target point $\bar{r}_T$. In our present formulation, the source is assumed to be normally incident on the phantom surface at $\bar{r}_0$ with direction $\hat{\Omega}_0$; it is monoenergetic at E_S with $\nu(E_S)$ incident photons. Thus the source is separable to spatial, energy, and spectral components, and it may be written as

$$S = \iiint S(\hat{P}_S)\delta(\bar{r} - \bar{r}_0)\delta(E - E_S)\delta(\hat{\Omega} - \hat{\Omega}_0)d\bar{r}\ dE\ d\hat{\Omega} = \nu(E_S), \tag{2.11}$$

with $\delta(\ldots)$ being the Dirac delta function. The dose in target region T, therefore, becomes:

$$D(S \to T) = \frac{1}{m_T} \int_{V_T} \rho(\bar{r}_T) \mathcal{G}(\bar{r}_0 \to \bar{r}_T) dV_T, \tag{2.12}$$

where the kernel in the above integral is defined as

$$\mathcal{G}(\bar{r}_0 \to \bar{r}_T) \equiv \sum_j \iiint \nu(E_S) R(\overline{P}_T) G_j(\hat{P}_S \to \hat{P}_T) dE_S \, dE_T \, d\hat{\Omega}_T. \tag{2.13}$$

This represents the total dose in target volume V_T. Here, we took advantage of the fact that the source is normally incident on the phantom at $\bar{r}_0$, and no integration with respect to source direction and volumetric distribution is necessary. If we further assume that the dose response function is independent of particle direction in the target volume, which is usually the case, we have

$$\mathcal{G}(\bar{r}_0 \to \bar{r}_T) \equiv \sum_j \iint \nu(E_S) R_i(E_T) \breve{G}_j(\bar{r}_S, E_S \to \bar{r}_T, E_T) dE_S \, dE_T, \tag{2.14}$$

where $\breve{G}_j(\bar{r}_S, E_S \to \bar{r}_T, E_T)$ is the scalar (non-angular) Green's function of radiation type j:

$$\breve{G}_j(\bar{r}_S, E_S \to \bar{r}_T, E_T) \equiv \iint G_j(\overline{P}_S \to \overline{P}_T) d\hat{\Omega}_S \, d\hat{\Omega}_T. \tag{2.15}$$

In a homogeneous medium, such as a small tally voxel of water or tissue may represent, $m_T = \rho V_T$, and for monodirectional source the integration with respect to $d\hat{\Omega}_S$ is not necessary. Further, in a relatively small energy range, the dose response function may be assumed constant, and we have:

$$D(S \to T) = \frac{1}{V_T} \int_{V_T} \mathcal{G}(\bar{r}_0 \to \bar{r}_T) dV_T \tag{2.16}$$

$$\begin{aligned} \mathcal{G}(\bar{r}_0 \to \bar{r}_T) &\equiv \sum_j R_j \iint \nu(E_S) \breve{G}_j(\bar{r}_0, E_S \to \bar{r}_T, E_T) dE_S \, dE_T \\ &= \int_{E_S} \nu(E_S) \left\{ \int_{E_T} \sum_j R_j \breve{G}_j(\bar{r}_0, E_S \to \bar{r}_T, E_T) dE_T \right\} dE_S \end{aligned}. \tag{2.17}$$

Here, the scalar Green's function is

$$\breve{G}_j(\bar{r}_0, E_S \to \bar{r}_T, E_T) \equiv \int_{\Omega} G_j(\bar{r}_0, E_S, \hat{\Omega}_0 \to \bar{r}_T, E_T \hat{\Omega}_T) d\hat{\Omega}_T. \tag{2.18}$$

By virtue of equation (2.8), the integral in the curly brackets above is equivalent to the total dose due to a single source particle having energy E_S. Therefore, we have:

$$\mathcal{G}(\bar{r}_0 \to \bar{r}_T) \equiv \int_{E_S} \nu(E_S) D(E_S) dE_S, \tag{2.19}$$

$$D(S \to T) = \frac{1}{V_T} \iint \nu(E_S) D(E_S) dE_S \, dV_T, \tag{2.20}$$

which, when discretized over energy bins E_i, becomes equivalent to equation (2.2). This formalism may be written for the dose in water with and without GNP present, hence the dose enhancement kernel given in equation (2.3) may be regarded as the Green's function of the dose enhancement ratio. Note that in general the assumption of normal incidence is not necessary. The doses and the DER may be written in discrete ordinates with $\hat{\Omega}_0$ in equation (2.10) replaced by $\hat{\Omega}_S$, leading to $\nu(E_S, \hat{\Omega}_S)$.

References

[1] Leung M K, Chow J C, Chithrani B D, Lee M J, Oms B and Jaffray D A 2011 Irradiation of gold nanoparticles by x-rays: Monte Carlo simulation of dose enhancements and the spatial properties of the secondary electrons production *Med. Phys.* **38** 624–31

[2] McMahon S J *et al* 2011 Biological consequences of nanoscale energy deposition near irradiated heavy atom nanoparticles *Sci. Rep.* **1** 18

[3] McMahon S J *et al* 2011 Nanodosimetric effects of gold nanoparticles in megavoltage radiation therapy *Radiother. Oncol.* **100** 412–6

[4] Lechtman E, Chattopadhyay N, Cai Z, Mashouf S, Reilly R and Pignol J P 2011 Implications on clinical scenario of gold nanoparticle radiosensitization in regards to photon energy, nanoparticle size, concentration and location *Phys. Med. Biol.* **56** 4631–47

[5] Cho S H 2005 Estimation of tumour dose enhancement due to gold nanoparticles during typical radiation treatments: a preliminary Monte Carlo study *Phys. Med. Biol.* **50** N163–73

[6] Cho S H, Jones B L and Krishnan S 2009 The dosimetric feasibility of gold nanoparticle-aided radiation therapy (GNRT) via brachytherapy using low-energy gamma-/x-ray sources *Phys. Med. Biol.* **54** 4889–905

[7] Jones B L, Krishnan S and Cho S H 2010 Estimation of microscopic dose enhancement factor around gold nanoparticles by Monte Carlo calculations *Med. Phys.* **37** 3809–16

[8] Zygmanski P, Liu B, Tsiamas P, Cifter F, Petersheim M, Hesser J and Sajo E 2013 Dependence of Monte Carlo microdosimetric computations on the simulation geometry of gold nanoparticles *Phys. Med. Biol.* **58** 7961–77

[9] Gadoue S M, Zygmanski P and Sajo E 2018 The dichotomous nature of dose enhancement by gold nanoparticle aggregates in radiotherapy *Nanomedicine* **13** 809–23

[10] Gadoue S M, Toomeh D, Zygmanski P and Sajo E 2017 Angular dose anisotropy around gold nanoparticles exposed to X-rays *Nanomedicine* **13** 1653–61

[11] Lorence L J J and Morel J E 1992 *CEPXS/ONELD: A One-dimensional Coupled Electron-photon Discrete Ordinates Code Package* (Albuquerque, NM: Sandia National Laboratories) SAND-92-0261C

[12] Bonhoff W J, Drumm C R, Fan W C, Pautz S D and Valdez G D 2016 *SCEPTRE: Sandia Computational Engine for Particle Transport for Radiation Effects, v. 1.7* (Albuquerque, NM: Sandia National Laboratories)

[13] Ngwa W, Makrigiorgos G M and Berbeco R I 2010 Applying gold nanoparticles as tumor-vascular disrupting agents during brachytherapy: estimation of endothelial dose enhancement *Phys. Med. Biol.* **55** 6533–48

[14] Ngwa W, Makrigiorgos G M and Berbeco R I 2012 Gold nanoparticle-aided brachytherapy with vascular dose painting: estimation of dose enhancement to the tumor endothelial cell nucleus *Med. Phys.* **39** 392–8
[15] Berbeco R I, Ngwa W and Makrigiorgos G M 2011 Localized dose enhancement to tumor blood vessel endothelial cells via megavoltage x-rays and targeted gold nanoparticles: new potential for external beam radiotherapy *Int. J. Radiat. Oncol. Biol. Phys.* **81** 270–6
[16] Tsiamas P, Sajo E, Cifter F, Theodorou K, Kappas C, Makrigiorgos G M, Marcus K and Zygmanski P 2013 Beam quality and dose perturbation of 6 MV flattening-filter-free linac *Eur. J. Med. Phys.* **30** 47–56
[17] Tsiamas P *et al* 2013 Impact of beam quality on megavoltage radiotherapy treatment techniques utilizing gold nanoparticles for dose enhancement *Phys. Med. Biol.* **58** 451–64
[18] Williams M L and Sajo E 2002 Deterministic calculations of photon spectra for clinical accelerator targets *Med. Phys.* **29** 1019–28
[19] Lorence L J J, Morel J E and Valdez G D 1990 *Results guide to CEPXS/ONELD: A one-dimensional coupled electron-photon discrete ordinates code package* (Albuquerque, NM: Sandia National Laboratories) SAND-89-2211
[20] Jordan T 2005 *Update of the CEPXS/ONEDANT coupled photon-electron deterministic transport code package* (Oak Ridge, TN: Oak Ridge National Laboratory)
[21] Lorence L J J 1988 Electron photoemission predictions with CEPXS/ONETRAN *IEEE Trans. Nucl. Sci.* **35** 1288–93
[22] Lorence L J J, Morel J E, Valdez G D, Los Alamos National Lab N and Applied Methods I 1989 *Physics guide to CEPXS: A multigroup coupled electron-photon cross-section generating code* (Albuquerque, NM: Sandia National Laboratories) SAND-89-1685
[23] Berger M J and Seltzer S M 1968 Electron and Photon Transport Programs (Program DATAPAC 4) *National Bureau of Standards* **Vol. NBS-9836**
[24] Berger M J and Seltzer S M 1968 Electron and Photon Transport Programs (Program ETRAN 15) *National Bureau of Standards* **Vol. NBS-9837**
[25] Biggs F and Lighthill R 1971 Analytical approximations for x-ray cross sections *Part II. Sandia National Laboratories* **Vol. SC-RR--710507**
[26] Biggs F and Lighthill R 1988 Analytical approximations for x-ray cross sections *Part III. Sandia National Laboratories* **Vol. SAND-87-0070** 137
[27] Halbleib J A, Kensek R P, Mehlhorn T A, Valdez G D, Seltzer S M and Berger M J 1992 *ITS Version 3.0: The integrated TIGER series of coupled electron/photon Monte Carlo transport codes*
[28] Basu S, Ghosh S K, Kundu S, Panigrahi S, Praharaj S, Pande S, Jana S and Pal T 2007 Biomolecule induced nanoparticle aggregation: effect of particle size on interparticle coupling *J. Colloid Interface Sci.* **313** 724–34
[29] Chithrani B D, Ghazani A A and Chan W C 2006 Determining the size and shape dependence of gold nanoparticle uptake into mammalian cells *Nano Lett.* **6** 662–8
[30] Rahman W N, Bishara N, Ackerly T, He C F, Jackson P, Wong C, Davidson R and Geso M 2009 Enhancement of radiation effects by gold nanoparticles for superficial radiation therapy *Nanomedicine* **5** 136–42
[31] Jaeger R G 1968 *Engineering Compendium on Radiation Shielding, Prepared by Numerous Specialists* (Berlin: Springer)

[32] Ngwa W, Tsiamas P, Zygmanski P, Makrigiorgos G M and Berbeco R I 2012 A multipurpose quality assurance phantom for the small animal radiation research platform (SARRP) *Phys. Med. Biol.* **57** 2575–86
[33] Tsiamas P, Seco J, Han Z, Bhagwat M, Maddox J, Kappas C, Theodorou K, Makrigiorgos M, Marcus K and Zygmanski P 2011 A modification of flattening filter free linac for IMRT *Med. Phys.* **38** 2342–52
[34] Davisson C M and Evans R D 1952 Gamma-ray absorption coefficients *Rev. Mod. Phys.* **24** 79–107
[35] Zygmanski P, Hoegele W, Tsiamas P, Cifter F, Ngwa W, Berbeco R I, Makrigiorgos G M and Sajo E 2013 A stochastic model of cell survival for high-Z nanoparticle radiotherapy *Med. Phys.* **40** 024102
[36] McMahon S J, Mendenhall M H, Jain S and Currell F 2008 Radiotherapy in the presence of contrast agents: a general figure of merit and its application to gold nanoparticles *Phys. Med. Biol.* **53** 5635–51
[37] Van den Heuvel F, Locquet J P and Nuyts S 2010 Beam energy considerations for gold nano-particle enhanced radiation treatment *Phys. Med. Biol.* **55** 4509–20
[38] Carter J D, Cheng N N, Qu Y, Suarez G D and Guo T 2007 Nanoscale energy deposition by X-ray absorbing nanostructures *J. Phys. Chem.* B **111** 11622–5
[39] Shultis J K and Faw R E 2000 *Radiation Shielding* (La Grange Park, IL: American Nuclear Society) p xvi 537

Chapter 3

Deterministic computation benchmarks of nanoparticle dose enhancement—part II. Microscopic to macroscopic scales

Erno Sajo, Fulya Cifter and Piotr Zygmanski

3.1 The effect of concentration distributions

There are many factors other than the physical properties of gold nanoparticles (GNPs) (e.g. size) that can affect the impact of energy deposition near and among GNPs. For example, the spectrum of the incident x-rays, the type of linac target, the irradiation technique, and the depth and location of the tumor with respect to the source were all shown to be key parameters for dose enhancement [1–7]. Another important factor is the heterogeneous biodistribution of GNPs inside the tumor volume [8]. In a radiobiological study by this research group the physical parameters that may effect the dose enhancement inside the tumor were investigated and it was shown that the 3D distribution of GNPs around the cellular target has a significant effect on cell survival [9]. This is because the nanoscopic dose enhancement is a stochastic variable, which leads to stochastic distribution of cell inactivation. In a separate study, it was demonstrated that the computed dose enhancement is sensitive to the microscopic geometry used in the MC simulations, and caution must be exercised in cross-comparing results of various Monte Carlo studies that used seemingly similar microbeam geometries [10].

It is important to understand the dosimetric consequences of the non-uniform accumulation and distribution of GNPs in tumors and their vasculature. Detailed analysis of doses and dose enhancement as a function of homogenized gold concentrations in target volumes at the microscopic to macroscopic scales versus individual GNP clusters at interfaces (nanoscopic scale) are presented in this section. This includes the effects of charged particle disequilibrium, self-shielding, effective ranges of significant dose enhancement, and the relation of dose to kerma for computational efficiency. An important distinction is made between the distal versus proximal sides with respect to the beam incident on the target. Simulation

doi:10.1088/978-0-7503-2396-3ch3

geometries and volumes rage from microvessels to tumor volumes, extending in spatial scales from nanometers (at interfaces) to microns and centimeters.

3.2 Radiation transport computations

Dose enhancement due to various regions of GNP clusters and uniform GNP concentrations (target volumes) embedded in water phantom and exposed to different monoenergetic photon beams (20, 80, 100, 400 keV) was calculated using the CEPXS/ONEDANT [11] deterministic computer code for coupled photon–electron radiation transport. In order to analyze the behavior of DER as a function of gold concentration, GNP clustering, simulation geometry and volume, we performed computations for two cases, as follows:

Case 1 simulates the effect of various homogeneous macroscopic concentrations of gold in defined volumes embedded in a water phantom, which may be the result of diffusion out of a target volume or due to pharmacokinetic mechanisms [12].

Case 2 simulates the effect of clustered GNPs separated by various distances and examines whether or not a volumetric homogenized approach, such as that used in case 1, is equivalent to the more realistic cluster geometry in terms of DER.

In both cases, computations were performed in 1D rectangular geometry, assuming lateral equilibria and that the lateral extent of the examined region (in y and z coordinate directions) is much greater compared to its size in the x-direction, which is also the direction of the incident beam. This is a realistic approach, as the literature reports that GNPs often form a layer on surfaces such as blood vessels or cell membranes, which can have a thickness of a few GNPs while their lateral size may be orders of magnitude greater [13, 14], while most of the dose enhancement is confined to the immediate vicinity of the GNP. Note that in this analysis, GNPs are not touching one-another. Coagulation of nanoparticles and the resultant agglomerates' effect on the DER distribution is a separate nanoscopic problem [15].

3.2.1 Case-1 geometries

The macroscopic dimensionless gold concentration, C, is defined as the ratio of the mass of gold to the total mass of gold-laden tumor or target volume (water–gold mixture), $C = m_{\text{Au}}/m_{\text{Au+Water}}$. Three geometries were investigated: (1) a fixed target volume with varying gold concentration embedded in a water phantom, figure 3.1(a); (2) a defined total mass of gold homogeneously distributed in varying target volumes whose beam-side boundary was located at a fixed distance from the phantom surface, figure 3.1(b); and (3) a defined total mass of gold homogeneously distributed in varying volumes whose center of mass was fixed with respect to the phantom surface, figure 3.1(c).

Geometry 1a examines the macroscopic DER effects in a constant-volume 200 μm-thick target at 2 cm depth while the gold concentration is varied between

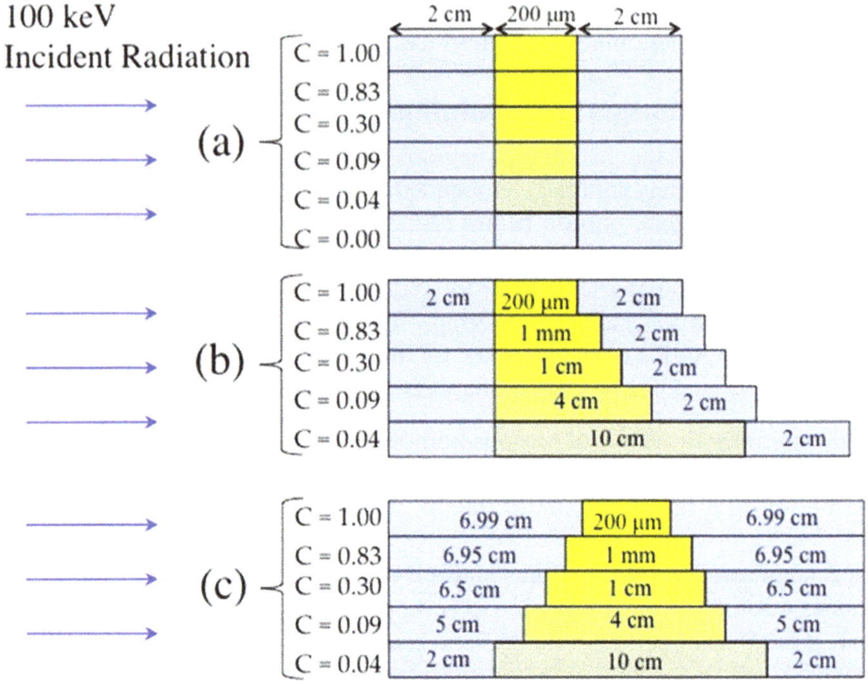

Figure 3.1. Geometries considered in case 1. (a) Fixed volume with varying GNP concentrations. (b) Defined mass of gold in varying volumes whose beam side is located at a fixed distance from the phantom surface. (c) Defined mass of gold in varying volumes whose center of mass is located at a fixed distance from the phantom surface.

two limiting cases, $C = 1$ (pure gold) and $C = 0$ (pure water). These limiting cases permit the analysis of the behavior of other gold concentrations in clinical applications when the aggregation of GNPs is unpredictable. They also provide natural physical limits of pure media (gold versus water).

In geometry 1b, the investigation of DER dependence extends to relatively large target volumes. The mass of gold inside the volume is kept constant while the region thickness is increased in steps such that the concentrations are the same as their counterparts shown in figure 3.1(a) but distributed over larger volumes. This represents a decreasing concentration, which may occur due to GNPs diffusing in one direction. The side of the target region facing the incident photon beam was kept at 2 cm from the surface of the phantom, therefore, for decreasing gold concentrations the center of the region shifts to greater phantom depths, and it reaches 7 cm when $C = 0.04$.

In geometry 1(c), the total mass of gold is again held constant while the center of target region is kept at a fixed depth $x = 7$ cm. Changing the thickness of the gold-laden region varied the gold concentration. Therefore, for decreasing concentrations the amount of water on the beam side of the target volume gradually decreased. The same parametric steps were used as in the first and second geometries. This corresponds to a case when an initial target volume is losing GNPs in two directions via, e.g. diffusion.

In each geometry, five parametric macroscopic gold concentrations were used: $C = 0.04, 0.09, 0.3, 0.83$ and 1. Note that geometries 1a and 1b are identical at $C = 1$, while geometries 1b and 1c are identical at $C = 0.04$. Computations were performed for 100 keV incident photon energy.

3.2.2 Case-2 geometries

These geometries consider periodically grouped GNPs versus homogeneously distributed gold atoms in the same phantom using the same total mass of gold (figure 3.2), exposed to four incident photon energies, 20, 80, 100, and 400 keV.

GNPs are modeled as cubic bodies with $\delta x = \delta y = \delta z$ sides. They form repeated parallel planar agglomerates with non-contiguous morphology (figures 3.2(a) and 3.3). In each agglomerate, the average particle density corresponding to a defined concentration is characterized by the GNP size δx and the average lateral nanoparticle separation of (Δy, Δz), as shown in figures 3.3(a) and (b). In this way, the agglomerate-plane forms a slab whose thickness is δx while its lateral size is substantially greater than δx. These parameters as well as the separation of planes (Δx) can be changed to adjust the gold concentration nanoscopically in the cluster-plane (figure 3.2(a)) or macroscopically by homogeneously distributing the same amount of gold in the target volume (figure 3.2(b)).

For example, in the case of 10 nm GNPs (δx = 10 nm) with a mean separation of 34 nm in y and z directions ($\Delta y = \Delta z$ = 34 nm) the homogenized concentration

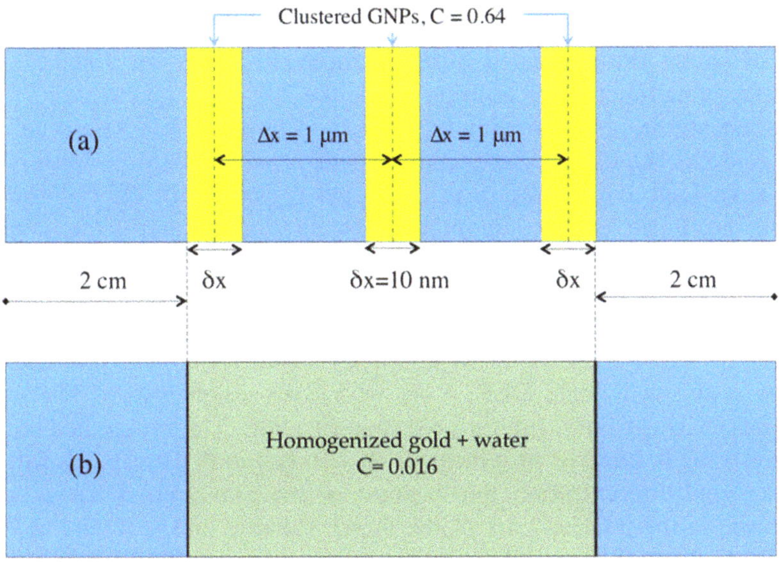

Figure 3.2. Periodic regions of GNP agglomerates in water (a), and when their mass is homogenized in the same volume (b). Dimensions are not to scale. The radiation source is a plane-parallel photon beam normally incident on the left side of the phantom with energies, 20, 80, 100, and 400 keV.

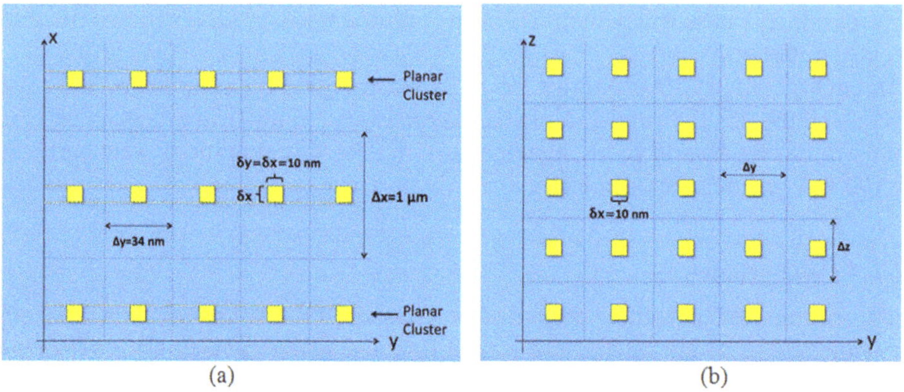

Figure 3.3. (a) x–y view of the three GNP planar clusters shown in figure 3.2(a). (b) y–z view of a single GNP planar cluster. The lateral size of the plane is substantially larger than δx. Dimensions are not to scale.

within a single agglomerate-plane becomes $C = 0.64 = 640$ mg g^{-1}. If within the entire target volume the separation of cluster-planes is $\Delta x = 1$ μm (figure 3.2(a)), the homogenized target concentration becomes 0.016, equivalent to 16 mg g^{-1} gold per gold–water mixture (figure 3.2(b)). The same target concentration can be achieved by appropriate variations of the above parameters. For example, $\delta x = 20$ nm with $\Delta y = \Delta z = 96$ nm or $\delta x = 2$ nm with $\Delta y = \Delta z = 9.7$ nm while the separation of the agglomerate-planes is kept constant at 1 μm.

3.3 Macroscopic DER effects in case-1 geometries

3.3.1 Dependence on concentration in a fixed tumor volume

Figure 3.4 shows the computed dose enhancement ratios for 100 keV incident photon energy as function of position inside the 200 μm target region for various gold concentrations, corresponding to geometry 1 in figure 3.1. As is seen, a region of pure gold has the highest dose enhancement proximally to the beam. This is a limiting case. High concentration in the target region is not only physiologically unfeasible but it also leads to suboptimal dose distribution across the target due to self-shielding, varying by a factor of 4 from proximal to distal in our example. Relatively homogeneous dose distribution can be achieved at and below $C = 0.3$. At this concentration the DER is nearly constant across much of the target volume at DER = ~28. At a more realistic tumor or vasculature gold concentration of $C = 0.04 = 40$ mg g^{-1} the DER = 4.6 within the target region. The maximum DER varies nearly linearly with the gold concentration. This is expected because the interaction rate is linearly proportional to the material density. However, with decreasing gold concentration the location of the maximum DER is gradually shifted towards the internal part of the target volume, and it occurs at its center when $C < 0.3$. Note that both the location and magnitude of the maximum value of DER are sensitive to the concentration in the target volume.

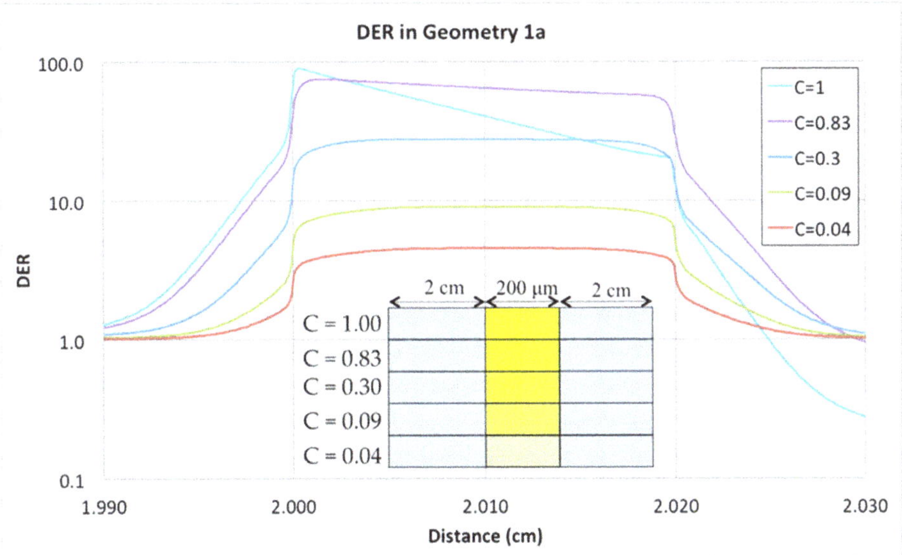

Figure 3.4. DERs versus depth for geometry 1a (figure 3.1(a)) using 100 keV incident photons. DER = 1 for $C = 0$.

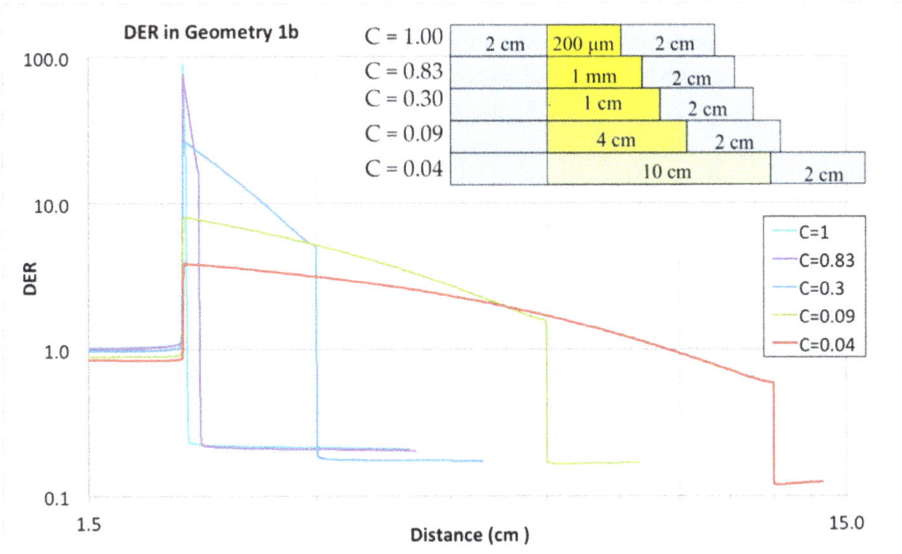

Figure 3.5. DER versus depth with gold concentration as parameter in geometry 1b (figure 3.1(b)). Incident photons are 100 keV.

3.3.2 Depth and volume dependence for diffusion in one direction

Figure 3.5 shows the DER as a function of position for geometry 1b (figure 3.1(b)). Here, the gold concentration is a parameter that is related to the volume of the target region, which varies across the simulations. This case corresponds to a physiological scenario when a gold-laden initial volume of 200 μm thickness with $C = 1$ (limiting case) experiences diffusion or other biodistribution mechanism towards the distal direction with respect to the beam. Table 3.1 compares the maximum DER values (DER_{MAX}) for the three geometries given in figure 3.1. Compared to geometry 1a, in this case the DER_{MAX} values are consistently lower due to beam attenuation with depth.

3.3.3 Depth and volume dependence for diffusion in two directions

Figure 3.6 shows a similar scenario as figure 3.5, except the biodistribution mechanism is allowed to take place in two directions, proximal and distal. The $C = 0.04$ case is identical to its counterpart in figure 3.5. Otherwise, the changing depth of the target region introduces a different phantom depth dependence compared to figure 3.5, due to photon attenuation in water, which results in lower DER_{MAX} values than seen in the latter scenario.

Important insights can be gained by examining the dependence of maximum DER values on the gold concentration and on the size and location of the gold-laden tumor region. In geometry 1a, varying amounts of gold are located in a constant 200 μm region at 2 cm depth, which has varying concentrations. Compared to geometry 1b, the depth of the mixture is the same, however, in the latter geometry the volume of the mixture is increased while the total mass of gold in the region is kept constant, which results in decreasing gold concentration. When the DER_{MAX} values of these two geometries are compared, we see that geometry 1a has slightly higher maximum DER values, even though the mass of gold is higher in geometry 1b (table 3.1). The difference in DER_{MAX} values is more pronounced in smaller concentrations. This is expected because while the gold atoms in geometry 1a are confined to the 200 μm region, the gold atoms in geometry 1b are spread into a larger volume that also includes more water, which has a non-trivial contribution to photon attenuation. When geometry 1c is compared to the first two geometries, we see that the DER_{MAX} values are even smaller because at increasing gold concentrations the mixture region is placed deeper in the phantom, thus photons undergo more attenuation before they reach the gold atoms.

Table 3.1. DER_{MAX} values for the three geometries in case 1 as a function of gold concentration.

Au concentration	Geometry 1a	Geometry 1b	Geometry 1c
$C = 0.04$	4.56	3.89	3.89
$C = 0.09$	9.04	8.06	7.53
$C = 0.30$	27.90	27.00	22.5
$C = 0.83$	75.17	75.15	58.8
$C = 1$ (limit)	90.10	90.10	69.9

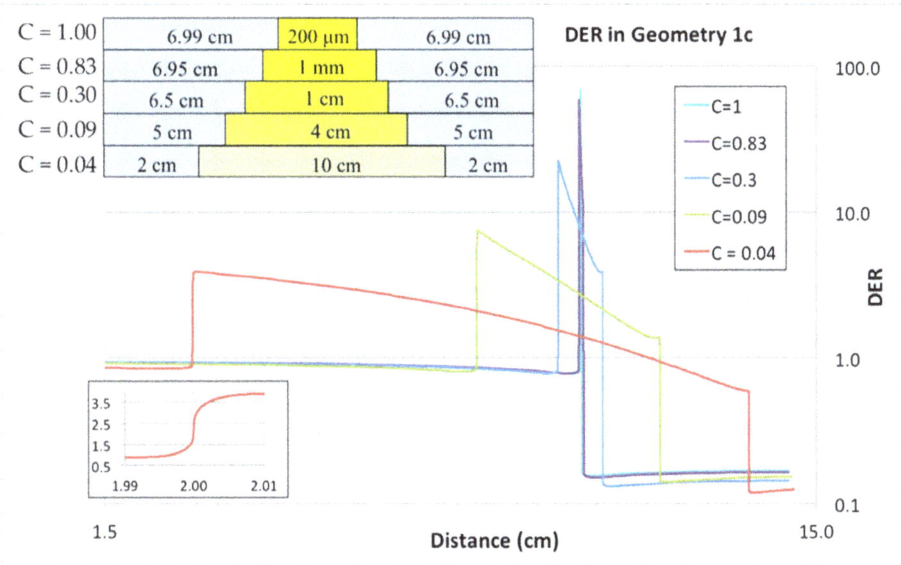

Figure 3.6. DER versus depth with gold concentration as parameter in geometry 1c (figure 3.1(c)). Inset shows the DER(C = 0.04) transition at 2 cm depth using linear scale. Incident photons are 100 keV.

3.3.4 Kerma approximation of dose

In detailed dose calculations an important reason for performing coupled electron–photon radiation transport computations is that charged particle equilibrium (CPE) does not exist in all regions of interest. At the interface of water and the gold-laden target CPE is reached at the range of the secondary electrons leaking from the target region. For example, the continuous slowing down approximation (CSDA) range of 100 keV electrons is 16 μm in gold and 143 μm in water. Therefore, there will be charged particle disequilibrium within 143 μm in the water outside the target region, and within a minimum of 16 μm inside the mixture depending on the gold concentration therein. The lower the GNP concentration, the deeper the CPE extends toward the center of mixture. One possible measure of the degree of CPE is the difference between the dose and kerma.

We wish to examine the extent and limitations of using kerma approximation of the dose in and in the vicinity of the homogenized gold-laden region. For this purpose, we calculated the kerma at proximal (at the point 500 nm in front of the GNP-laden region), center and distal sides (at the point 500 nm past the GNP-laden region) in case 1. From the computer simulations we extracted the energy spectrum and the corresponding photon flux at those points. The mass energy absorption coefficients were taken from the NIST XCOM database [16]. Kerma was computed using equation (3.1), where ψ_i is the photon flux in energy interval E_i:

$$KERMA = \sum_i \left(\frac{\mu_{en}}{\rho}\right)_i \psi_i E_i. \tag{3.1}$$

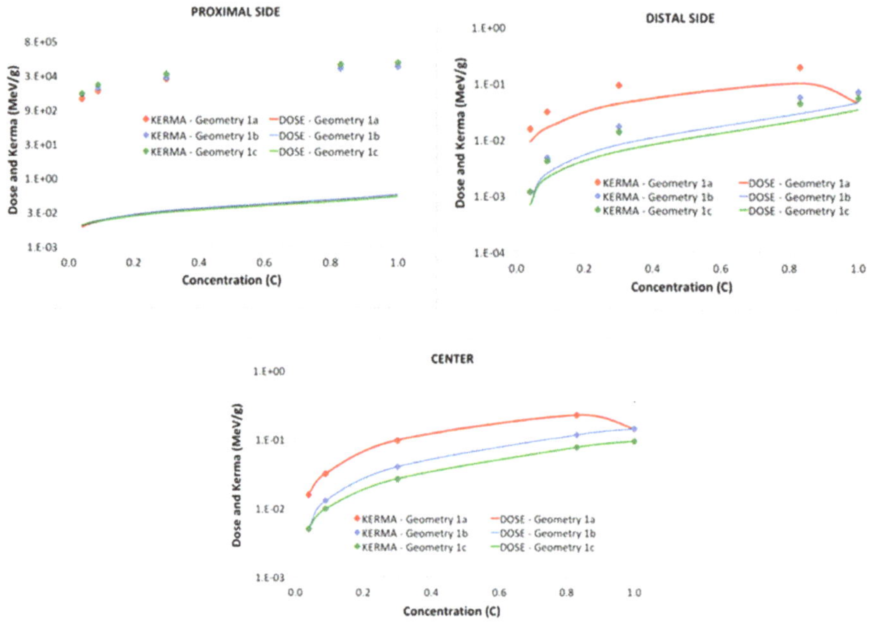

Figure 3.7. Dose and kerma at the proximal and distal sides, and in the center of the target volume as a function of concentration for the three geometries of case 1. Incident photons are 100 keV.

Figure 3.7 shows the computed dose and kerma values at the points of interest. Because the range of secondary electrons leaking from the gold-laden region is much greater than 500 nm, charged particle disequilibria exist at the boundaries of the target, at which points the differences between dose and kerma are the greatest. In the proximal side, the difference between dose and kerma is nearly constant and nearly linearly varies with the concentration regardless of geometry. In the distal side, geometry 1a exhibits greater nonlinearity at high concentrations compared to the other two geometries, where the situation reverses. The difference between the dose and kerma is greater at the proximal side, nearly six orders of magnitude, where the photon flux is much greater leading to higher interaction rate and higher degree of charged particle disequilibrium. That difference is significantly lower at the distal side because of the decrease in the ranges of secondary electrons. Note that at the distal side CPE is approached when $C = 1$, but this does not occur at the proximal side. At the center of the target region, nearly complete CPE exists, as seen by the coincidence of collisional kerma and dose.

3.3.5 The effective distance of dose enhancement

An important metric is the gradient of the DER adjacent to the GNP-laden region, which may be significant from the perspective of normal tissue sparing. We investigated the distance in water, away from the GNP-laden region, in which the DER drops below a cut-off value of 1.05. Within this range the presence of gold has

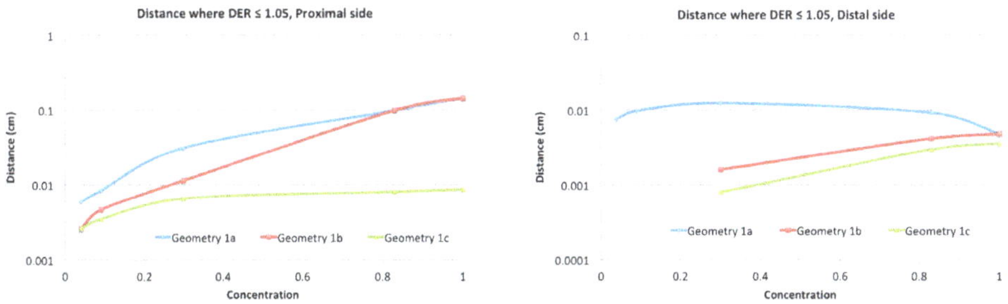

Figure 3.8. Effective distance of dose enhancement (d_{eff}) as a function of gold concentration on the proximal side (left) and distal side (right). Values for $d_{eff} < 0$ are not shown. Incident photons are 100 keV.

a significant influence, therefore, we term it as effective distance, or d_{eff}. Figure 3.8 shows the effective distances at which the DER falls below 1.05 in the proximal and distal sides as a function of gold concentration. Depending on the concentration and simulation geometry, d_{eff} varies between 26 μm–0.15 cm. There is a general tendency for d_{eff} to increase with concentration, except for the proximal side of geometry 3 and the distal side of geometry 1a.

At the proximal side, both geometries, 1a and 1b, show increasing d_{eff} with increasing gold concentration, whereas d_{eff} is almost constant in geometry 1c for all but the lowest concentrations. The data suggests that the similarity between geometries 1a and 1b in this regard is due in large part to the same photon fluence and spectra incident on the target region and because at high concentrations, the geometries start to converge. At small concentrations, there is a significant difference between their volumes, which gives rise to the observed differences in d_{eff}. In geometry 1c, as the concentration increases the location of the target is progressively deeper in the phantom with commensurate decrease in the photon fluence. This may provide an explanation for the relatively constant d_{eff}, as the increased amount of water is compensating for the effect of the increased gold concentration.

For the distal side, both geometries 1b and 1c exhibit increasing d_{eff} with concentration, whereas in geometry 1a d_{eff} first increases then decreases with concentration, becoming identical to geometry 1b at $C = 1$. In geometries 1b and 1c, the linear increase of d_{eff} with concentration is due to the combined effect of increasing the amount of gold in the target volume and decreasing distance of the distal side from the phantom surface. For the first geometry, we see that d_{eff} is increasing until C reaches 0.3, which is also the dose uniformity limit, as shown for the case of fixed tumor volume above. Above $C = 0.3$ the dose distribution in the target volume becomes non-uniform due to self-shielding, resulting in a gradual decrease of d_{eff}.

The dose enhancement effect is confined to a very narrow region about the gold-laden target due to low-energy electrons. Beyond this immediate vicinity, the DER drops below 1.0 at both the proximal and distal sides for all gold concentrations in geometries 1a and 1b and on the distal side of geometry 1a, which is due to a non-trivial shielding effect. However, the nature of this effect is different for the proximal versus distal sides.

At the distal side, DER is always less than 1.0 outside the target volume. This can be clearly seen in geometries 1b and 1c (figures 3.5 and 3.6, respectively). Here, when the gold is distributed in large volumes with low concentrations, the DER falls below 1.0 even inside the target volume, making $d_{\text{eff}} < 0$, which is not plotted in figure 3.8. This is because the larger target volume also contains water in addition to gold, which has an added shielding effect.

A notable effect takes place on the proximal side of the target volume, which also results in DER < 1 but farther away from the target volume. In the case of pure water, the dose at any depth is due to a superposition of forward and backscattered photons and electrons from various other depths. When a gold-laden region replaces a volume of water, many particles that otherwise would backscatter from this volume and reach this depth will be absorbed by gold atoms or their energies will be reduced due to increased scattering. Hence, these particles do not contribute to the dose farther away from the target, while the DER is restricted to the immediate vicinity of the target. In geometry 1a, and in high concentrations of geometry 1b, the gold-laden volume is very small; therefore, relatively few of these particles are lost. In addition, these volumes are relatively close to the phantom surface and many backscattered photons are lost with or without the presence of gold-laden volume. Thus, in these cases the DER remains above 1.0.

3.4 Microscopic effects in case-2 geometries—the inadequacy of spatial homogenization

Figure 3.9 plots the DER versus depth for the geometries shown in figures 3.2 and 3.3 using 20, 80, 100 and 400 keV incident photon energies. The blue line corresponds to the geometry where the GNPs form repeated planar groups or agglomerates, each of which is embedded in a Δx thick water layer (figure 3.2(a)). The red line corresponds to the case where the same amount of gold is homogenized within Δx (figure 3.2(b)). In these computations, the GNP sizes and their separations were chosen such that $C = 0.64 = 640$ mg g^{-1} inside each cluster, and $C = 0.016 = 16$ mg g^{-1} when the gold is homogenized over $\Delta x = 1$ μm.

The significance of the distinction between dose enhancements due to planar groups versus homogenized gold is that GNPs are more likely to agglomerate than remain solitary, and they never form a homogenized atomic mixture with tissue [12, 14]. When the dose is computed in such a mixture, some of the energy deposition occurs in gold, which does not contribute to cell inactivation potential. In reality, the radiobiologically important energy deposition occurs in tissue. Therefore, a dose enhancement computed using a homogeneous atomic or molecular mixture of gold and water gives an incorrect representation of the dose enhancement in tissue. This series of computations aims to show the difference between the DERs obtained using a homogeneous mixture versus groups of GNPs.

When the GNPs are considered in planar clusters, the DER has a sharp rise in the water approaching the cluster (figure 3.9, blue line). 20 keV and 100 keV incident photons provide the highest DER due to their respective proximity to the L- and K-shells of gold. But irrespective of the incident photon energy, the variation of

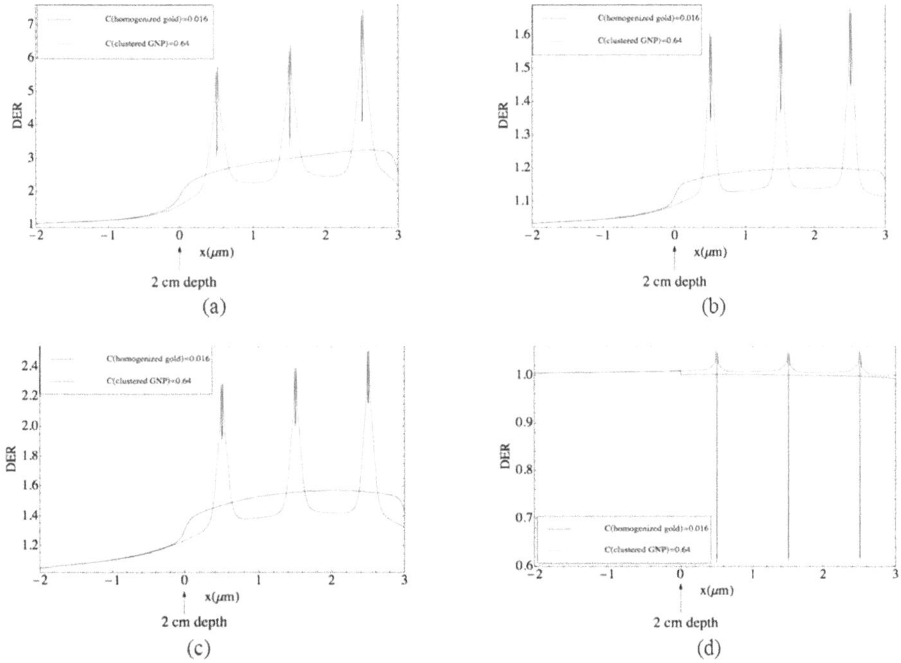

Figure 3.9. DER variation with depth for isolated GNP clusters (blue, cf figure 3.2(a)) versus homogenized gold–water mixture containing the same mass of gold (red, cf figure 3.2(b)) for the geometries of case 2 using incident photon energies (a) 20 keV, (b) 80 keV, (c) 100 keV and (d) 400 keV. Here, the gold concentration inside the cluster is $C = 0.64$, which becomes $C = 0.016$ when the clusters are homogenized over the entire target volume.

DER with depth has significant non-uniformity. In contrast, when the same amount of gold is homogenized in the target volume, the computed DER appears to provide a more uniform dose coverage of the target, including near the edge of the target region (figure 3.9, red line). But because atomic mixture of gold–water concentration following administration of GNPs is not likely to occur, it is clearly seen that spatial homogenization of the GNPs in the target region may give erroneous results for the computed dose enhancement. The relative error increases for energies where the incoherent scattering cross section of gold becomes comparable with or greater than its photoelectric cross section. In this case, homogenization shows DER $\leqslant 1$ due to the inclusion of gold in the medium where DER is computed (figure 3.9(d)). In reality, DER should be computed in tissue (or water), where it is greater than one, rather than in an atomic mixture of gold and water.

3.5 Discussion

The literature that focuses on the dependence of DER on macroscopic GNP concentration invariably uses homogenized atomic mixtures of gold and water. But disparate phantom geometries, incident beam energies and computational simulation methods hinder the cross-comparison of the results. A common finding in all studies, including ours, is that the maximum DER value is increasing with increasing concentration of gold and GNPs can be used as radiation enhancers in clinical applications. Apart from a deterministic study that considered the effect of coagulated GNPs at the nanoscale [15], none of the literature makes the distinction between proximal and distal effects, including the effective dose enhancement distances, and the differences between clustered versus homogenized GNP distributions.

Several studies may be compared to our results for case 1, albeit to a limited extent. For example, Cho found that for a concentration of 18 mg g^{-1} in a simulated tumor at 0.075 cm depth the average DER was 3.8 using 140 kVp x-rays [17]. Our study shows that for 16 mg g^{-1} homogenized gold concentration in a tumor at 2 cm depth the average DER is between 1.2 and 3.0 for energies ranging from 20 keV to 100 keV (figure 3.9). Further, for the same geometry and energy but for 30 mg g^{-1} concentration Cho's average DER value was 5.6, whereas in our work, using 40 mg g^{-1} concentration at 2 cm depth with 100 keV photons, the DER is approximately 4.0 (figure 3.4). In a separate but related work, Cho and colleagues used a ^{169}Yb (average 93 keV) brachytherapy source (among others) and they reported a dose enhancement factor (DEF) of 108% (equivalent to DER = 2.08) for 18 mg g^{-1} gold concentration [18]. Our work using 100 keV photons with 16 mg g^{-1} homogenized concentration region at 2 cm shows DER = 1.6 (figure 3.9(c)), which may be due to the difference in the phantom depth used.

Mesbahi *et al* simulated 18 mg g^{-1} Au homogeneously distributed in a tumor at $x = 0$ cm depth of a water phantom [19]. In their Monte Carlo computations they used 50–120 keV monoenergetic photons, a ^{60}Co beam, and 6 and 18 MV clinical beams. For 80 and 100 keV incident energies their DER values were in the range of 2.0–2.5. In comparison, for the same two incident photon energies, our study shows that the DER varies between 1.2–1.6 when 16 mg g^{-1} concentration is used in a region at 2 cm depth.

Amato *et al* studied the potential anti-angiogenetic effects of GNP-diffusion from the tumor vasculature [20]. Average DERs were computed as function of target depth and homogeneous gold concentration within the investigated volume. For $C = 0.09$ at 3 cm and 5 cm depths with incident beam energy of 150 kVp, the DER was computed as ~5. This may be compared to our case 1, geometry 1b with $C = 0.09$, which shows DER = 8. The discrepancy is most likely due to the different incident photon energies and phantom depths used in the studies.

Our results showing values of DER < 1 agree with the observations of Guidelli and Baffa who studied how silver and gold nanoparticles affect the dose deposition in alanine dosimeters at several different concentrations [21]. Their computational evaluation uses the assumption of charged particle equilibrium, and they report that while homogeneous size distribution of GNPs gives rise to DER values greater than 1, large and segregated concentrations of silver shield the radiation, resulting in DER < 1. For 100 keV incident energy, their theoretical DER values for $C = 0.01$ and $C = 0.03$ were 1.8 and 3.5, respectively, while experimental results for the same concentrations and 107 keV effective energy showed DER = 1.7 and DER = 2.5, respectively. In comparison, in our study we find that for $C = 0.016$ and $C = 0.04$

with 100 keV incident energy DER = 1.4–1.6 (case 2, homogenized) and DER = 2.9–4.5 (case 1, geometry 1a), respectively, depending on the location inside the target volume.

These results demonstrate a relatively good agreement considering the differences in concentrations, phantom depths and incident energies. Our results show that the dosimetric properties of the region of interest significantly vary as a function of gold concentration, tumor size and the depth in tissue. For large volumes and low gold concentrations the role of water is significant and it prevents dose homogeneity inside the tumor. Even for relatively small volumes, the concentration of GNPs should be small if a uniform dose distribution is needed. Separately, if a distinct peak in the dose distribution is desired at a defined location in the tumor while the GNPs are homogeneously distributed, it can be achieved only at the proximal side of the region of interest and it can be modulated by changing the gold concentration. This will also lead to less dose uniformity within the region and a higher DER_{MAX} with a sharp dose fall-off that will prevent any unwanted dose in regions, which are out of interest.

Unlike case 1 of our study, which is relatively simple and whose results may be compared to data in the literature, case 2 presents a more realistic geometry, which has not been extensively studied. The presence of individual GNP clusters results in sharp peaks and valleys in the DER distribution across the targeted volume. When the DER is computed using the simplifying assumption of homogeneous atomic gold concentration, the results can significantly underpredict or overpredict the actual DER values. Further, the total dose deposited in tumor volume is also overpredicted because the dose computation includes gold atoms rather than only water (or tissue). Despite this shortcoming of the homogenization method in predicting the magnitude of the DER, evaluation of the dosimetric impact of the presence of GNPs in a macroscopic volume is not feasible by nanoscopic computations of dose distribution about individual or even clusters of GNPs. Dose computations in homogenized gold–water or gold–tissue mixtures may be used as surrogate for the superposition of energy deposition at the nanoscale about GNPs. This work contributes to the understanding of this concept and its limitations.

Understanding the variability of dose distribution inside and in the proximity of the volume of interest is important in many respects, especially from the perspective of normal tissue sparing and when the tumor volume has heterogeneous structure, including radio-resistant regions. Studies are underway on 'dose painting', which includes delivering a non-uniform dose distribution to the tumor so that radio-resistant cells receive more radiation. Our results would play a critical role in a possible future GNP-aided dose painting, such as studied by Ngwa and Hao who present a particular application of radiotherapy with *in situ* dose painting via inhalation delivery as one of the chapters in this book.

3.6 Conclusions

In this work we showed that in the microscopic to macroscopic spatial scale, GNP concentration, biodistribution, and target volume have a strong impact on the magnitude of DER, dose uniformity, and the distance within which DER > 1 or DER < 1. Additionally, distinction must be made between DER effects at the proximal versus distal sides of the gold-laden volume, with respect to the incident beam direction.

In small gold concentrations confined to a small volume (case 1, geometry 1a) dose uniformity is nearly achieved throughout the volume, except for its edges. In contrast, varying volumes having the same mass of gold but commensurately different concentrations (case 1, geometries 1a and 1b) cannot yield uniform DER distribution.

A significant difference exists between the proximal and distal sides in terms of DER and the range within which DER is greater than unity. The role of self-shielding by both gold and water (the latter for larger volumes) is important. The effective distance from the edge of the target volume at which DER > 1.05 varies by more than an order of magnitude, depending on the geometry and gold concentrations, ranging from 30 μm to 1400 μm on the proximal and 8.0 μm to 120 μm on the distal sides. Outside of the immediate vicinity of the gold-laden region where large DERs are observed, DER becomes less than unity on both the proximal and distal sides. For large volumes, the depth at which DER < 1 may be inside the gold-laden target volume.

Kerma is a good predictor of the dose in the center of the target volume. Therefore, when the DER is to be determined at the center, no detailed coupled electron–photon radiation transport computations are necessary. Towards the edges of the target volume, the charged particle equilibrium is rapidly lost, where there is a precipitous departure of dose from kerma. The discrepancy between kerma and dose at the distal side of the target volume is smaller than a factor of 2 for all concentrations except for $C = 1$, However, there is a very large charged particle disequilibrium at the proximal side of the volume, reaching many orders of magnitude.

The more realistic clustering effect that GNPs experience gives rise to sharp peaks and valleys of DER. The assumption of homogeneous atomic gold distribution versus individual GNP clusters can significantly under- or overestimate the computed DER in tumor subvolumes and near vascular deposits of GNPs.

References

[1] Tsiamas P *et al* 2013 Impact of beam quality on megavoltage radiotherapy treatment techniques utilizing gold nanoparticles for dose enhancement *Phys. Med. Biol.* **58** 451–64

[2] Tsiamas P, Mishra P, Cifter F, Berbeco R I, Marcus K, Sajo E and Zygmanski P 2014 Low-Z linac targets for low-MV gold nanoparticle radiation therapy *Med. Phys.* **41** 021701

[3] Tsiamas P, Sajo E, Cifter F, Theodorou K, Kappas C, Makrigiorgos M, Marcus K and Zygmanski P 2014 Beam quality and dose perturbation of 6 MV flattening-filter-free linac *Phys. Med.* **30** 47–56

[4] Detappe A, Tsiamas P, Ngwa W, Zygmanski P, Makrigiorgos M and Berbeco R 2013 The effect of flattening filter free delivery on endothelial dose enhancement with gold nanoparticles *Med. Phys.* **40** 031706

[5] Robar J L 2006 Generation and modelling of megavoltage photon beams for contrast-enhanced radiation therapy *Phys. Med. Biol.* **51** 5487–504
[6] Robar J L, Riccio S A and Martin M A 2002 Tumour dose enhancement using modified megavoltage photon beams and contrast media *Phys. Med. Biol.* **47** 2433–49
[7] Garth J C, Critchfield K L, Turinetti J R and Beutler D E 1996 A comprehensive comparison of CEPXS/ONELD calculations of dose enhancement with the Co-60 data set of Wall and Burke *IEEE Trans. Nucl. Sci.* **43** 2731–41
[8] Jain S *et al* 2011 Cell-specific radiosensitization by gold nanoparticles at megavoltage radiation energies *Int. J. Radiat. Oncol. Biol. Phys.* **79** 531–9
[9] Zygmanski P, Hoegele W, Tsiamas P, Cifter F, Ngwa W, Berbeco R, Makrigiorgos M and Sajo E 2013 A stochastic model of cell survival for high-Z nanoparticle radiotherapy *Med. Phys.* **40** 024102
[10] Zygmanski P, Liu B, Tsiamas P, Cifter F, Petersheim M, Hesser J and Sajo E 2013 Dependence of Monte Carlo microdosimetric computations on the simulation geometry of gold nanoparticles *Phys. Med. Biol.* **58** 7961–77
[11] Lorence L J 1991 CEPXS/ONELD version 2. 0; A discrete ordinates code package for general one-dimension coupled electron-photon transport *IEEE Trans. Nucl. Sci.* **39** 1031–5
[12] Perry J L, Reuter K G, Kai M P, Herlihy K P, Jones S W, Luft J C, Napier M, Bear J E and DeSimone J M 2012 PEGylated PRINT nanoparticles: the impact of PEG density on protein binding, macrophage association, biodistribution, and pharmacokinetics *Nano Lett.* **12** 5304–10
[13] Shukla R, Bansal V, Chaudhary M, Basu A, Bhonde R R and Sastry M 2005 Biocompatibility of gold nanoparticles and their endocytotic fate inside the cellular compartment: a microscopic overview *Langmuir* **21** 10644–54
[14] Basu S, Ghosh S K, Kundu S, Panigrahi S, Praharaj S, Pande S, Jana S and Pal T 2007 Biomolecule induced nanoparticle aggregation: effect of particle size on interparticle coupling *J. Colloid Interface Sci.* **313** 724–34
[15] Gadoue S M, Zygmanski P and Sajo E 2018 The dichotomous nature of dose enhancement by gold nanoparticle aggregates in radiotherapy *Nanomedicine* **13** 809–23
[16] Berger M J, Hubbell J H, Seltzer S M, Chang J S, Coursey R, Sukumar R, Zucker D S and Olsen K 2010 NIST Standard Reference Database 8 (XGAM) https://dx.doi.org/10.18434/T48G6X
[17] Cho S H 2005 Estimation of tumour dose enhancement due to gold nanoparticles during typical radiation treatments: a preliminary Monte Carlo study *Phys. Med. Biol.* **50** N163–73
[18] Cho S H, Jones B L and Krishnan S 2009 The dosimetric feasibility of gold nanoparticle-aided radiation therapy (GNRT) via brachytherapy using low-energy gamma-/x-ray sources *Phys. Med. Biol.* **54** 4889–905
[19] Mesbahi A, Jamali F and Garehaghaji N 2013 Effect of photon beam energy, gold nanoparticle size and concentration on the dose enhancement in radiation therapy *Bioimpacts* **3** 29–35
[20] Amato E, Italiano A, Leotta S, Pergolizzi S and Torrisi L 2013 Monte Carlo study of the dose enhancement effect of gold nanoparticles during X-ray therapies and evaluation of the anti-angiogenic effect on tumour capillary vessels *J. X-ray Sci. Technol.* **21** 237–47
[21] Guidelli E J and Baffa O 2014 Influence of photon beam energy on the dose enhancement factor caused by gold and silver nanoparticles: an experimental approach *Med. Phys.* **41** 032101

IOP Publishing

Nanoparticle Enhanced Radiation Therapy
Principles, methods and applications
Erno Sajo and Piotr Zygmanski

Chapter 4

Mechanisms of low energy electron interactions with biomolecules: relationship to gold nanoparticle radiosensitization

Yi Zheng and Léon Sanche

Electrons are abundantly emitted from the interaction of high-energy particles or photons with gold nanoparticles (GNPs). These electrons have a broad energy range, but the electron distribution in the vicinity of GNPs lies essentially at low energies (0–30 eV), since those directly emitted produce further generations of lower energy electrons (LEEs). All LEEs have ranges of about 10 nm and strongly react with the surrounding medium, mainly via resonances, which lead to their temporary capture by molecules or moieties of large biomolecules. This capture leads to the formation of molecular transient anions that decay by re-emitting the captured electron (i.e. autoionization) or by dissociating (i.e. dissociative electron attachment). Since autoionization can leave the target molecule in a dissociative electronic state, both channels can break bounds and damage biomolecules. In complex molecules, such as DNA, electron transfer between fundamental units increases the complexity of the process. In this review article, these mechanisms are explained with reference to LEEs created within nanometer distances of GNPs. It is generally concluded that, in radiotherapy, efficient use of the selective deposition of radiation energy, due to increased absorption coefficient of gold in comparison to soft tissue, is limited by the nanoscale range of most emitted and generated electrons. Unless targeted to vital molecules in the cell, like DNA, GNPs only serve to increase the energy deposited and the amount of radicals randomly created.

4.1 Introduction

4.1.1 Gold nanoparticle (GNP) radiosensitization

The potential use of GNPs as radiosensitizers in the treatment of cancer with ionizing radiation has attracted considerable interest [1–3]. Several *in vitro* and *in vivo* experiments have demonstrated enhancement of radiation damage due to the presence of GNPs in cells [4–13]. The role of GNPs in the radiosensitization process has been essentially understood from models developed to account for dose enhancement induced by an increase in radiation energy deposition [14–20], due to the higher energy-absorption coefficient of gold, compared to that of tissue [15, 17, 18, 21].

4.1.2 Primary mechanisms

The physics behind dose enhancement using high-Z metal nanoparticles can be understood from well-established basic phenomena. If the initial interaction with biological matter is that of a high-energy photon, the primary energy-loss phenomena involve Compton scattering, the photoelectric effect and pair production, which are all well explained in the literature [22, 23]. Figure 4.1(a) shows the dependence of the mass absorption coefficient of gold and tissue and their ratio as a function of photon energy [24]. It clearly shows that at certain energies GNPs should absorb many more photons compared to biological tissue. In figure 4.1(b) the enhancement of SSBs induced by the presence of GNPs in a plasmid DNA solution is plotted as a function of the energy of irradiating x-rays [25]. As shown in figure 4.1(b), the ratio of x-ray-induced biological damage with and without the presence of GNPs (i.e. the enhancement factor EF) may follow a more complex energy dependence than that of figure 4.1(a), but maximum radiosensitization still lies well within the range 20–60 keV.

The most efficient energy-loss mechanisms in the keV range (i.e. Compton scattering and the photoelectric effect) depend on photon energy [24]. In the energy range of 10–100 keV, used in certain cancer radiotherapy protocols [26, 27], the photon absorption coefficient of high-Z metals, including that of GNPs, is one to two order magnitudes larger compared to the coefficient of soft tissues (figure 4.1(a)). In this range, the photoelectric effect and Compton scattering contribute in different proportions to energy deposition depending on primary-photon energy. In both materials at 10 keV, essentially all photon energy is transferred through the photoelectric effect. At 100 keV, however, 90% of the photon energy is initially transferred by Compton scattering [22]. In the photoelectric effect, an inner shell electron is usually ejected from a gold atom, which leaves the atom unstable with a positive hole. In order to get to a stable lower energy state, the atom goes through a relaxation process, resulting first in the ejection of a secondary electron or a characteristic x-ray. When the atom relaxes to a lower energy state, i.e. an outer shell electron fills the inner shell vacancy, either a secondary electron, known as an Auger electron, or a characteristic x-ray is released. If the secondary electron is not from the outermost shell, intra-atomic relaxation can continue until all vacancies are transferred to the outer shell, allowing for the creation of multiple Auger electrons and x-rays [23, 24, 28]. The Auger process generates copious amounts of electrons with energies below 300 eV [29]; in addition, within a GNP, further ionization of other gold atoms by electrons or photons and electron energy losses, contribute to the emitted low energy electron (LEE)

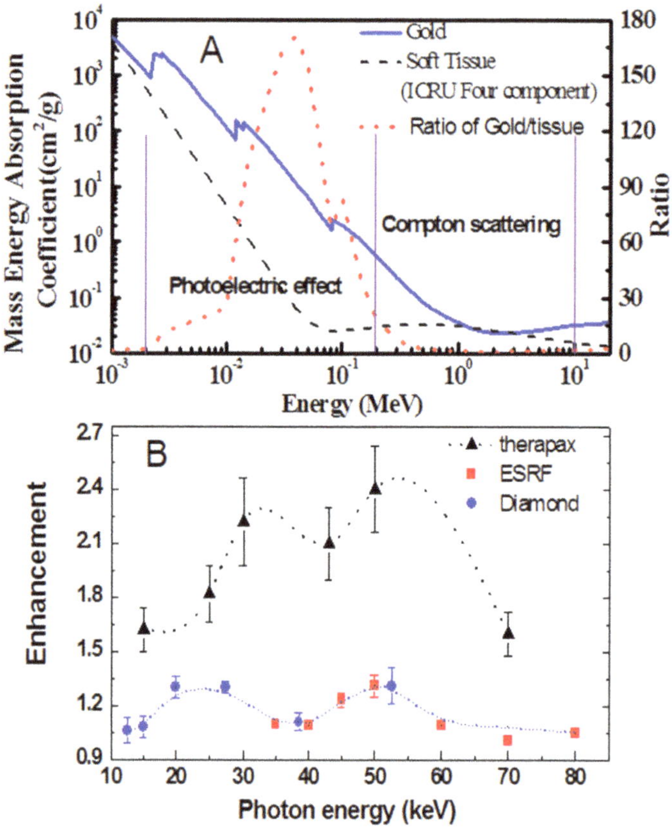

Figure 4.1. (a) Mass absorption coefficients of gold and biological tissue as a function of x-ray energy [24]. The red dashed line denotes the ratio of these two coefficients and vertical lines delineate regions dominated by the photoelectric effect and Compton scattering. (b) Energy dependence of GNP enhancement factor (EF) for inducing SSBs by 10–80 keV photon irradiation of a plasmid DNA solution. The data were produced by a therapax x-ray unit with energy filters (▲) and monochromatic photons from the European Synchrotron Radiation Facility (ESRF) (■) and Diamond (●) synchrotrons [25].

distribution. Furthermore, any higher-energy Auger electron escaping a GNP generates along its path an intense distribution of LEEs, as does any fast charged particle. However, in the case of a GNP, the LEE density decreases more rapidly from the radiation source, than the usual exponential dependence on attenuation length.

Above 200 keV photon energy, Compton scattering dominates up to 10 MeV. Thus, in this radiotherapeutic range, subsequent events likely involve the interactions of relatively fast-electrons within GNPs and/or the biological medium, as well as lower-energy photons undergoing Compton scattering or inducing photoelectron emission. Thus, the energy degradation process can produce lower-energy photons with a high absorption coefficient for gold. Moreover, the fast electrons from Compton scattering behave like broad-band electromagnetic radiation leading mostly to ionization and thus further emission of LEEs from GNPs [30, 31] and soft tissue [32]. In principle, the electron energy distribution arising from these multiples processes can be evaluated by Monte Carlo codes, but the accuracy of these distributions is limited by the availability of the energy-dependence of many interaction cross sections (CSs), especially those related to LEE scattering, ionization and attachment [33]. Figure 4.2(a) depicts the results of a Monte Carlo calculation using the Geant4 software [34]. It shows the electron emission spectrum from 5–300 nm GNPs produced by 40 keV x-rays. Clearly, large amounts of electrons with energies below 300 eV are emitted from the GNPs. Other models [4–20] take into account localized effects of Auger-electron cascades and local generation of photoelectrons and characteristic x-rays [17, 28, 35, 36]. As expected, absorption and electron emission is inversely proportional to the diameter of the GNP [28, 37, 38] which is correlated to relative biological effectiveness [39].

Even though many calculations exist on photon and electron emission from GNPs, no data can be found from experiments on *isolated GNPs* irradiated with high energy particles or photons. As a substitute, we show in figure 4.2(b), an example of the secondary electron distribution produced by 1.5 keV photons striking a clean gold surface in vacuum. More than 96% of the emitted electrons lie below 30 eV [40]. They have a maximum in the distribution lying around 1.4 eV and an average energy of 4 eV. A shift of this spectrum toward higher energies is expected to be inversely proportional to the GNP diameter [35]. According to the experimental results of Casta *et al* [41] a surface consisting of layers of GNPs produces slightly higher yields of secondary electrons. Other experiments have consistently generated distributions of secondary electron emission from gold or GNP surfaces produced by x-rays, which were similar to those of figure 4.2 [36, 41, 42].

GNPs can also sensitize biological damage induced by fast charged particles [2]. In the case of electron irradiation, secondary electrons are ejected in collisions governed by the relativistic Möller CS [43], which can also provide the number of collisions within the nanoparticle. However, fast charged particles do not need to directly hit a GNP to produce secondary electron emission. When they pass close to any molecule or nanoparticle, they act as broad-band electromagnetic radiation, causing emission of essentially LEEs, whose numbers and energies are determined according to the oscillator strengths of the target [23, 32]. According to recent calculations, the number of LEEs produced by high-energy protons interacting with GNPs would be about an order of magnitude higher than that from an equivalent water volume and not very dependent on the primary particle energy [44]. Due to electron production via the excitation of plasmons in GNPs, by fast initial charged particles, the secondary electron distribution lies essentially in the 0–30 eV range [44]. Radiosensitization of various EFs has been observed from irradiation by high-energy electrons and protons [2, 45–50].

4.1.3 Biological damage induced by low energy electrons (LEEs)

The interaction between GNPs and cells is determined by many factors including the nanoparticle dimensions (size and shape), charge, type of ligand and density, receptor expression levels and cellular internalization mechanisms [2, 51]. GNPs

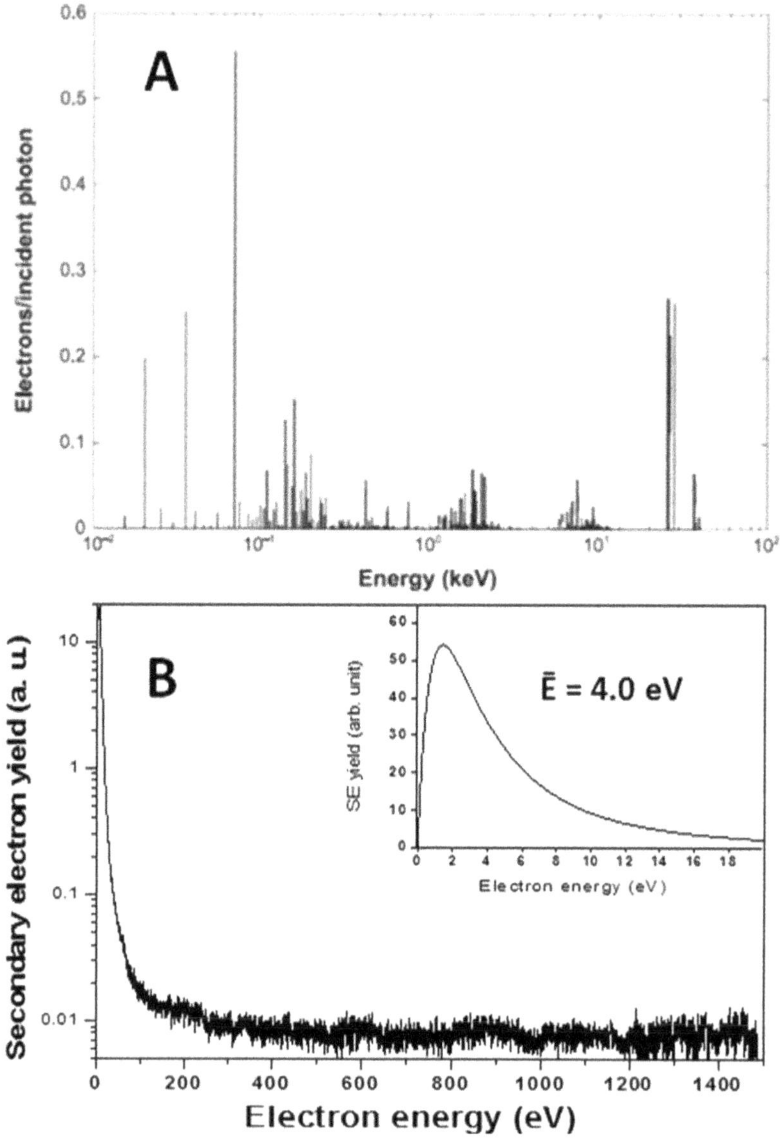

Figure 4.2. (a) Electron emission spectrum from 5–300 nm diameter GNPs irradiated by 40 keV x-rays. The peaks around 10 keV and above are photoelectrons and those at lower energies are Auger electrons [34]. Reprinted with permission from [34]. Copyright 2020 Radiation Research Society. (b) Secondary electron energy distribution from a gold surface irradiated with 1.48 keV photons. The photoelectrons have an average energy of 4.0 eV [40]. Reprinted with permission from [40].

bound to ligands, such as polyethylene glycol (PEG), have been shown to be favorably taken up by tumor cells [52]. Although nuclear DNA is the principal target in radiotherapy, most *in vitro* [3, 4, 8, 9, 12] and *in vivo* [5, 7, 53] studies have shown that destruction of cancer cells is enhanced by GNPs that do not enter the nucleus. There are several cellular perturbations that can be induced by irradiated GNPs outside the nucleus [2, 12, 50]. For example, the efficient functioning of the endoplasmic reticulum is essential for most cellular activities and survival. Around irradiated GNPs in the cellular cytoplasm, LEEs and radiation-induced radicals may modify biomolecules. Subsequently, this modification could interfere with endoplasmic reticulum function, leading to the accumulation and aggregation of unfolded proteins [54]. Such accumulation can induce stress-associated programmed cell death [52], i.e. apoptosis.

On the other hand, when GNPs enter the nucleus, they lie close to DNA, where LEEs most efficiently damage the molecule due to their large number and short range, causing maximal destruction of cancer cells (e.g. cytokinesis arrest and apoptosis) [50, 55]. Many investigations with LEEs have focused on DNA damage for this reason, but also because the molecule is the main target in radiotherapy and because it is possible to target GNPs to the nucleus by linking coded peptides to their surface [10]. Studies on LEE-induced damage to DNA have provided a basic understanding of the physics and chemistry involved in the action of radiation in cells. This information can explain mechanisms of GNP radiosensitization. The species produced by LEEs near DNA or within the molecule itself, can inflict severe lesions to the molecule, including single and double strand breaks (SSBs and DSBs) [56], crosslinks [57], base deletion [58] and base and clustered [59, 60] damage. Such damage within the cell nucleus can cause mutagenic, recombinogenic, and other potentially lethal lesions [61, 62], leading to chromatin remodeling, apoptosis and cell cycle arrest [63]. Many experimental and theoretical studies indicate that even at subionization energies, electrons play a significant role in inducing DNA damage [64–69].

In this chapter, we first provide a general overview of the interaction of LEEs with molecular solids and condensed biomolecules. Our goal is to provide basic concepts needed to describe the phenomena related to the damage induced in cellular biomolecules by electrons emitted from GNPs and the LEEs generated along their tracks, when GNPs are irradiated by high energy charged particles or photons. Afterwards, we describe the interactions of LEEs with the cell's most biologically relevant components, i.e. water and DNA. Examples are provided of biomolecular damage induced by GNP-generated LEEs. We restrict our description to the 0–30 eV range, since above 30 eV, electron scattering from biomolecules leads essentially to ionization and thus the production of lower energy electrons. This review is centered on GNP radiosensitization, but it is reasonable to assume that the data and the mechanisms presented broadly apply to any high-Z metallic nanoparticle.

4.2 Interaction of LEEs with condensed-phase biomolecules

4.2.1 Basic principles of interaction of LEEs with molecules

The dynamics of LEE scattering in a dilute gas or within condensed material must be described in terms of wave functions. For each interaction, a wave that is the sum of simpler waves called 'partial waves' is associated with an electron of certain energy. Thus, intra- as well as inter-molecular interferences of electron waves play a dominant role in LEE scattering within condensed matter. LEEs of energy below 30 eV have wavelengths comparable to the size of molecules and the distances between molecules in biological media. Hence, intra- and inter-molecular coherent scattering modulate electron energy losses via localized (e.g., vibrational and electronic excitation) [70, 71] and delocalized processes [72, 73], including phonon [74, 75] and exciton [76] creation and charge transfer [77, 78]. However, electrons scattering within biological material rapidly lose their long-range coherence due to the random orientation of the biomolecules and rapid energy losses. Consequently, long-range coherent scattering causing diffraction of the electron waves is diminished considerably and short-range and intra-molecular phenomena become dominant [79, 80]. Thus, descriptions of scattering processes in terms of the basic principles of isolated electron–molecule interactions are still valid. However, modifications to the electron–molecule potential and the effect of the band structure of the condensed phase introduced by the presence of other neighboring targets must be properly taken into account [81–83].

As a general rule, it has been found desirable for understanding the essential physics, to divide LEE scattering into resonant and direct processes [84]. In a resonance, there are always one or more partial waves that undergo constructive interference within the target. The amplitudes of the electron waves scattered from molecules may then be seen as derived from a competition between resonant and non-resonant (i.e. direct) contributions. When at a given energy, the time-dependent amplitude of a LEE wave function does not increase significantly in the vicinity of a particular molecular site, the scattering process is considered to be direct. Insight into the physical phenomenon may be gained from analysis of the interaction potential. In other words, by estimating the magnitude of the various terms, in the expansion of this potential, it may be possible to sort out the dominant ones, from which the main scattering mechanism may be deduced. Such considerations are helpful in calculating the probabilities of LEE energy losses to a target molecule, particularly those leading to molecular dissociation and hence to the production of reactive radicals. Usually, electrons of energy less than about 30 eV can damage biomolecules by direct or resonance scattering [82, 85]. However, below 15 eV, the scattering or capture CS for a given LEE-induced process is often controlled by resonances, i.e. by the formation of transient molecular anions (TMAs).

Direct scattering occurs at all energies above the energy threshold for an electron energy loss, because the interaction potential between the electron and the molecule is always present. Since this latter interaction changes slowly with incident electron energy, direct scattering produces a smooth and usually rising signal that does not exhibit any particular feature in the electron energy dependence of the measured CSs or yields of molecular fragments (i.e. the yield function). In contrast, resonance scattering occurs only when the incoming electron occupies a previously unfilled orbital of the target molecule [82]. This orbital exists at a precise energy [84, 85], corresponding to that of the TMA state. At the resonance energy, the scattering CS and/or product yields are enhanced, exhibiting a pronounced maximum often superimposed on an increasing monotonic background arising from direct scattering.

4.2.2 Transient molecular anions (TMAs) and their decay channels

The formation of TMAs is well described and reviewed in the literature [80, 82, 84–86]. They occur at specific energies, when an incoming electron occupies a previously unfilled orbital of a molecule, during a time exceeding the usual scattering time [80, 85, 87]. According to the uncertainty principle, the TMA state has a width in energy, which can be identified in the dependence on incident electron energy of particular energy-loss processes or in yield functions. There are two major types of TMAs [80, 85, 87]. The one known as a single-particle anion or shape resonance occurs when the additional electron occupies an otherwise unfilled orbital of the molecule in its ground state. Such temporary electron capture can also occur at the site of a subunit of a large biomolecule [88]. In shape resonances, the angular momentum barrier of the electron–molecule potential temporarily traps the additional electron. Another category of TMAs consists of core-excited resonances or 'two-particle, one-hole' states. These are formed when the scattering electron is captured by the positive electron affinity of an excited state of the molecule, or a basic subunit of a large biomolecule, such as a base, sugar, or phosphate group in the DNA molecule. If a momentum barrier in the electron–molecule or electron–subunit potential contributes to the retention of the additional electron by the electronically excited state, the TMA is referred to as core-excited shape resonance.

Repulsive TMA states can either dissociate or re-emit the electron into vacuum or within the scattering medium. The latter phenomenon (i.e. autoionization) may leave the target molecule in the ground state or in excited rotational, vibrational and electronically excited states. In condensed media, TMAs can also decay into phonon modes. When a TMA is associated with a repulsive interatomic potential surface (in the Franck–Condon region) and its lifetime is greater than about half of the vibration period of the anion, then it may dissociate. *This trapping of an electron to form a TMA that dissociates into neutral and anionic fragments is called dissociative electron attachment (DEA).* Thus, for such dissociative anion states there is competition between dissociation and autoionization. These two processes are very sensitive to the environment, because they depend exponentially on the lifetime of the TMA [82], which in turn is highly sensitive to the band structure of the medium and perturbations of the electron-target potential arising from neighboring molecules [81].

4.2.3 Modification of electron capture and decay of transient anions in biological media

In molecular solids, such as biological matter, molecules retain their intrinsic properties [89]. The weak inter-molecular interaction between the constituents of such materials is characterized by a lack of a chemical bonds between molecules, so that the electronic structure and vibrational frequencies of condensed molecules are essentially unchanged from those in the gas phase [80, 89]. Due to the weak intermolecular interaction, the formation and decay of TMAs of condensed-phase molecules can be described by modified isolated electron–molecule models, that take into account changes in the properties of TMAs [80, 90]. For example, in the gas phase the incoming electron wave function is a plane wave, but scattering events in the condensed phase modify its partial wave content. The latter changes the electron capture CS responsible for the formation of the TMAs. Furthermore, a TMA's lifetime changes in the condensed media, since new decay channels (e.g. phonon modes) appear and the TMA is formed at lower energy due to the polarization potential induced by the temporary localization of the negative charge [80, 88] and possible lowering of the symmetry of the anion state [82, 90, 91]. Reviews reporting experiments showing the results of the transformation of electron scattering and properties of TMAs due to a phase change are available in the literature [82, 88, 92, 93]. Here, we provide a simple example of relevance to the presence of a metal near the site of interaction of an electron with a condensed molecule.

Figure 4.3 shows the result of a simple experiment, in which 0.1 monolayer (ML) of CH_3Cl was condensed onto a 20 ML thick Kr film deposited on a polycrystalline platinum substrate held at 20 K in ultra-high vacuum [94]. In this experiment, the film is bombarded for a pre-determined duration with monoenergetic LEEs and the surface charge accumulated is measured. The experiment is repeated at different

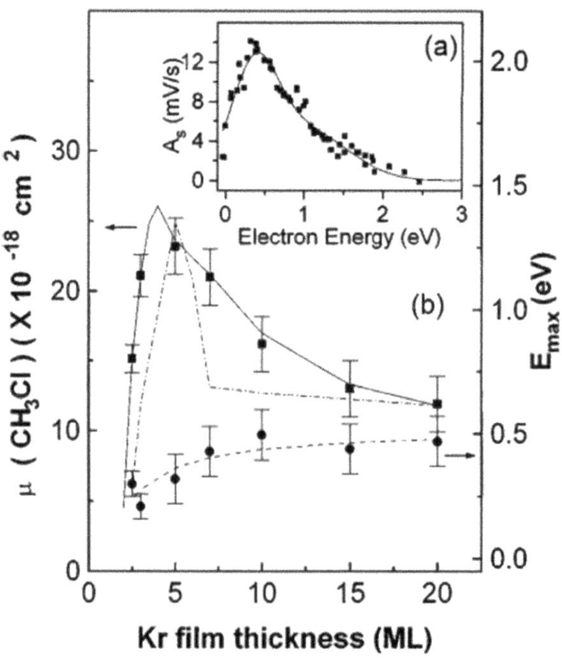

Figure 4.3. Temporary CH_3Cl^- formation and dissociation induced by electrons of 0–2.5 eV incident on 0.1 monolayer of CH_3Cl physisorbed on a multilayer film of Kr deposited on platinum [94]. (a) Variation with electron energy of the charging coefficient A_s of the film, due to CH_3Cl^- dissociation into CH_3 and Cl^-. (b) Variation with film thickness of: (■) the amplitude of the maximum in the inset (i.e. in A_s) expressed as a charging cross section (CS) μ; (-·-·) the amplitude of the maximum in μ calculated with the R-matrix method; (•) variation of the energy of maximum in μ; (---) a parametric fit of this energy using the image charge model [95]. Reprinted with permission from [94]. Copyright 1995 by the American Physical Society.

electron energies for the same duration. The accumulated negative charge can be expressed as a coefficient A_S, which in this example is directly proportional to the absolute CS (μ) for the 0–2.5 eV reaction $e^- + CH_3Cl \rightarrow CH_3Cl^- \rightarrow CH_3 + Cl^-$, shown in the inset of figure 4.3. In this reaction, CH_3Cl captures an incoming electron of a precise energy generated in the front of the surface by an electron monochromator. Within the 0–2.5 eV range, there exists a single structure in the A_S energy dependence, the maximum of which lies at approximately 0.5 eV for large Kr coverage of the platinum substrate. The peak denotes the energy of the TMA CH_3Cl^-. As the Kr film thickness is reduced, the transitory CH_3Cl^- anion moves closer to the metal substrate and the energy of the maximum in A_S in the inset, decreases owing to the larger polarizability of the metal compared to that of Kr [95]. The lower curve in figure 4.3 shows this shift of CH_3Cl^- to smaller energy with decreasing thickness [94]. As the energy of transitory CH_3Cl^- on the Kr film lowers, the number of decay channels diminishes and the TMA becomes more stable, causing an increase in its lifetime. Thus, as seen in the experimental curve with the full squares in figure 4.3, the magnitude of the peak in μ for Cl^- production via DEA increases with decreasing thickness of the Kr film. When CH_3Cl^- is formed too close to the metal, the additional electron can transfer to the metal, causing μ to sharply decrease. The same fundamental behavior is expected for TMA formed close to any metal nanoparticle. Thus, these results suggest that (1) LEE reactions with a ligand coating a metallic nanoparticle cannot be neglected, (2) the presence of a metal can enhance DEA reactions, unless the molecule is too close to the surface and (3) only partial coverage of a metallic nanoparticle with a ligand may be preferable under physiological conditions, if possible.

4.2.4 Short range and high damage efficiency of LEEs

The penetration depth of 1–30 eV electrons in liquid water or amorphous ice lies in the range of 1–20 nm (figure 4.4) [96] and has been determined to be ~11–16 nm in DNA films [57]. LEEs are also highly destructive as demonstrated by the values of absolute CSs for DNA damage [57]. *These two characteristics are responsible for their nanoscopic damage efficiency.* As an example, absolute CSs for producing DNA crosslinks, SSBs, DSBs and loss of the initial supercoiled (LS) configuration, induced by electrons of 2–20 and 100 eV [57, 97] are shown in figure 4.5. Open points in figure 4.5 represent the directly measured absolute CSs and solid points those deduced from effective yields [98]. One striking observation is that 10 eV and high energy-transfer 100 eV electrons have similar absolute CSs to damage supercoiled DNA (LS) and form SSBs. Thus, electrons of 10 eV damage DNA with a probability of the same order as 100 eV electrons, which are known to have the highest efficiency to damage biomolecules [99], principally due to their high ionization yields. However, according to the distribution from a gold surface (figure 4.2(b)), electrons emitted with energy below 15 eV are orders of magnitude more numerous than those of 100 eV and higher energies. In other words, the considerable damage produced by LEE emission from GNPs can be essentially confined within a range of a few nearby biomolecules (e.g. the DNA of cancer cells

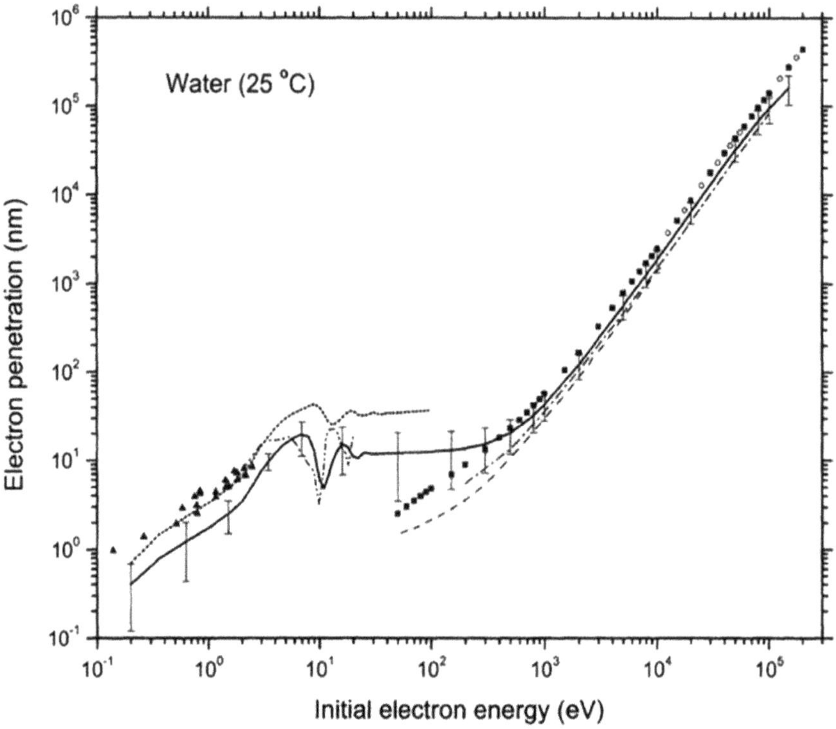

Figure 4.4. Variation of the electron penetration range in liquid water at 25 °C as a function of initial electron energy between 0.2 eV and 150 keV [96]. The data were taken from various Monte Carlo simulations; below 20 eV the solid line was obtained using solid-phase scattering CSs. Reprinted with permission from [96]. Copyright 2020 Radiation Research Society.

and nearby water and proteins). *More generally, considering the range of 0–300 eV electrons* (figure 4.4) *and the geometry of electron emission from GNPs, radiosensitization is expected to result from the large amount of additional energy deposited by high energy radiation in cells within nanometer range of the creation of the photoelectrons.* The latter have considerable efficiency to break nearby biomolecules and produce multiple damage sites, which are particularly cytotoxic, if the biomolecule is DNA. *Thus, GNPs possess the necessary characteristics to relocate radiation energy within nanoscopic volumes*, increasing within this space the radiation dose by orders of magnitude. In other words, controlling the local density of LEEs with metallic nanoparticles and the reactions they induce should result in the control, within a short range, of a large amount of the energy deposited by high-energy radiation in cells.

4.3 Interaction of LEEs with water and DNA

4.3.1 LEE interaction with water and the indirect effect of radiation

Because cells contain 70%–80% water by weight, the latter represent along with genomic DNA, the most biologically relevant molecules. DNA radiolysis has been

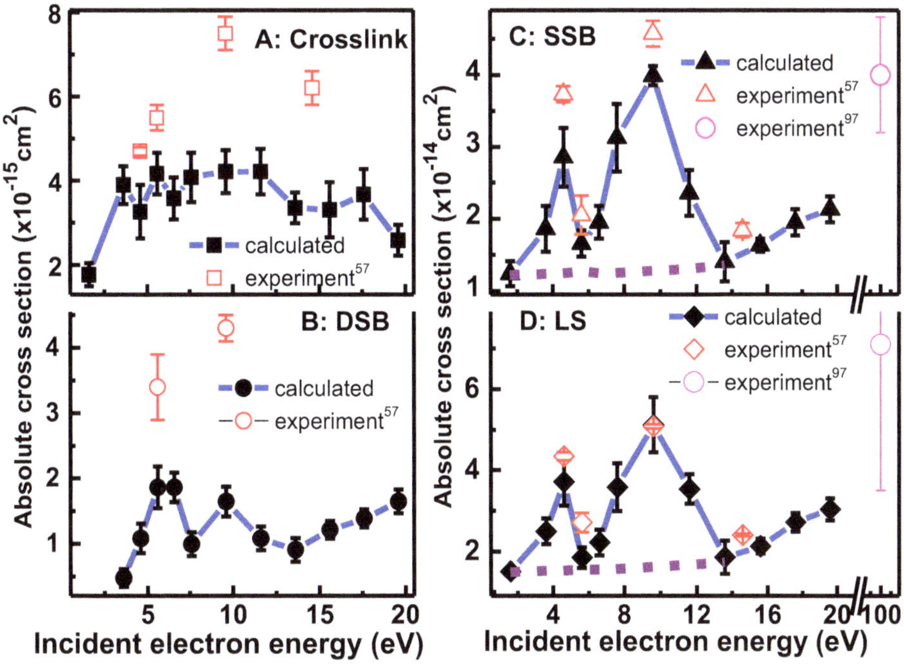

Figure 4.5. The open characters in frames (a)–(d) are measured absolute CSs for crosslink, DSB, SSB and loss of supercoiled form (LS), respectively, induced in pGEM-3Zf (-) plasmid DNA by 2–20 and 100 eV electrons. The black full characters between 2–20 eV were generated mathematically from experimentally measured effective yields. The error bars are the standard deviations.

classified into two categories: the direct effect, when radiation energy is deposited directly into the molecule and the indirect effect, when damage results from reaction with DNA of new species created by the radiation within the local molecular environment surrounding DNA [100], e.g. water, salts, proteins, and oxygen.

During the last two decades considerable research has been focused on the direct interaction of LEEs with DNA and its different subunits [58–60, 64–66, 88, 91, 97, 98, 101, 102]. More recently, the indirect effects of x-ray induced photoelectrons from a tantalum surface have been investigated by Alizadeh *et al* [103]. These authors reported the effect of hydration (i.e. humidity) level on the DNA damage yields induced by 1.5 keV x-rays that produce a photoelectron distribution similar to that shown in figure 4.2(b). Films of plasmid DNA, maintained at atmospheric pressure and room temperature, were deposited on the metal surface. Conformational damage increased by about 50% as the DNA environment approached bulk-like hydration conditions, indicating that the indirect effect of the emitted low-energy photoelectrons should constitute a substantial contribution to the radiosensitivity conferred by metallic particles. This contribution was found to arise principally from reactive dissociated-water species, such as H^-, OH•, and H•, created within the outmost bulk-like water layer covering DNA [91, 103, 104].

Fragmentation by LEE impact of condensed-phase H_2O has been mainly investigated by electron stimulated desorption (ESD) from amorphous ice. The yield functions for desorption of H^- [105–107], H_2 [108, 109], $H(^2S)$, $O(^3P)$, and O $(^1D2)$ [110, 111] from ice films were recorded in the range 5–30 eV. Most of these functions exhibit broad peaks below 15 eV, characteristic of TMA formation. DEA to condensed H_2O was found to lead principally in the formation of H^- and $OH^\bullet$ radicals from dissociation of the transient $^2B_1$ state of H_2O^- in the 7–9 eV region. Smaller contributions arise from the $^2A_1$ and $^2B_2$ anionic states, near 9 and 11 eV, respectively [105, 106]. At higher energies, non-resonant processes, such as dipolar dissociation (e.g. $H_2O^* \rightarrow H^+ + OH^-$ or $H^- + OH^+$) fragment H_2O, with the assistance of a broad resonance that extends from 20 to 30 eV [106] Kimmel *et al* [110, 111] measured $D_2(X^1\ \Sigma_g^+)$, $D(^2S)$, $O(^3Pj = 2,1,0)$, and $O(^1D2)$ ESD yields from nanoscale-thick D_2O films versus incident electron energy. The threshold lies around ~6.5 eV and all yield function follow a steadily increasing intensity. The $D(^2S)$ yield function exhibits a broad resonance around ~14–21 eV. Above 7 eV, direct electronic excitation of the $^{3,1}B$ states lead to $H^\bullet$ and $OH^\bullet$ desorption. Beyond 10 eV, ionization progressively takes over and dominates energy losses. The ensemble of these reactions leads to an abundant production of OH and H radicals and H_2 molecules. Books on radiation chemistry [112, 113] can be consulted to learn about the following water radiolysis and the reactions of initial radicals with DNA. More specifically, Sicard-Roselli *et al* [114] investigated the complex chemistry at the water–GNP interface arising from 20 keV x-ray irradiated solutions of GNPs. The authors reported massive additional production of hydroxyl radicals, capable of inducing DNA damage via the indirect effect [114]. When GNPs are bound to ligands, however, such hydroxyl radical production considerably decreases [115].

Absolute CSs for elastic collisions, phonon, vibrational and electronic excitations, DEA and ionization induced by 1–100 eV electron scattering in amorphous ice condensed at a temperature of 14 K were reported by Michaud *et al* [116–119]. Within the energy range 0–30 eV, the CSs for excitation of the electronic states leading to $OH^\bullet$, $H^\bullet$ and H_2 production varies from 10^{-19} to about 10^{-17} cm^2 [116, 120–122]. These values are comparable with CSs of ~1–7 × 10^{-18} cm^2 per nucleotide for inducing strand breaks in DNA with LEEs [57, 123]. The CSs reported by Michaud *et al* are now used for detailed modeling in radiation dose assessment via Monte Carlo calculations [124].

With respect to irradiated GNPs in cell nuclei, the emitted electrons and the LEEs created along their tracks can interact either directly with DNA or with nearby biomolecules. The latter interactions may form radicals that could react with DNA; thus, LEEs from GNPs participate to the direct and indirect effects of radiation on DNA. Meanwhile, the ions or holes produced from ionization within the GNPs remain on the nanoparticle. *In tissue initial creation of a positive ion or hole by ionization contributes considerably to high-energy radiation damage* [112, 113], *however, this damage is quenched in the case of metallic nanoparticle irradiation by positive charge retention within the nanoparticle. This phenomenon should therefore increase the relative contribution and importance of LEEs in the radiosensitization process and additional radiation dose.*

4.3.2 Mechanisms of LEE-induced DNA and cellular damage

DNA damage has been identified as a key element regulating radiation response. The experimental results obtained from LEE-irradiated supercoiled plasmid DNA, short single DNA strands (i.e. oligonucleotides) and DNA basic constituents are well described in the literature and summarized in authoritative review articles [82, 88, 91, 92, 101, 125]. Several papers also review theoretical advances on LEE interaction with basic DNA constituents and oligonucleotides [86, 102, 126–128]. Various DNA damage induced by 2–20 eV electrons to different DNA-related configurations is compared in figure 4.6. Figure 4.6(a) represents the loss (LS) of the initial supercoiled DNA (pUC21, 3151 base pairs (bp)), uniformly deposited on highly oriented pyrolytic graphite by intercalating between each DNA doubly charged 1–3 diaminopropane (Dap^{2+}) molecules [129]. The results of frame (b) exhibit the yield functions corresponding to release of thymine (T) and strand breaks producing pT and pCAT, from a short DNA strand, i.e. the tetramer GCAT, where G represents guanine, C cytosine, A adenine, and p the sugar-phosphate group [130]. The curve in C represents the yield of H^- anions desorbed by electron impact on a film composed of synthetic 25 bp doubly-stranded DNA and the pGEM 3199-bp plasmid [131]. (d) and (e) show, respectively, the yield function for the formation of DSBs and SSBs from pGEM-3Zf(-) plasmid DNA [98] These results indicate that most yield functions for DNA damage exhibit two strong maxima, associated from the formation of core-excited resonances (i.e. TMAs) [98].

Figure 4.6(f) shows the loss of transformation efficiency of *E. coli* JM109 bacteria (i.e. the decrease in the number of bacterial colonies growing in an antibiotic ampicillin environment) after insertion into the cells of the pGEM-3Zf(-) plasmid [132]. When undamaged, this plasmid confers to *E. coli* JM109, resistance to the antibiotic [133]. Before insertion into the cells, the plasmids were irradiated with electrons of specific energies in the range 0.5–25 eV. Cells that receive plasmids severely damaged by LEEs, multiply less in the ampicillin environment, leading to a decrease in transformation efficiency. Strikingly, the transformation efficiency reveals minima at 5.5 and 9.5 eV, coincident with the maxima observed in the yields of DNA DSBs [60, 98]. As local multiple damage sites, DSBs are potentially lethal or mutagenic lesions compared to SSBs and related to diverse human diseases [63, 134]. The results of figure 4.6 indicate that the effects of TMAs are observable in the electron-energy dependence of biological processes with negative consequences for cell viability. The comparison of direct DNA damage with cell survival provided evidence that LEEs play an important role in cell mutagenesis and death during radiotherapeutic cancer treatment [91, 135].

Below 15 eV, damage to biological DNA results essentially from initial electron capture by a base [60, 68, 91, 98, 128, 136, 137] to form a shape resonance below 5 eV [65] or a core-excited anion above this energy [98]. The former can decay by DEA, whereas the other type can decay by DEA or autoionization. DEA can lead only to base release or a single bond dissociation on the base. However, multiple lesions are possible from decay via autoionization, since the departing electron and the electronic excitation can separate, with each of them creating a lesion [60, 98].

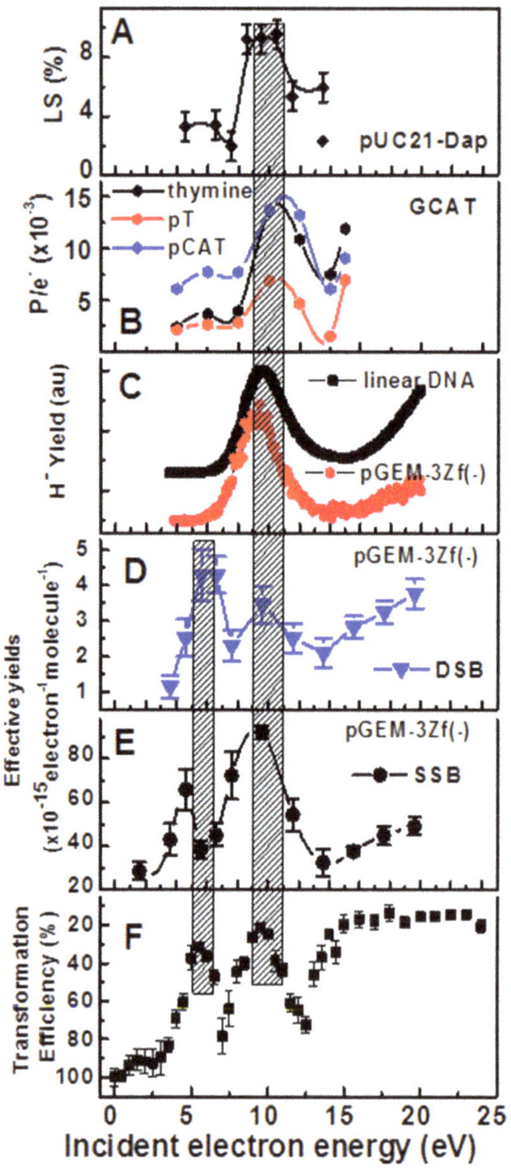

Figure 4.6. Comparison of DNA damage induced by 2–20 eV electron impact on DNA films composed of (a) plasmid–diaminopropane cation complexes (pUC21–Dap^{2+}); (b) oligonucleotides GCAT integrating one of each of the four DNA bases; (c) linear DNA composed of 40 base pairs (black squares) and pGEM-3Zf(-) plasmid DNA (red dots); (d) and (e) pGEM-3Zf(-) plasmid DNA [98]. Curve F is the inverse of the transformation efficiency of *E. coli* containing pGEM-3Zf(-) plasmids needed for their survival. The plasmids were irradiated with 0.2–25 eV electrons at a fluence of 27×10^{13} electrons cm^{-2} [132]. The detected damage was (a) loss of supercoiled (LS), (b) fragment products identified in the legend, (c) H^- electron stimulated desorption yields, (d) DSBs and (e) SSBs. (a)–(e) reprinted with permission from [98], copyright 2015 American Chemical Society. (f) Reprinted with permission from [132], copyright 2017 American Chemical Society.

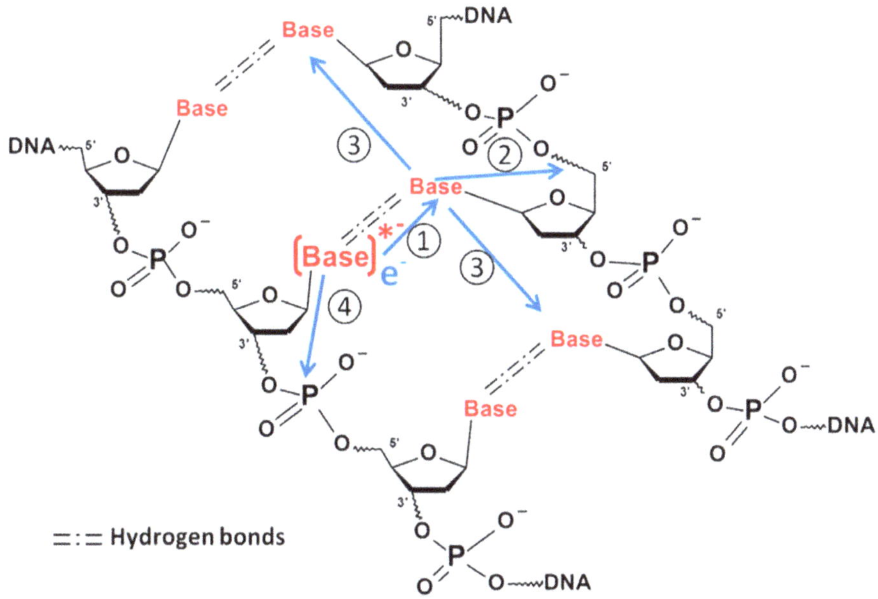

Figure 4.7. Scheme of possible electron (e⁻) pathways, following the formation of a core-excited transient anion on a DNA base. When dissociation of the electronically excited state occurs the following pathways lead to a local multiple damaged site. (1) e⁻ transfer to the base on the opposite strand produces two adjacent BDs. (2) e⁻ transfer to the phosphate unit, causes a strand break via C–O bond breakage (SSB with opposite BD). (3) The subsequent e⁻ hops between bases, giving BD or SSB at a farther location with opposite BD. (4) e⁻ transfer to the phosphate unit of the strand hosting the TMA, leading to C–O bond scission (i.e. SSB with nearby BD on the same strand). Reprinted with permission from reference [59].

It is for this reason that LEE-induced DSBs have been observed only at electron energies above 5 eV in pure DNA films [138]. *A priori*, either the excitation or electron can transfer to the opposite strand, but electron transfer is much more probable [77]. Figure 4.7 illustrates how multiple DNA damage can be formed from an initial core-excited TMA on a base [59], represented by an electronically excited base between brackets and an additional electron in subscript. Autoionization of the TMA can occur via electron transfer to another base or the phosphate group of the same strand (path 4) or to the adjacent base (path 1). Electron transfer to another base repeats the initial condition, whereas pathways 4 and 1 can produce either a TMA on the phosphate group or on the adjacent base, respectively. When these latter anion states are dissociative, the respective rupture of the C–O bond (i.e. a single strand break) or base damage (BD) occurs via DEA. If the initial base is left in a dissociative state, pathway 4 results in dissociation of a base and a strand break occurs within a single strand, as observed experimentally by Li *et al* [139]. Alternatively, if the autoionizing electron follows pathway 1 and the initial base dissociates, two adjacent BDs can be created: one formed by dissociation of the electronic excited state on one strand and the other via DEA of the electron transferred to the opposite base. Transfer of the additional electron from the base to the phosphate group of the complementary strand (path 2) can produce a BD on one strand and a strand break by rupture of the C–O bond via DEA on the opposite strand. If the transferred electron hops from base to base (path 3), any damage created as the result of a dissociative base or phosphate group anion is considered a local multiply damaged site, if the reactions occur within 20 bp from the initial electron capture. The reaction of a base radical with a nearby DNA can produce an inter-duplex crosslink [60, 98].

4.3.3 DNA damage from GNP-generated LEEs and LEE-bombarded GNP–DNA complexes

Several studies have compared high-energy electron [45, 140] and x-ray [25, 141–145] induced DNA damage in the presence and absence of nanoparticles or of an electron-emitting gold surface. For *monolayer* DNA adsorbed on a gold substrate and bombarded with 60 keV electrons, the damage per DNA molecule was enhanced by an order of magnitude compared to that measured in 2.9 μm thick films [45]. Most of the energy of 60 keV electrons was absorbed by the thick DNA film, whereas for only one-monolayer, essentially all the energy was absorbed by the gold substrate. As with x-rays (figure 4.2(b)), the gold surface when exposed to high-energy electrons, generates secondary electrons having essentially energies below 30 eV [30]. Thus, the increase in damage per DNA molecule, in going from thick to thin films deposited on a gold substrate, could be understood as arising from a higher effective density of LEEs in the thinner film due to electrons emitted from gold.

DNA damage induced by LEEs emitted from GNPs bombarded with 60 keV electrons [42] was also measured with films of plasmid DNA electrostatically bound to GNPs and compared to the results obtained under the same conditions without GNPs [45]. The yields of SSBs and DSBs following the exposure of 1:1 and 2:1 GNP:plasmid mixtures to fast electrons were measured by agarose gel electrophoresis [45, 140]. The EF for production of these lesions was about 2.5. Xiao *et al* [42] repeated these experiments [45, 140] with 5 nm diameter GNPs coated with ligands of different lengths. The corresponding EFs were reduced from 2.3 to 1.6 and 1.2, depending on the length of ligands, which ranged from 0 to 2.5 to 4 nm (figure 4.8) [146]. With 200 keV x-ray irradiation of 5–30 nm diameter PEG-coated GNPs, larger differences in length of ligand (~11 nm) were needed to obtain a similar reduction (60%) in EF [145]. In both experiments, attenuation by the coating of the number of emitted short-range LEEs that could reach the DNA was proposed to explain the decreasing radiosensitization with increasing ligand length. *From this perspective, to achieve the highest possible levels of radiosensitization, GNPs should either be coated with the shortest possible ligand or should only be partially coated.* In all cases, the high density of emitted LEEs from GNPs is expected to *produce radicals that could result in both chemical modifications of the ligand and the local cellular environment*; the new species could induce reactions detrimental to cell function from the presence of only a few GNPs within the nucleus, or at larger quantities in the cytoplasm.

The other non-exclusive radiosensitizing property of a GNP lies in its capacity to alter the chemical sensitivity of the target. In other words, the GNP can enhance

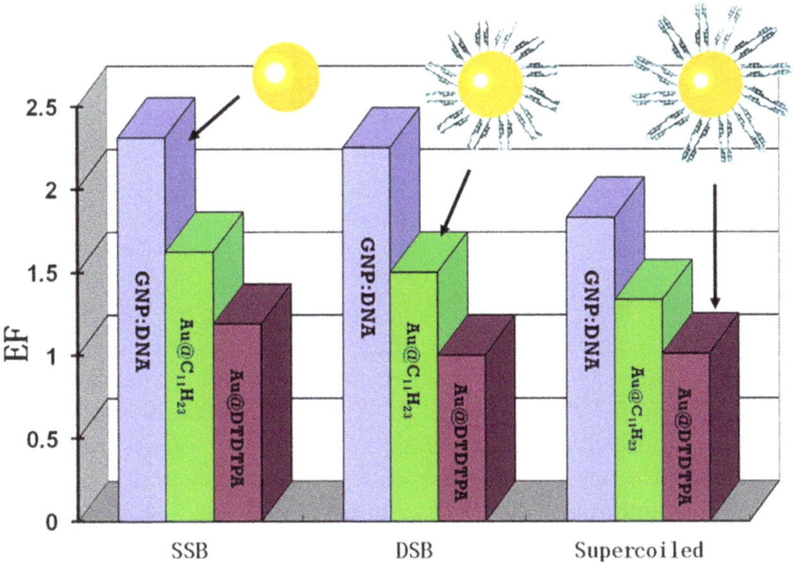

Figure 4.8. EFs for the formation of SSBs, DSBs and LS induced by 60 keV electrons in GNP–DNA complexes with ratio 1:1 [42, 146]. The groups of three histograms, respectively, represent SSBs, DSBs and LS. In each group, the EFs correspond to enhancement factors for specific DNA damage, when GNPs of 5 nm diameter bound to DNA are bare or coated with $C_{11}H_{23}$ or DTDTPA (i.e. dithiolated diethylenetriamine-pentaacetic) ligands. The corresponding ligand lengths are 2.5 and 4 nm, respectively.

radiation damage solely by binding to a target molecule, without any contribution from secondary-particle emission. When the EFs induced by naked GNPs electrostatically bound to plasmid DNA were measured after irradiation with 1, 10, 100 and 60 000 eV electrons, the largest EF value (3.2), was found at 10 eV [140]. At this energy, secondary electron emission is expected to be very low [147]. Therefore, the large enhancement of damage in DNA–GNPs complexes could only be caused by a modification of the DNA sensitivity to electron irradiation (i.e. by a chemical mechanism of radiosensitization). As seen from figure 4.6, at 10 eV there is a maximum in DNA damage corresponding to the formation of TMAs. It was conjectured that TMA parameters or bond strengths could be modified by the presence of the metal, which would increase bond breaking within DNA via formation of TMAs [140] In similar experiments with 10 eV electrons, Yao *et al* [148] investigated in more detail this hypothesis. Conformational damage was measured with DNA-bound GNPs of different diameters in films having different nanoparticle–DNA ratios. Positively-charged 5 nm GNPs, which bind strongly to DNA, resulted in a nearly constant increase of damage as a function of nanoparticle–DNA ratio up to an optimum EF at a ratio of 1:1. The same 10 eV electron bombardment of negatively-charged GNPs of 15 nm diameter, which bind weakly and randomly to DNA, resulted in much less chemical radiosensitization compared to the smaller GNPs. Thus, it appeared that the type of site and strength of binding of GNPs to DNA could significantly influence the efficiency of the chemical radiosensitization mechanism. This type of radiosensitization was also demonstrated to depend on the A and B conformations of DNA [149]. A is the common configuration at neutral pH and physiological salt concentration; the B form is similar, but has a shorter distance between base pairs compared to A. During transcription the DNA–RNA duplexes adopt the A form [150]. Thus, GNPs could be genotoxic, which suggest that they may have potential as chemotherapeutic agents if conjugated to nuclear targeting ligands [10].

4.4 Conclusions and future trends

In this chapter, we reviewed the results of experiments and calculations, indicating that radiation damage to DNA and cell sensitivity to radiation can be considerably increased by binding GNPs to nuclear DNA. This electrostatic binding causes an increase in the production of short-range LEEs having thermalization distances approximately four times the diameter of the DNA helix and hence capable of depositing a large amount of their energy into the molecule. Moreover, binding of GNPs to DNA modifies its morphology and/or its chemical structure, inducing radiosensitization independently of electron emission. This may at least partly explain the radiosensitization observed with fast charged particles and 0.3–20 MeV photon beams [26], regularly used in radiotherapy, whose absorption coefficients are much smaller than those of 10–200 keV x-rays. Thus, when bound to DNA, GNPs are unusual radiosensitizers in that they increase damage by two distinctive processes: modification of the DNA and increasing the absorption of ionizing radiation energy close to the molecule. Considering ongoing refinement in the methods of targeting GNPs to cancer cells via intravenous injection of carriers [55, 151–153] or convention enhanced delivery (i.e. direct intratumoral injection) [53, 154, 155] these particles could become highly efficient for treating tumors and their metastasis.

With GNPs, the best radiosensitization is obtained with 10–200 keV photons as expected from the high mass absorption coefficient ratios of gold to biological tissue (figure 4.1) in this energy range. However, in treatments with external beams, this high level of radiosensitization remains restricted to superficial tumors, due to the short penetration depths of x-rays in biological tissue (~ mm). On the other hand, a GNP can be delivered bound to (or with) a radioactive isotope to deep cancer sites via targeted radionuclide therapy [156–159] or convention enhanced delivery [53, 155, 160, 161]. In patient treatments with targeted Auger emitters of high atomic number [156], the radionuclide decays by electron capture or internal conversion processes, both of which create a cascade ejection of many Auger electrons (e.g. 5 and 25 electrons are released on average per decay of ^{67}Ga and ^{125}I, respectively) [162]. Most of these electrons have energies less than a few hundreds of eV and ranges on the order of 10 nm in biological media (figure 4.4) [96]. Those with energies above the ionization potential of cellular biomolecules generate another high-density distribution of LEEs. The local density of LEEs becomes even larger, if the targeted radionuclides are combined with GNPs [158, 160] or embedded in gold nanocages [163]. Under such conditions, most of the radiation energy absorbed by gold is transformed into kinetic energy of LEEs [164], thus further enhancing local damage [53, 135]. Depending on our ability to localize nanoparticles at specific sites in cells, these methods are promising not only for nanoparticle-aided radiotherapy, but more generally in extending the field of radiobiology to the nanoscopic level.

4.5 Abbreviations

BD	Base damage
Bp	Base pairs
CS	Cross section
DEA	Dissociative electron attachment
DNA	Deoxyribonucleic acid
DSB	Double strand break
EF	Enhancement factor
ESD	Electron stimulated desorption
GNP	Gold nanoparticle
LEE	Low energy electron
LS	Loss of supercoiled
PEG	Polyethylene glycol
SSB	Single strand break
TMA	Transient molecular anion

Acknowledgments

Financial support was provided by the Canadian Institute of Health Research (PJT-162325), the Natural Sciences and Engineering Research Council of Canada (NSERC), National Key Technologies R & D Program of China (2014BAC13B03), the State Key Laboratory of Photocatalysis on Energy and Environment (SKLPEE-2017B03) and the National Natural Science Foundation of China (21673044). The authors are indebted to Dr Andrew Bass for discussions and critical evaluation of this manuscript.

References

[1] Su X, Liu P, Wu H and Gu N 2014 Enhancement of radiosensitization by metal-based nanoparticles in cancer radiation therapy *Cancer Biol. Med.* **11** 86–91

[2] Haume K, Rosa S, Grellet S, Śmiałek M, Butterworth K, Solovyov A, Prise K, Golding J and Mason N 2016 Gold nanoparticles for cancer radiotherapy: a review *Cancer Nano* **7** 8

[3] Chithrani D, Jelveh S, Jalali F, van Prooijen M, Allen C, Bristow R, Hill R and Jaffray D 2010 Gold nanoparticles as radiation sensitizers in cancer therapy *Radiat. Res.* **173** 719–28

[4] Coulter J A, Jain S, Forker J, McMahon S J, Schettino G, Prise K M, Currell F J and Hirst D G 2010 Evaluation of cytotoxicity and radiation enhancement using 1.9 nm gold particles: potential application for cancer therapy *Nanotechnology* **29** 295101

[5] Chang M Y, Shiau A L, Chen Y H, Chang C J, Chen H H and Wu C L 2008 Increased apoptotic potential and dose-enhancing effect of gold nanoparticles in combination with single-dose clinical electron beams on tumor-bearing mice *Cancer Sci.* **99** 1479–84

[6] Coulter J A, Hyland W B, Nicol J and Currell F J 2013 Radiosensitising nanoparticles as novel cancer therapeutics—pipe dream or realistic prospect? *Clin. Oncol.* **25** 593–603

[7] Hainfeld J F, Slatkin D N and Smilowitz H M 2004 The use of gold nanoparticles to enhance radiotherapy in mice *Phys. Med. Biol.* **49** N309–15
[8] Jain S *et al* 2011 Cell-specific radiosensitization by gold nanoparticles at megavoltage radiation energies *Int. J. Radiat. Oncol. Biol. Phys.* **79** 531–9
[9] Liu C J *et al* 2010 Enhancement of cell radiation sensitivity by pegylated gold nanoparticles *Phys. Med. Biol.* **55** 931–45
[10] Kang B, Mackey M A and El-Sayed M A 2010 Nuclear targeting of gold nanoparticles in cancer cells induces DNA damage, causing cytokinesis arrest and apoptosis *J. Am. Chem. Soc.* **132** 1517–9
[11] Hébert E, Debouttière P J, Lepage M, Sanche L and Hunting D J 2010 Preferential tumor accumulation of gold nanoparticles, visualized by magnetic resonance imaging: radiosensitization studies *in vivo* and *in vitro Int J Radiat Biol.* **86** 692–700
[12] Schuemann J, Berbeco R, Chithrani D B, Cho S H, Kumar R, McMahon S J, Sridhar S and Krishnan S 2016 Roadmap to clinical use of gold nanoparticles for radiation sensitization *Int. J. Radiat. Oncol. Biol. Phys.* **94** 189–205
[13] Rieck K, Bromma K, Sung W, Bannister A, Schuemann J and Chithrani D B 2019 Modulation of gold nanoparticle mediated radiation dose enhancement through synchronization of breast tumor cell population *Br. J. Radiol.* **92** 20190283
[14] Cho S H, Jones B L and Krishnan S 2009 The dosimetric feasibility of gold nanoparticle-aided radiation therapy (GNRT) via brachytherapy using low-energy gamma-/x-ray sources *Phys. Med. Biol.* **54** 4889–905
[15] Lechtman E, Mashouf S, Chattopadhyay N, Keller B M, Lai P, Cai Z, Reilly R M and Pignol J P 2013 A Monte Carlo-based model of gold nanoparticle radiosensitization accounting for increased radiobiological effectiveness *Phys. Med. Biol.* **58** 3075–85
[16] McMahon S J, Mendenhall M H, Jain S and Currell F 2008 Radiotherapy in the presence of contrast agents: a general figure of merit and its application to gold nanoparticles *Phys. Med. Biol.* **53** 5635–51
[17] McQuaid H N *et al* 2016 Imaging and radiation effects of gold nanoparticles in tumour cells *Sci. Rep.* **6** 19442
[18] Cho S 2005 Estimation of tumour dose enhancement due to gold nanoparticles during typical radiation treatments: a preliminary Monte Carlo study *Phys. Med. Biol.* **50** N163–73
[19] Rahman W N 2009 Enhancement of radiation effects by gold nanoparticles for superficial radiation therapy *Nanomedicine* **5** 136–42
[20] Carter J D, Cheng N N, Qu Y, Suarez G D and Guo T 2007 Nanoscale energy deposition by x-ray absorbing nanostructures *J. Phys. Chem.* B **111** 11622–5
[21] Hainfeld J F, Slatkin D N, Focella T M and Smilowitz H M 2006 Gold nanoparticles: a new x-ray contrast agent *Br. J. Radiol.* **7** 248–53
[22] Johns H E and Cunningham J 1983 *The Physics of Radiology* (Springfield, IL: Charles C. Thomas)
[23] Mozumder A and Hatano Y 2004 *Charged Particle and Photon Interactions with Matter, Chemical, Physicochemical, and Biological Consequences with Applications* (New York: Marcel Dekker)
[24] Hubbell J and Seltzer S 1996 *NIST Report. Table of X-ray Mass Attenuation and Mass Energy Absorption Coefficients*
[25] McMahon S *et al* 2011 Energy dependence of gold nanoparticles radiosensitisation in plasmid DNA *J. Phys. Chem.* C **115** 20160–7

[26] Connell P and Hellman S 2009 Advances in radiotherapy and implications for the next century: a historical perspective *Cancer Res.* **69** 383–92
[27] Matar J R, Coffey C and Maruyama Y 1988 Rectal carcinoma: treatment with Papillon technique and fiberoptic-guided methods *Radiology* **168** 562–4
[28] Casta R, Champeaux J P, Moretto Capelle P, Sence M and Cafarelli P 2015 Electron and photon emissions from gold nanoparticles irradiated by x-ray photons *J. Nanopart. Res.* **17** 3
[29] Michaud M, Bazin M and Sanche L 2013 Nanodosimetry of Auger electrons: a case study from the decay of 125 I and 0–18-eV electron stopping cross sections of cytosine *Phys. Rev.* E **87** 032701
[30] Reimers L and Drescher H 1977 Secondary electron emission of 10–100 keV electrons *J. Phys.* D **10** 805–15
[31] Verkhovtsev A V, Korol A V and Solov'yov A V 2015 Electron production by sensitizing gold nanoparticles irradiated by fast ions *J. Phys. Chem.* C **2015** 11000–13
[32] Pimblott S M and LaVerne J A 2007 Production of low-energy electrons by ionizing radiation *Radiat. Phys. Chem.* **76** 1244
[33] Liamsuwan T, Emfietzoglou D, Uehara S and Nikjoo H 2012 Microdosimetry of low-energy electrons *Int. J. Radiat. Biol.* **88** 899–907
[34] Wardlow N, Polin C, Villagomez-Bernabe B and Currell F 2015 A simple model to quantify radiolytic production following electron emission from heavy-atom nanoparticles irradiated in liquid suspensions *Radiat. Res.* **184** 518–32
[35] Casta R, Champeaux J P, Cafarelli P, Moretto-Capelle P and Sence M 2014 Model for electron emission of high-Z radio-sensitizing nanoparticle irradiated by x-rays *J. Nanopart. Res.* **16** 2480
[36] Casta R, Champeaux J P, Sence M, Moretto-Capelle P, Cafarelli P, Amsellem A and Sicard-Roselli C 2014 Electronic emission of radio-sensitizing gold nanoparticles under x-ray irradiation: experiment and simulations *J. Nanopart. Res.* **16** 2348
[37] Chow J, Leung M and Jaffray D A 2012 Monte Carlo simulation on a gold nanoparticle irradiated by electron beams *Phys. Med. Biol.* **57** 3323–31
[38] Leung M K, Chow J C, Chithrani B D, Lee M J, Oms B and Jaffray D A 2011 Irradiation of gold nanoparticles by x-rays: Monte Carlo simulation of dose enhancements and the spatial properties of the secondary electrons production *Med. Phys.* **38** 624–31
[39] McMahon S J *et al* 2011 Biological consequences of nanoscale energy deposition near irradiated heavy atom nanoparticles *Sci. Rep.* **1** 18
[40] Brun E, Cloutier P, Sicard-Roselli C, Fromm M and Sanche L 2009 Damage induced to DNA by low-energy (0–30 eV) electrons under vacuum and atmospheric conditions *J. Phys. Chem.* B **113** 10008–13
[41] Casta R, Champeaux J P, Sence M, Moretto-Capelle P and Cafarelli P 2015 Comparison between gold nanoparticle and gold plane electron emissions: a way to identify secondary electron emission *Phys. Med. Biol.* **60** 9095–105
[42] Xiao F, Zheng Y, Cloutier P, He Y, Hunting D and Sanche L 2011 On the role of low-energy electrons in the radiosensitization of DNA by gold nanoparticles *Nanotechnology* **22** 465101
[43] Barkas W H, Deutsch R W, Gilbert F C and Violet C E 1952 High energy electron-electron scattering *Phys. Rev.* **86** 59
[44] Verkhovtsev A V, Korol A V and Solov'yov A V 2015 Electron production by sensitizing gold nanoparticles irradiated by fast ions *J. Phys.* C **119** 11000–13

[45] Zheng Y, Hunting D J, Ayotte P and Sanche L 2008 Radiosensitization of DNA by gold nanoparticles irradiated with high-energy electrons *Radiat. Res.* **169** 19
[46] Mousavi M, Nedaei H A, Khoei S, Eynali S, Khoshgard K, Robatjazi M and Iraji Rad R 2017 Enhancement of radiosensitivity of melanoma cells by pegylated gold nanoparticles under irradiation of megavoltage electrons *Int. J. Radiat. Biol.* **93** 214–21
[47] Heuskin A C, Gallez B, Feron O, Martinive P, Michiels C and Lucas S 2017 Metallic nanoparticles irradiated by low-energy protons for radiation therapy: are there significant physical effects to enhance the dose delivery? *Med. Phys.* **44** 4299–312
[48] Li S *et al* 2016 LET-dependent radiosensitization effects of gold nanoparticles for proton irradiation *Nanotechnology* **27** 455101
[49] Torrisi L 2015 Gold nanoparticles enhancing proton herapy efficiency *Recent Pat. Nanotechnol.* **9** 51–60
[50] Kuncic Z and Lacombe S 2017 Nanoparticle radio-enhancement: principles, progress and application to cancer treatment *Phys. Med. Biol.* **63** 02TR01
[51] Albanese A, Tang P and Chan W 2012 The effect of nanoparticle size, shape, and surface chemistry on biological systems *Annu. Rev. Biomed. Eng.* **14** 1–16
[52] Chithrani D 2010 Intracellular uptake, transport, and processing of gold nanostructures *Mol. Membr. Biol.* **17** 299–311
[53] Shi M, Paquette B, Thippayamontri T, Gendron L, Guérin B and Sanche L 2016 Increased radiosensitivity of colorectal tumors with intra-tumoral injection of low dose of gold nanoparticles *Int. J. Nanomed.* **11** 5323–33
[54] Fribley A, Zhang K Z and Kaufman R J 2009 Regulation of apoptosis by the unfolded protein response *Methods Mol. Biol.* **559** 191–204
[55] Yang C and Chithrani D 2016 Nuclear targeting of gold nanoparticles for improved therapeutics *Curr. Top. Med. Chem.* **16** 271–80
[56] Huels M A, Boudaïffa B, Cloutier P, Hunting D and Sanche L 2003 Single, double, and multiple double strand breaks induced in DNA by 3–100 eV electrons *J. Am. Chem. Soc.* **125** 4467–77
[57] Chen W, Chen S, Dong Y, Cloutier P, Zheng Y and Sanche L 2016 Absolute cross sections for DNA strand breaks and crosslinks induced by low energy electrons *Phys. Chem. Chem. Phys.* **18** 32762–71
[58] Choofong S, Cloutier P, Sanche L and Wagner J 2016 Base release and modification in solid-phase DNA exposed to low-energy electrons *Radiat. Res.* **186** 520–30
[59] Shao Y, Dong Y, Hunting D, Zheng Y and Sanche L 2017 Unified mechanism for the generation of isolated and clustered DNA damages by a single low energy (5–10 eV) electron *J. Phys. Chem.* C **121** 2466–72
[60] Dong Y, Gao Y, Liu W, Gao T, Zheng Y and Sanche L 2019 Clustered DNA damage induced by 2–20 eV electrons and transient anions: general mechanism and correlation to cell death *J. Phys. Chem. Lett.* **10** 2985–90
[61] Fucarelli A F and Zimbrick J D (ed) 1995 *Radiation Damage in DNA: Structure/Function Relationships at Early Times* (Columbus, OH: Battelle)
[62] Becker D and Sevilla M D 1993 The chemical consequences of radiation damage to DNA *Advances in Radiation Biology* ed J Lett vol 17 (New York: Academic) pp 121–80
[63] Jackson S and Bartek J 2009 The DNA-damage response in human biology and disease *Nature* **461** 1071–8

[64] Boudaiffa B, Cloutier P, Hunting D, Huels M A and Sanche L 2000 Resonant formation of DNA strand breaks by low-energy (3 to 20 eV) electrons *Science* **287** 1658

[65] Martin F, Burrow P D, Cai Z, Coultier P, Hunting D and Sanche L 2004 DNA strand breaks induced by 0–4 eV electrons: the role of shape resonances *Phys. Rev. Lett.* **93** 068101

[66] Zheng Y, Cloutier P, Hunting D J, Sanche L and Wagner J 2005 Chemical basis of DNA sugar– phosphate cleavage by low-energy electrons *J. Am. Chem. Soc.* **127** 16592

[67] Berdys J, Anusiewicz I, Skurski P and Simons J 2004 Damage to model DNA fragments from very low-energy (<1 eV) electrons *J. Am. Chem. Soc.* **126** 6441

[68] Barrios R, Skurski P and Simons J 2002 Mechanism for damage to DNA by low-energy electrons *J. Phys. Chem.* B **106** 7991

[69] Kumar A and Sevilla M D 2012 Low energy electron (LEE) induced DNA damage: theoretical approaches to modeling experiment *Handbook of Computational Chemistry, Vol. III: Applications Biomolecules* ed M Shukla and J Leszczynski (Berlin: Springer)

[70] Sanche L and Michaud M 1984 Interaction of low-energy electrons (1–30 eV) with condensed molecules: II. Vibrational-librational excitation and shape resonances in thin N_2 and CO films *Phys. Rev.* B **30** 6078–92

[71] Michaud M, Bazin M and Sanche L 2012 Measurement of inelastic cross sections for low-energy electron scattering from DNA bases *Int. J. Radiat. Biol.* **88** 15–21

[72] Liljequist D 2012 A model calculation of coherence effects in the elastic backscattering of very low energy electrons (1–20 eV) from amorphous ice *Int. J. Radiat. Biol.* **88** 50–3

[73] Sambe H, Ramaker D E, Parenteau L and Sanche L 1987 Electron-stimulated desorption enhanced by coherent scattering *Phys. Rev. Lett.* **59** 505–8

[74] Michaud M, Cloutier P and Sanche L 1991 Phonon excitations in low-energy-electron scattering from solid Ar, Kr, and Xe films: direct observation of conduction-band density of states *Phys. Rev.* B **44** 10485–92

[75] Michaud M, Cloutier P and Sanche L 1994 Phonon excitations in low-energy electron resonant scattering from solid films of N_2 *Phys. Rev.* B **49** 8360–6

[76] Michaud M and Sanche L 1994 Low-energy electron-energy-loss spectroscopy of solid films of argon: surface and bulk valence excitons *Phys. Rev.* B **50** 4725–32

[77] Rowntree P, Sambe H, Parenteau L and Sanche L 1993 Formation of anionic excitations in the rare-gas solids and their coupling to dissociative states of adsorbed molecules *Phys. Rev.* B **47** 4537–54

[78] Bass A D and Sanche L 2003 Dissociative electron attachment and charge transfer in condensed matter *Radiat. Phys. Chem.* **68** 3–13

[79] Fano U and Stephens J A 1986 Slow electrons in condensed matter *Phys. Rev.* B **34** 438

[80] Sanche L 1991 Primary interactions of low-energy electrons in condensed matter *Excess Electrons in Dielectric Media* ed J-P Jay-Gerin and C Ferradini 1st edn (Boca Raton, FL: CRC Press)

[81] Michaud M, Lepage M and Sanche L 1998 Lifetime of negative ion resonances and the density of free electron states: O_2 isolated in an argon matrix *Phys. Rev. Lett.* **81** 2807–10

[82] Alizadeh E, Ptasińska S and Sanche L 2016 Transient anions in radiobiology and radiotherapy: from gaseous biomolecules to condensed organic and biomolecular solids *Radiation Effects in Materials* ed W Monterio (London: InTech)

[83] Hedhili M N, Parenteau L, Huels M A, Azria R, Tronc M and Sanche L 1997 The effects of different substrates on the electron stimulated desorption dynamics of $\overline{O}$ from physisorbed O_2 *J. Chem. Phys.* **107** 7577–81

[84] Schulz G J 1973 Resonances in electron impact on diatomic molecules *Rev. Mod. Phys.* **45** 423–86

[85] Allan M 1989 Study of the triplet-states and short-lived negative-ions by means of electron impact spectroscopy *J. Electron. Spectrosc. Relat. Phenom.* **48** 219–351

[86] Kohanoff J, McAllister M, Tribello G and Gu B 2017 Interactions between low energy electrons and DNA: a perspective from first-principles simulations *J. Phys.: Condens. Matter* **29** 383001

[87] Sanche L 1990 Low-energy electron scattering from molecules on surfaces *J. Phys.* B **23** 1597–624

[88] Sanche L 2012 Nanoscale dynamics of radiosensitivity: role of low energy electrons *Radiation Damage in Biomolecular Systems* ed G G Gomez-Tejedor and M C Fuss 1st edn (New York: Springer)

[89] Torchia D A 2011 Dynamics of biomolecules from picoseconds to seconds at atomic resolution *J. Magn. Reson.* **21** 1–10

[90] Palmer R E and Rous P 1992 Resonances in electron-scattering by molecules on surface *Rev. Mod. Phys.* **64** 383–479

[91] Alizadeh E, Orlando T M and Sanche L 2015 Biomolecular damage induced by ionizing radiation: the direct and indirect effects of low-energy electrons on DNA *Ann. Rev. Phys. Chem.* **66** 379–98

[92] Arumainayagam C R, Lee H L, Nelson R B, Haines D R and Gunawardane R P 2010 Low-energy electron-induced reactions in condensed matter *Surf. Sci. Rep.* **65** 1–44

[93] Smyth M and Kohanoff J 2012 Excess electron interactions with solvated DNA nucleotides: strand breaks possible at room temperature *J. Am. Chem. Soc.* **134** 9122–5

[94] Sanche L, Bass A D, Ayotte P and Fabrikant I I 1995 Effect of the condensed phase on dissociative electron attachment: CH_3Cl condensed on a Kr surface *Phys. Rev. Lett.* **75** 3568

[95] Michaud M and Sanche L 1990 The $^2\Pi g$ shape resonance of N_2 near a metal surface and in rare gas solids *J. Electron. Spectrosc. Relat. Phenom.* **51** 237–48

[96] Meesungnoen J, Jay-Gerin J P, Filali-Mouhim A and Mankhetkorn S 2002 Low-energy electron penetration range in liquid water *Radiat. Res.* **158** 657–60

[97] Rezaee M, Cloutier P, Bass A D, Hunting D J and Sanche L 2012 Absolute cross section for low energy electron damage to condensed macromolecules: a case study of DNA *Phys. Rev.* E **86** 031913

[98] Luo X, Zheng Y and Sanche L 2014 DNA strand breaks and crosslinks induced by transient anions in the range 2–20 eV *J. Chem. Phys.* **140** 155101

[99] Inokuti M 1995 *Atomic and Molecular Data for Radiotherapy and Radiation Research* (Vienna: International Atomic Energy Agency)

[100] Douki T and Cadet J 2008 *Radiation Chemistry, From Basics to Applications in Material and Life Sciences* ed M Spotheim-Maurizot, M Mostafavi, T Douki and J Belloni (Cedex France: EDP Sciences) pp 177–89

[101] Baccarelli I, Bald I, Gianturco F A, Illenberger E and Kopyra J 2011 Electron-induced damage of DNA and its components: experiments and theoretical models *Phys. Rep.* **508** 1–44

[102] Sevilla M D and Bernhard W A 2008 Mechanisms of direct radiation damage to DNAM *Radiation Chemistry: From Basics to Applications in Material and Life Sciences* ed M Spotheim-Maurizot, M Mostafavi, T Douki and J Belloni 1st edn (Les Ulis: EDP Sciences) pp 191–201

[103] Alizadeh E, Sanz A G, García G and Sanche L 2013 Radiation damage to DNA: the indirect effect of low-energy electrons *J. Phys. Chem. Lett.* **4** 820–5
[104] Alizadeh E and Sanche L 2012 Precursors of solvated electrons in radiobiological physics and chemistry *Chem. Rev.* **112** 5578–602
[105] Rowntree P, Parenteau L and Sanche L 1991 Electron stimulated desorption via dissociative attachment in amorphous H_2O *J. Chem. Phys.* **94** 8570
[106] Simpson W C, Sieger M T, Orlando T M, Parenteau L, Nagesha K and Sanche L 1997 Dissociative electron attachment in nanoscale ice films: Temperature and morphology effects *J. Chem. Phys.* **107** 8668
[107] Simpson W C, Orlando T M, Parenteau L, Nagesha K and Sanche L 1998 Dissociative electron attachment in nanoscale ice films: thickness and charge trapping effects *J. Chem. Phys.* **108** 5027
[108] Kimmel G A and Orlando T M 1996 Observation of negative ion resonances in amorphous ice via low-energy (5–40 eV) electron-stimulated production of molecular hydrogen *Phys. Rev. Lett.* **77** 3983
[109] Kimmel G A, Orlando T M, Vezina C and Sanche L 1994 Low-energy electron-stimulated production of molecular hydrogen from amorphous water ice *J. Chem. Phys.* **101** 3282
[110] Kimmel G A and Orlando T M 1995 Low-energy (5–120 eV) electron-stimulated dissociation of amorphous D_2O ice: D (^2S), O ($^3P_{2,1,0}$), and O ($^1D_2$) yields and velocity distributions *Phys. Rev. Lett.* **75** 2606
[111] Kimmel G A, Orlando T M, Cloutier P and Sanche L 1997 Low-energy (5–40 eV) electron-stimulated desorption of atomic hydrogen and metastable emission from amorphous ice *J. Phys. Chem.* B **101** 6301
[112] von Sonntag C 1987 *The Chemical Basis for Radiation Biology* (London: Taylor and Francis)
[113] O'Neil P 2001 *Radiation Chemistry: Present Status and Future Trends* (Amsterdam: Elsevier)
[114] Sicard-Roselli C, Brun E, Gilles M, Baldacchino G, Kelsey C, McQuaid H, Polin C, Wardlow N and Currell F 2014 A new mechanism for hydroxyl radical production in irradiated nanoparticle solutions *Small* **10** 3338–46
[115] Gilles M, Brun E and Sicard-Roselli C 2014 Gold nanoparticles functionalization notably decreases radiosensitization through hydroxyl radical production under ionizing radiation *Colloids Surf. B: Biointerfaces* **123** 770–7
[116] Michaud M, Wen A and Sanche L 2003 Cross sections for low-energy (1–100 eV) electron elastic and inelastic scattering in amorphous ice *Radiat. Res.* **159** 3–22
[117] Michaud M and Sanche L 1987 Total cross section for slow electrons (1–20 eV) scattering in solid H_2O *Phys. Rev.* A **36** 4672–83
[118] Michaud M and Sanche L 1987 Absolute vibrational excitation cross sections for slow electron (1–18 eV) scattering in solid H_2O *Phys. Rev.* A **36** 4684–99
[119] Bader G, Chiasson J, Caron L G, Michaud M, Perluzzo G and Sanche L 1988 Absolute scattering probabilities for subexcitation electrons in condensed H_2O *Radiat. Res.* **114** 467–79
[120] Ness K F and Robson R E 1988 Transport properties of electrons in water vapor *Phys. Rev.* A **38** 1446–56
[121] Djuric N L, Cadez I M and Kupera M V 1988 H_2O and D_2O total ionization cross-sections by electron impact *Int. J. Mass Spectrom. Ion Process.* **83** R7–10

[122] Bolorizadeh M A and Rudd M E 1986 Angular and energy dependence of cross sections for ejection of electrons from water vapor. I. 50–2000-eV electron impact *Phys. Rev.* A **33** 882–7

[123] Panajotovic R, Martin F, Cloutier P, Hunting D and Sanche L 2006 Effective cross sections for production of single-strand breaks in plasmid DNA by 0.1 to 4.7 eV electrons *Radiat. Res.* **165** 452

[124] Nikjoo H, Emfietzoglou D, Liamsuwan T, Taleei R, Liljequist D and Uehara S 2016 Radiation track, DNA damage and response—a review *Rep. Prog. Phys.* **79** 116601

[125] Zheng Y and Sanche L 2019 Clustered DNA Damages induced by 0.5 to 30 eV electrons *Int. J. Mol. Sci.* **20** 3749

[126] Winstead C and McKoy V 2006 Interaction of low-energy electrons with the purine bases, nucleosides, and nucleotides of DNA *J. Chem. Phys.* **125** 244302

[127] Caron L G and Sanche L 2012 Theoretical studies of electron interactions with DNA and its subunits: from tetrahydrofuran to plasmid DNA *Low Energy Electron Scattering from Molecules, Biomolecules and Surfaces* ed P Čársky and R Čurík 1st edn (Boca Raton, FL: CRC Press) pp 161–230

[128] Gu J, Leszczynski J and Schaefer F III 2012 Interactions of electrons with bare and hydrated biomolecules: from nucleic acid bases to DNA segments *Chem. Rev.* **112** 5603–40

[129] Boulanouar O, Fromm M, Bass A D, Cloutier P and Sanche L 2013 Absolute cross section for loss of supercoiled topology induced by 10 eV electrons in highly uniform/DNA/1, 3-diaminopropane films deposited on highly ordered pyrolitic graphite *J. Chem. Phys.* **139** 055104

[130] Zheng Y, Cloutier P, Hunting D J, Wagner J R and Sanche L 2006 Phosphodiester and N-glycosidic bond cleavage in DNA induced by 4–15 eV electrons *J. Chem. Phys.* **124** 064710

[131] Pan X, Cloutier P, Hunting D and Sanche L 2003 Dissociative electron attachment to DNA *Phys. Rev. Lett.* **90** 208102

[132] Sahbani S, Sanche L, Cloutier P, Bass A D and Hunting D J 2015 Electron resonance decay into a biological function: decrease in viability of *E. coli* transformed by plasmid DNA irradiated with 0.5–18 eV electrons *J. Phys. Chem. Lett.* **6** 3911–4

[133] Sahbani S, Sanche L, Cloutier P, Bass A and Hunting D 2014 Loss of cellular transformation efficiency induced by DNA irradiation with low-energy (10 eV) electrons *J. Phys. Chem.* B **118** 13123–31

[134] Khanna K K and Jackson S P 2001 DNA double-strand breaks: signaling, repair and the cancer connection *Nat. Genet.* **27** 247–54

[135] Rezaee M, Hill R and Jaffray D 2017 The exploitation of low-energy electrons in cancer treatment *Radiat. Res.* **188** 123–43

[136] Zheng Y, Wagner J R and Sanche L 2006 DNA damage induced by low-energy electrons: electron transfer and diffraction *Phys. Rev. Lett.* **96** 208101

[137] Li Z, Zheng Y, Cloutier P, Sanche L and Wagner J 2008 Low energy electron induced DNA damage: effects of terminal phosphate and base moieties on the distribution of damage *J. Am. Chem. Soc.* **130** 5612–3

[138] Sanche L 2009 Low-energy electron interaction with DNA: bond dissociation and formation of transient anions, radicals and radical anions *Radicals and Radical Ion Reactivity in Nucleic Acid ChemistryWiley Series on Reactive Intermediates in Chemistry and Biology* ed M Greenberg (New York: Wiley)

[139] Li Z, Cloutier P, Sanche L and Wagner J 2011 Low energy electron induced DNA damage in a trinucleotide containing 5-bromouracil *J. Phys. Chem.* B **115** 13668–73

[140] Zheng Y, Cloutier P, Hunting D J and Sanche L 2008 Radiosensitization by gold nanoparticles: comparison of DNA damage induced by low and high-energy electrons *J. Biomed. Nanotech.* **4** 469
[141] Butterworth K T, Wyer J A, Brennan-Fournet M, Latimer C J, Shah M B, Currell F J and Hirst D G 2008 Variation of strand break yield for plasmid DNA irradiated with high-Z metal nanoparticles *Radiat. Res.* **170** 381–7
[142] Foley E A *et al* 2005 Enhanced relaxation of nanoparticle-bound supercoiled DNA in x-ray radiation *Chem. Commun.* 3192–4
[143] Brun E, Sanche L and Sicard-Roselli C 2009 Parameters governing gold nanoparticle x-ray radiosensitization of DNA in solution *Colloids Surf. B-Biointerfaces* **72** 128–34
[144] Berbeco R, Korideck H, Ngwa W, Kumar R, Patel J, Sridhar S, Johnson S, Price B, Kimmelman A and Makrigiorgos G 2012 DNA damage enhancement from gold nanoparticles for clinical MV photon beams *Radiat. Res.* **178** 604–8
[145] Spaas C *et al* 2016 Dependence of gold nanoparticle radiosensitization on functionalizing layer thickness *Radiat. Res.* **185** 384–92
[146] Zheng Y and Sanche L 2013 Low energy electrons in nanoscale radiation physics: relationship to radiosensitization and chemoradiation therapy *Rev. Nanosci. Nanotechnol.* **2** 1–28
[147] Bruining H and Fry D 1962 *Physics and Applications of Secondary Electron EmissionPergamon Science Series: Electronics and Waves—a Series of Monographs* (Oxford: Pergamon)
[148] Yao X, Huang C, Chen X, Zheng Y and Sanche L 2015 Chemical radiosensitivity of DNA induced by gold nanoparticles *J. Biomed. Nanotechnol.* **11** 478–85
[149] Huang C, Bao Q, Hunting D, Zheng Y and Sanche L 2013 Conformation-dependent DNA damage induced by gold nanoparticles *J. Biomed. Nanotechnol.* **9** 856–62
[150] Florentiev V L and Ivanov V I 1970 RNA polymerase: two-step mechanism with overlapping steps *Nature* **228** 519
[151] Ajith T A 2015 Strategies used in the clinical trials of gene therapy for cancer *J. Exp. Ther. Oncol.* **11** 33–9
[152] Brazzale C *et al* 2017 Control of targeting ligand display by pH-responsive polymers on gold nanoparticles mediates selective entry into cancer cells *Nanoscale* **9** 11137–47
[153] Kong L, Qiu J, Sun W, Yang J, Shen M, Wang L and Shi X 2017 Multifunctional PEI-entrapped gold nanoparticles enable efficient delivery of therapeutic siRNA into glioblastoma cells *Biomater. Sci.* **5** 258–66
[154] Lai P, Lechtman E, Mashouf S, Pignol J P and Reilly R 2016 Depot system for controlled release of gold nanoparticles with precise intratumoral placement by permanent brachytherapy seed implantation (PSI) techniques *Int. J. Pharm.* **515** 729–39
[155] Bobyk L *et al* 2013 Photoactivation of gold nanoparticles for glioma treatment *Nanomedicine* **9** 1089–97
[156] Reilly R M 2005 *Modern Biopharmaceuticals: Design, Development and Optimization* ed J Knaeblein and R Mueller (Weinheim: Wiley) pp 497–526
[157] Ngwa W, Kumar R, Sridhar S, Korideck H, Zygmanski P, Cormack R A, Berbeco R and Makrigiorgos G M 2014 Targeted radiotherapy with gold nanoparticles: current status and future perspectives *Nanomedicine* **9** 1063–82
[158] Ngwa W, Korideck H, Kassis A, Kumar R, Sridhar S, Makrigiorgos G M and Cormack R A 2013 *In vitro* radiosensitization by gold nanoparticles during continuous low-dose-rate gamma irradiation with I-125 brachytherapy seeds *Nanomedicine* **9** 25–7

[159] Yook S, Cai Z, Lu Y, Winnik M, Pignol J-P and Reilly R 2016 Intratumorally injected ^{177}Lu-labeled gold nanoparticles—gold nanoseed brachytherapy with application for neoadjuvant treatment of locally advanced breast cancer (LABC) *J. Nucl. Med.* **115** 168906
[160] Shi M and Sanche L 2019 Convection-enhanced delivery in malignant gliomas: a review of toxicity and efficacy *J. Oncol.* **2019** 9342796
[161] Ngwa W, Makrigiorgos G and Berbeco R 2010 Applying gold nanoparticles as tumor-vascular disrupting agents during brachytherapy: estimation of endothelial dose enhancement *Phys. Med. Biol.* **55** 6533–48
[162] Pomplun E 2012 Monte Carlo-simulated Auger electron spectra for nuclides of radiobiological and medical interest—a validation with noble gas ionization data *Int. J. Radiat. Biol.* **88** 108–14
[163] Sanche L 2015 Cancer treatment: low-energy electron therapy *Nat. Mater.* **14** 861–3
[164] Pronschinske A, Pedevilla P, Murphy C J, Lewis E, Lucci F, Brown G, Pappas G, Michaelides A and Sykes E 2015 Enhancement of low-energy electron emission in 2D radioactive films *Nat. Mater.* **14** 904–7

Chapter 5

Monte Carlo models of electron transport for dose-enhancement calculations in nanoparticle-aided radiotherapy

Dimitris Emfietzoglou and Sebastien Incerti

The physical origin of the radiosensitizing effect of nanoparticles (NP) stems from the increased energy deposition (and radiation dose) in their vicinity due to the enhanced emission of secondary electrons. Monte Carlo radiation transport codes are presently considered the gold standard for dose calculations in radiotherapy, so they have naturally become the main theoretical tool for studying the dose enhancement effect in NP-aided radiotherapy (NRT). Depending on the approach used for simulating the transport of electrons in irradiated matter, Monte Carlo models are generally divided into two major classes, namely, condensed-history models and track-structure models. To understand the advantages and limitations of each simulation approach for application to NRT, as well as some of the essential differences among the available Monte Carlo codes, the most used physical models in electron transport simulations will be reviewed. In particular, we will restrict our discussion to inelastic electron scattering (leading to ionizations and electronic excitations) which is the physical process mainly responsible for the secondary electron emission of NPs and their dose enhancement effect.

5.1 Introduction

The physical origin of the radiosensitizing effect of high atomic number (high-Z) NP stems from the increased energy deposition (and radiation dose) in their vicinity [1]. This increase is mainly due to the enhanced emission of secondary electrons that are generated via the interaction of the incoming beam with the electronic subsystem of the NP. An increased number of fluorescent and bremsstrahlung photons may also be emitted from the NP but their contribution to the radiosensitizing effect is generally considered to be small since they lead to an enhanced energy deposition at

doi:10.1088/978-0-7503-2396-3ch5

relatively large distances from the NP where the absorbed dose has decreased considerably.

A very popular physical metric for assessing the radiotherapeutic efficacy of NP is the *dose enhancement ratio* (DER)[1] which can be generally defined as

$$\text{DER} = \left.\frac{\text{dose to the medium with NP}}{\text{dose to the medium w/o NP}}\right|_{\text{same irradiation}}, \tag{5.1}$$

where the dose is averaged over some macro- or microscopic target volume of the medium. This target volume is typically considered to be made of liquid water, as a surrogate to cellular medium (this assumption will also be used hereafter). Thus, a common distinction in the literature is between the *microscopic* DER, i.e. the dose enhancement that takes place at the nm–μm scale, and the *macroscopic* DER which usually refers to the mm–cm scale [2]. Although this distinction is not strict, it is operationally useful and particularly instructive in the present context because different Monte Carlo models are suitable in the two cases.

Following the general definition of equation (5.1), the microscopic DER can be defined as

$$\text{DER}_{\text{micro}}(\vec{r}) = \frac{D_{\text{NP}}(\vec{r})}{D_{\text{water}}(\vec{r})}, \tag{5.2}$$

where $D_{\text{NP}}(\vec{r})$ is the dose in an infinitesimal mass of water centered at distance $\vec{r}$ from the NP, and $D_{\text{water}}(\vec{r})$ is the dose at the same point in the absence of NP. In practice, the 3D dose distribution is approximated (assuming it is spherical symmetric) by a 1D distribution by interpreting $D_{\text{NP}}(\vec{r})$ as a radial distribution function of the 'local' radiation dose around the NP. The radial distance r may be measured from the center or the surface of the NP. In the context of Monte Carlo simulations, the radial DER is essentially a histogram with bin-widths ($\delta\, r$) of the order of nm. The microscopic DER is (mainly) due to low-energy electrons below few keV which deposit all of their energy within distances of less than about 100 nm in water. The main source of low-energy electrons are either Auger electrons following photoelectric absorption (and less often Compton scattering) by the inner-shell electrons of the NP atoms with their subsequent non-radiative de-excitation, or outer-shell secondary electrons following ionization by inelastic scattering of charged-particles. Higher-energy electrons (>1 keV) are also contributing to the microscopic DER but to a much lesser degree due to their smaller energy-loss rate and higher penetration distance.

On the other hand the *macroscopic* DER is defined as

$$\text{DER}_{\text{macro}}(\vec{r}) = \frac{\int_{V(\vec{r})} D_{\text{NP}}(\vec{r})dV}{\int_{V(\vec{r})} D_{\text{water}}(\vec{r})dV}, \tag{5.3}$$

[1] Also called dose enhancement factor (DEF).

where the integration is over a macroscopic volume of water (centered at distance $\vec{r}$ from the NP) with linear dimensions in the mm–cm scale (e.g. representing the tumor volume). The macroscopic DER is mainly due to high-energy photoelectrons and Compton electrons or high-energy delta rays that may reach distances in a water medium of the order of mm–cm away from the NP. Thus, the electron energies of interest to the macroscopic DER exceed ~10–100 keV (which excludes most of the Auger electrons).

Translating the DER to a radiobiological outcome is not straightforward, since the radiosensitizing effect of NP depends also on a number of pharmacological (NP targeting, concentration, and intracellular localization) and biological (cell and tissue type) factors [3]. Nevertheless, the practical importance of DER is that it can be easily implemented into some biophysical dose-response models to predict cell survival probabilities [4]. For example, the macroscopic DER is often used within the linear-quadratic (LQ) model to predict the reduced cell survival in NRT through the expression

$$S_{\mathrm{NP}} \approx \exp[-\alpha(D + D_{\mathrm{enhance}}) - \beta(D + D_{\mathrm{enhance}})^2] \tag{5.4}$$

where $\alpha(\mathrm{Gy}^{-1})$ and $\beta(\mathrm{Gy}^{-2})$ are, respectively, the one-hit and two-hit LQ coefficients which are assumed not to change in the presence of NP. As in the conventional use of the LQ model, $D = D_{\mathrm{water}}$ is the average radiation dose to the cell (assumed to be made of water), and $D_{\mathrm{enhance}} = D_{\mathrm{NP}} - D_{\mathrm{water}}$ is the enhanced radiation dose to the cell due to the presence of NP calculated from the macroscopic DER of equation (5.3). On the other hand, the microscopic DER can be conveniently implemented into the local-effect-model (LEM) using the expression:

$$S_{\mathrm{NP}} \approx \exp\left\{-\frac{1}{V}\int_V \ln\left[S_{\mathrm{X}}(D(r) + D_{\mathrm{enhance}}(r))\right]dV\right\}, \tag{5.5}$$

where S_{NP} is the cell survival probability in the presence of NP, $S_{\mathrm{X}}(D)$ is the cell survival probability at a radiation dose D obtained from low-LET radiation (typically high-energy x-rays), $D(r) = D_{\mathrm{water}}(r)$ is the local radiation dose to water at distance r from the NP (but in the absence of it), $D_{\mathrm{enhance}}(r) = D_{\mathrm{NP}}(r) - D_{\mathrm{water}}(r)$ is the enhanced radiation dose at distance r from the NP obtained from the microscopic DER of equation (5.2), and V is the target volume (usually assumed to be the cell nucleus). The LQ model (or its LQ-L high-dose extension) is commonly used to describe $S_{\mathrm{X}}(D)$ in equation (5.5).

In general, the microscopic DER may be orders of magnitude larger than the macroscopic DER. This huge difference is due to the strong dose gradient near the NP whereby the energy deposition peaks near its surface and drops rapidly within the first 100 nm [2]. So, the large discrepancies on DER values reported in the literature may be partly attributed to the different spatial scale of the examined DER. Given the large difference in magnitude, the distinction between macroscopic and microscopic DER has important implications to the design and optimization of NRT. For example, in pursuing active NP targeting methodologies whereby the NPs are localized to the surface (or internally) of tumor cells, the microscopic DER is a more pertinent physical metric because it allows more accurate estimates of the energy deposition within the nucleus of the targeted cells. In this case, the magnitude of NP radiosensitization might be grossly underestimated by the use of the macroscopic DER. The opposite holds when NPs are passively targeted in tumors (due to their leaky vasculature) and remain in the extracellular matrix. In this case, one is generally interested in the dose enhancement at longer distances from the NPs [5].

5.2 The challenge

The exact spectrum of secondary particles emitted from the NP, which is responsible for its dose enhancement, depends upon both the incoming beam (type and energy) as well as the physical characteristics of the NP (atomic composition, size and shape). The interplay of these factors is not straightforward [6]. One of the aims of Monte Carlo transport simulations in NRT is to reliably determine the DER for different primary beams, NP compositions, sizes, shapes, concentrations, and localizations. The above task faces several challenges, both computational and physical. In general, the source of these challenges can be traced to the *multiscale* nature of the problem which, in principle, involves the simulation of both the macroscopic (incoming or primary) beam as it propagates between the surface of the patient (or the phantom) and the NP-loaded target regions, as well as the microscopic beam of secondary particles generated within the NP and leaking out [2]. The transition from a macroscopic to microscopic beam simulation is accompanied by a corresponding transition of the spatial resolution of the simulation, i.e. from ~mm–cm down to ~nm–μm volumes. It is also a transition from high-event probability (macroscopic regions) to low-event probability (microscopic regions) simulations which may lead to (prohibitively) long simulation times. The varied spatial resolution and statistical uncertainty present distinctive challenges to Monte Carlo codes applied to NRT. Although deterministic codes may offer some advantages under particular circumstances because of their short simulation times and lack of statistical uncertainty, Monte Carlo transport simulations are presently the most widely used approach in NRT dosimetry.

Comparisons between experimental data and theoretical predictions of S_{NP} have pointed out that the microscopic DER better correlates with the radiosensitizing effect of NP, likely because of its closer association to radiation-induced damage at critical biological structures (e.g. cell nucleus, DNA) [6, 7]. At a more fundamental level, the high local dose around NP resembles the effects of high-LET radiations which are associated with high relative biological effectiveness (RBE). These effects are inherently 'microscopic' since they arise from the spatial pattern of energy deposition (inelastic collisions) at the nanometer scale.

Key challenges in Monte Carlo modeling of the *microscopic* dose enhancement include: (i) Describing the microscopic beam produced within the NP which is comprised by the initial energy spectrum of all secondary electrons generated in the NP. This step requires consideration of the electronic structure of the NP atoms (excitation levels, ionization shells) as well as their de-excitation process (e.g. the Auger electron cascade). (ii) Describing the 'outgoing' microscopic beam that leaks out from the NP. This requires event-by-event simulation of the transport of secondary electrons within the NP, including consideration of various low-energy energy-loss processes, such as plasmon excitations (and their decay mode) which further enhance secondary electron generation. (iii) Simulating the transport of the emitted electrons in the surrounding liquid water medium with nanometer resolution. This step of the simulation essentially yields the (microscopic/macroscopic) dose enhancement.

The above level of detail far exceeds the capabilities offered by the conventional (macroscopic) Monte Carlo codes used for radiotherapy applications [8]. For example, the second and third points are entirely beyond the scope of the physics models used in conventional Monte Carlo codes, whereas the first point is only partly addressed since, at the most, only high-energy secondary electrons are included in those codes. The third point also represents an important research topic in the context of radiation biophysics and microdosimetry [9].

5.3 Monte Carlo simulation of electron transport

Monte Carlo radiation transport simulations are presently considered the gold standard for dose calculations in radiotherapy [8]. A number of Monte Carlo based software packages have been developed and optimized specifically for clinical dosimetry in conventional external-beam radiotherapy (e.g. DPM, VMC++, ORANGE, PEREGRINE). Some of these software packages have already been implemented in commercial treatment planning systems. It is therefore natural that Monte Carlo simulations have been widely used to calculate the dose enhancement in NRT [2].

The essence of the Monte Carlo technique is the sampling, through computer-generated (pseudo) random numbers, of probability distributions that describe the various interaction processes that take place as the radiation beam propagates in matter. It is the combination of suitable single- or multiple-scattering physics models with random sampling algorithms which enables the simulation of radiation transport in matter by the Monte Carlo method [10].

In radiotherapy applications (including NRT) energy deposition is primarily due to the secondary electrons that are abundantly generated in the irradiated tissue as a consequence of ionization processes. Thus, simulating the transport of secondary electrons represents an important consideration in the development of Monte Carlo codes for dosimetry applications. This is particularly true in NRT where secondary electrons are (mainly) responsible for the dose enhancement effect. However, contrary to photon (and neutron) transport, in which all interactions can be simulated in a chronological order, electrons undergo a large number of electromagnetic interactions before they come to rest, e.g. an 1 MeV electron may undergo more than a million collisions before it practically stops. Therefore, simulating electron transport collision-by-collision may become computer intensive [5, 10].

The 'tracking cutoff energy' (hereafter simply tracking cut) and the 'production cutoff energy' (hereafter simply production cut) are two simulation parameters of particular importance to Monte Carlo models of electron transport. The tracking cut, T_{cut}, is the kinetic energy below which electrons (primary and secondary) are 'killed' and their residual kinetic energy is assumed to be deposited at the spot. The production cut, E_{prod}, is the kinetic energy above which secondary electrons are explicitly simulated. In practice, $E_{prod} \geqslant T_{cut}$ since it is 'expensive' to simulate the production of particles that will not be followed. All things being equal, the lower the T_{cut} and E_{prod} the longer the simulation time.

The spatial resolution of a Monte Carlo simulation essentially depends on the adopted T_{cut} (assuming $E_{prod} = T_{cut}$). This is not only because of the neglect of the finite penetration range of sub-threshold electrons, but also because of the different physics models which are used to transport electrons at the low- and high-energy regime (see below). Aside quantum mechanical uncertainties due to the wave-particle duality (coherent scattering), the lower the tracking (and production) cuts the higher the spatial resolution of the simulation. In the NRT context, it is clear that the calculation of the microscopic DER requires electron transport simulations down to much lower energies than the macroscopic DER. However, a major problem for low-energy electron transport is that the physics models that describe the interaction of sub-keV electrons with matter become increasingly more complicated and have a larger uncertainty margin [11]. Thus, applications where the tracking (and production) cuts must be set at low energies (below ~1 keV) present challenges that are *not* encountered in 'conventional' radiotherapy where electron transport is commonly terminated at the 1–100 keV energy range (depending on the problem).

Monte Carlo models of electron transport refer to the physics models used to describe the transfer of energy and momentum to matter. These models may refer to a single collision or to many collisions. In the former case we talk about single-scattering (cross-section) models, whereas in the latter case we talk about multiple-scattering models [10]. It suffices to distinguish between two types of electron interactions: elastic collisions with atomic nuclei which result in large momentum-transfer (q) but negligible energy-transfer (E), and inelastic collisions with atomic electrons which result in sizeable E but small q. Although elastic collisions play an important role in electron transport simulations since they are (mainly) responsible for the tortuous path of electrons in matter (with multiple elastic scattering models being the main source of uncertainty in high-energy Monte Carlo codes [12]), we will here limit our discussion to inelastic collisions associated with the various energy-loss processes which are directly relevant to radiation dosimetry. The corresponding Monte Carlo models are commonly classified as condensed-history (CH) or track-structure (TS) models.

5.4 Condensed-history models (class I code)

In CH models the electron track is divided into segments, called 'steps', sufficiently long compared to the mean free path, so that many interactions take place along each step. Thus, rather than simulating all interactions, the number of which is often prohibitively large, the net energy-loss and the net angular deflection (along with corrections for the longitudinal and lateral displacements) at the end of each step are calculated based on multiple-scattering models. According to Berger's classification [13], this method defines the class I codes. The ETRAN (Electron Transport) code developed at the National Institute of Standards and Technology (NIST) is a typical example of class I code [14]. The ETRAN code is essentially the electron transport engine in the well-known MCNP (Monte Carlo N-Particle) code developed (and maintained) at the Los Alamos National Laboratory (LANL). Although original a neutron code, the incorporation of ETRAN to MCNP version 4 in 1990, through the ITS (Integrated TIGER Series) code of the Sandia National Laboratory, opened up MCNP's application range to medical physics [15].

In CH models, the energy-loss is based on the concept of the stopping-power of the medium. The latter is formally defined from the *first moment* of the differential inelastic cross section, $d\sigma/dE$, as follows [16]

$$-\frac{dT}{dx} = NZ\int_0^{E_{\max}} E\frac{d\sigma}{dE}dE, \tag{5.6}$$

where T is the projectile kinetic energy, N is the number of atoms per unit volume, and Z is the atomic number of the medium. For electrons the upper integration limit in equation (5.1) is commonly set at $E_{\max} = \frac{1}{2}(T + B)$, where B is the binding energy of the target electron, or $E_{\max} = \frac{1}{2}T$ when $B \ll T$. The electron kinetic energy is $T = \frac{1}{2}mv^2$ where $v = c\beta = c\sqrt{\frac{T(T+2mc^2)}{(T+mc^2)^2}}$ with m being the electron rest mass and c the speed of light. Assuming that the projectile energy (T) remains approximately constant along the step length (s), the average energy-loss (Δ_{av}) along the step can be calculated from

$$\Delta_{\text{av}} = \left|\frac{dT}{dx}\right| s \tag{5.7}$$

The assumption of a constant T is justified when $\Delta_{\text{av}} \ll T$, i.e. when s is small compared to the range of the projectile. If, in addition, T is much larger than the mean excitation energy of the material (the so-called I-value), then equation (5.7) can be approximated by

$$\Delta_{\text{av}} = \left|\frac{dT}{dx}\right|_{\text{Bethe}} s, \tag{5.8}$$

where $(-\frac{dT}{dx})_{\text{Bethe}}$ is the celebrated Bethe stopping-power formula. Note that equation (5.8) does not apply at low energies (practically below ~1–10 keV for electrons) since the Bethe formula is valid only for $T \gg I$. The advantage of the approximation of equation (5.8) is that the Bethe stopping-power formula, $(-\frac{dT}{dx})_{\text{Bethe}}$, has a rather simple analytic form and can be calculated accurately (to the % level) for many materials, whereas the calculation of $(-\frac{dT}{dx})$ from the (generally unknown) inelastic cross section $d\sigma/dE$ through equation (5.6) is not always possible (or accurate enough). The use of either equation (5.7) or (5.8) is commonly referred to as the

continuous-slowing-down-approximation (CSDA). In this approximation, it is assumed that the energy-loss is dissipated in *continuous* manner along the track over many relatively closely-spaced inelastic collisions. The finite range of secondary electrons is entirely ignored (i.e. $E_{\text{prod}} = \infty$). The main advantage of adopting the CSDA in Monte Carlo simulations is that it significantly reduces the computational time. Unfortunately, the CSDA has proven to be inadequate for many dosimetry applications.

At the next level of sophistication one must take into account the stochastic variation (called ***straggling***) of energy-loss along the step. Then, the actual energy-loss (Δ) along the step must be determined by sampling an appropriate energy-loss straggling function, $F(\Delta, s)$. For sufficient long track-segments (but not too long, so that T can still be considered constant) the straggling function can be approximated (through the central limit theorem) by a Gaussian distribution [17]

$$F(\Delta T, s) = (\Omega\sqrt{2\pi})^{-1} \exp[-(\Delta - \Delta_{\text{av}})^2/(2\Omega^2)], \tag{5.9}$$

where $\Omega^2 = \langle(\Delta - \Delta_{\text{av}})^2\rangle$ is the variance of the energy-loss defined by the *second moment* of the differential inelastic scattering cross section

$$\Omega^2 = \left(NZ\int_0^{E_{\max}} E^2\frac{d\sigma}{dE}dE\right)s \tag{5.10}$$

If, in addition, the $d\sigma/dE$ is approximated by the Rutherford formula which ignores binding effects (the target electrons are assumed to be free and at rest), the variance is given by the simple Bohr expression

$$\Omega^2_{\text{Bohr}} = \xi\, s\, E_{\max}, \tag{5.11}$$

where $\xi = \frac{8\pi\, a_0^2 \text{Ry}^2 NZ}{mc^2\beta^2}$ with a_0 being the Bohr radius and Ry the Rydberg constant. The product $\xi\, s$ in equation (5.11) represents an approximate estimate of the average energy-loss along the step. In practice, the Gaussian distribution is applied when the condition $\kappa \gg 1$ (with $\kappa = \frac{\xi\, s}{E_{\max}}$) holds. For short track-segments (but long enough that $\xi\, s \gg I$) the Gaussian approximation to $F(\Delta, s)$ is not suitable since the most probable energy-loss (Δ_{prob}) differs from the average energy-loss, i.e. $\Delta_{\text{av}} \neq \Delta_{\text{prob}}$. In this case, $F(\Delta, s)$ may be computed from either the Landau or Vavilov distributions which exhibit a high-energy tail (being Poisson-like). The straggling function in the Landau model may be expressed in terms of a universal function of a single variable (λ) as [17]

$$F(\Delta, s)d\Delta = F_{\text{L}}(\lambda)d\lambda, \tag{5.12}$$

where $F_{\text{L}}(\lambda)$ is a tabulated function and

$$\lambda = \frac{\Delta}{\kappa} - \left\{\ln\left[\xi\frac{2mc^2\beta^2}{(1-\beta^2)I^2}\right] - \beta^2 + 1 - C - \delta\right\}, \tag{5.13}$$

with δ being the density effect correction and $C \approx 0.577$ (Euler's constant). The Landau distribution assumes $E_{\max} = \infty$. In the Vavilov distribution this restriction is removed by setting $E_{\max}$ equal to the maximum energy-transfer in a single collision. This provides a more accurate straggling distribution to the expense of losing the convenient analytic properties of the Landau function. The Vavilov distribution reduces to the Landau distribution for $\kappa \leqslant 0.01$ and to the Gaussian distribution for $\kappa \gg 1$.

It is important to highlight that to obtain a tractable form of the straggling function through any of the above models (Gaussian, Landau, Vavilov), the single-scattering inelastic cross section must be approximated by the Rutherford (or Thomson) formula [18]

$$\frac{d\sigma_{\mathrm{Ruth}}}{dE} = \frac{8\pi\, a_0^2 \mathrm{Ry}^2}{mc^2\beta^2}\frac{1}{E^2} \tag{5.14}$$

which assumes that the target electrons are unbound (and at rest). In this approximation, inelastic collisions lead to ionizations (excitations are neglected) and the energy-loss E in equation (5.14) is equivalent to the energy of the ejected electron. Therefore, strictly speaking, equation (5.14) is only valid for hard ionization collisions. To extend the applicability of these straggling functions to shorter track-segments or to lower energies, where soft collisions become dominant, the binding of target electrons has to be considered. However, the transition from the simple Rutherford-like single-scattering model to a more realistic inelastic cross section wipes out all the analytic properties underlying the above straggling functions. In practice, a useful approximation is the Blunck–Leisegang correction to the Landau distribution (its application to the Vavilov distribution is less practical). The Landau/Blunck–Leisegang straggling distribution is being used by ETRAN (and MCNP).

It is clear from the above discussion that the multiple-scattering models for the energy-loss are based on some severe simplifications (Rutherford model) to the *single-scattering* inelastic cross section. These simplifications, however, yield physics models which have a very simple material-dependence, e.g. through the mass density or the atomic number of the material, which is particular advantageous for Monte Carlo simulations. For example, the mean excitation energy (or I-value) in Bethe's stopping-power formula (and in the straggling distributions) is the only non-trivial material parameter, whereas the exact material-dependence of $d\sigma/dE$ is far more complicated and difficult to implement into a Monte Carlo code. This property makes CH models applicable to different transport media, thus, rendering them suitable for a wide range of applications.

One of the drawbacks of CH models (of class I) is that the spatial resolution is practically limited by the length of the step (s) which is typically in the macroscopic scale (~mm). Although, in principle, the step can be shortened to improve the spatial resolution, there is a limit to that since multiple-scattering models fail when the number of collisions to be grouped is small. For example, the multiple-scattering models of Landau and Vavilov fail for very short steps involving less than

~100 collisions (on average). In addition, they neglect the binding of electrons in the atoms which drive molecular aggregation and condensed-phase effects. For very short steps (plural-scattering regime), where soft-collisions dominate the energy-loss spectrum, binding effects cannot be ignored and a more realistic description of inelastic electron scattering is required [19].

In summary, by ignoring the fact that energy-loss takes place in discrete inelastic collisions, class I CH models cannot properly account for the microscopic spatial distribution of energy deposition in irradiated matter.

5.5 Mixed condensed-history models (class II codes)

For improving the spatial resolution, some CH models adopt a 'mixed' approach whereby 'soft' collisions are still treated by multiple-scattering models but 'hard' collisions (often termed 'catastrophic') are simulated individually by single-scattering cross sections. The reasoning behind the distinction of soft and hard collisions is that the latter may cause large angular deflections and/or energy losses which may have a strong impact on the particle trajectory [10]. This mixed approach to electron transport defines the class II codes according to Berge's classification [13]. The most used codes in medical physics applications are class II codes and include the EGS4 (Electron-Gamma-Shower version 4) code [20] developed at Stanford Linear Acceleration Center (SLAC), and later evolved to EGSnrc [21] at Canada's National Research Council (NRC), the Geant4 (Geometry And Tracking version 4) code [22–24] originally developed at CERN and presently maintained by an International Collaboration, and the PENELOPE (Penetration and Energy Loss of Positrons and Electrons) code [25] developed (and maintained) at the University of Barcelona. The FLUKA (Flukturiende Kaskade) code [26] developed (and maintained) by both CERN and INFN is also a class II code, but it is much less used in medical physics (apart perhaps from hadron therapy applications) compared to the above codes.

In class II codes, energetic secondary electrons (called δ-rays or knock-on electrons) liberated in hard inelastic collisions are followed along with the primary beam. The production cut (E_{prod}) separates the continuous ($E < E_{\text{prod}}$) from the discrete ($E > E_{\text{prod}}$) part of the energy-loss spectrum. Specifically, the contribution of the continuous energy-loss associated with soft inelastic collisions is calculated from a restricted stopping-power expression using the relation [6, 16]

$$\Delta_{\text{cont}} = \left|\frac{dT}{dx}\right|_{\text{soft}} s = \left(NZ\int_0^{E_{\text{prod}}} E\frac{d\sigma}{dE}dE\right) s. \qquad (5.15)$$

In contrast, the contribution of the discrete energy-loss associated with individual hard inelastic collisions (producing δ-rays) is determined by sampling the differential ionization cross section in the interval (E_{prod}, E_{max}]. A popular single-scattering model (e.g. used in EGS4) is based on the Møller formula [18]

$$\left.\frac{d\sigma_{\text{Moller}}}{dE}\right|_{E>E_{\text{prod}}} = \frac{8\pi\, a_0^2 \text{Ry}^2}{mc^2\beta^2}\left(\frac{1}{E^2} + \frac{1}{(T-E)^2} - \frac{1-b_0}{E(T-E)} + \frac{b_0}{T^2}\right), \tag{5.16}$$

with $b_0 = [T/(T + mc^2)]^2$. The Møller formula is a high-energy approximation obtained within the (relativistic) plane-wave Born approximation (PWBA). Similar to equation (5.14), it assumes that the target electrons are free (and at rest) so the energy-loss exactly equals the secondary electron energy. Thus, the Møller formula should be a good approximation only for the hard ionization collisions ($E_{\text{prod}} \gg B$) of high-energy electrons ($T \gg B$). Since $E_{\max} \approx \frac{1}{2}T$, δ-rays can be generated only when $T > 2 \times E_{\text{prod}}$. It is therefore important that the setting of E_{prod} is carefully considered. An important property of equation (5.16) is that, contrary to equation (5.14), it includes exchange effects in electron–electron scattering and, therefore, it is more accurate than the Rutherford formula for large E.

In the limit $E_{\text{prod}} \to 0$ a class II code simulates all inelastic collisions individually. In the opposite limit ($E_{\text{prod}} \to \infty$), a class II CH model becomes a class I CH model. In practice, (most) class I codes do not carry out 'pure' CH simulation because they consider δ-ray production through an expression similar to equation (5.16). The important difference is that, in class I codes, the energy-loss along the step is strictly calculated from a continuous model, that is, the δ-ray energy is not subtracted. Thus, straggling is considered over the entire energy-loss spectrum, from threshold to $E_{\max}$ (e.g. via the Landau, Vavilov, or Gaussian distributions). In contrast, energy-loss straggling in class II codes is accounted for *only* in hard collisions through the sampling of $d\sigma_{\text{ioniz}}/dE$ in the interval $(E_{\text{prod}}, E_{\max}]$. This means that electron transport in class II codes below E_{prod} is carried out in the CSDA. This may compromise the performance of class II codes as the incident electron energy approaches E_{prod} (this might be the case for electrons below, say, 100 keV).

The *correlation* of the energy-loss in soft and hard inelastic collisions is an important issue in CH simulations and underlines the essential distinction between class I and class II codes. Specifically, in class I codes (e.g. ETRAN/MCNP) this correlation is ignored by assuming that the primary electron remains unaffected by a δ-ray production, that is, the generation of δ-rays does not alter the energy or direction of the primary. As mentioned above, this approach has the advantage that it preserves straggling to the expense of occasional artifacts. In class II codes (e.g. EGS4), on the other hands, this correlation is explicitly considered to the expense of ignoring straggling for the soft collisions. The development of a 'restricted' straggling function associated with soft inelastic collisions remains a challenge for class II codes owing to the dominant role of binding effects which render any binary (Rutherford-like) model inappropriate.

5.6 The case of PENELOPE and Geant4

PENELOPE and Geant4 are class II codes that use a more sophisticated approach to calculate the energy-loss which allows them to simulate *all* inelastic collisions (both soft and hard) in a discrete manner by a suitable choice of the production cut.

PENELOPE treats inelastic collisions from first-principles within the PWBA whereby the double differential inelastic cross section is proportional to the generalized-oscillator-strength (GOS):

$$\frac{d^2\sigma_{\text{PWBA}}}{dEdq} \propto \frac{df(E, q)}{dE}, \tag{5.17}$$

with q being the momentum transfer and $df(E, q)/dE$ the GOS. To simplify calculations, PENELOPE adopts the Sternheimer–Liljequist (or 'δ-oscillator') model for the GOS which reads [27]

$$df_i(Q, E)/dE = N_i[\delta(E - E_i)\Theta(B_i - Q) + \delta(E - Q)\Theta(Q - B_i)], \tag{5.18}$$

where Θ is the Heaviside step function, E_i is the resonant energy of the ith transition, N_i is the number of electrons in the ith shell, and $Q = q^2/2m$ is the free-electron recoil energy. The resonant energies E_i are obtained by assuming that $E_i = a\ B_i$ with the parameter a being determined by the condition that the $df(E, q = 0)/dE$ yields the proper mean excitation energy (I) of the medium (note that I is defined through $df(E, q = 0)/dE$). In equation (5.18) the first term on the right-hand-side corresponds to soft collisions and the second term to hard collisions. It follows from equations (5.17) and (5.18) that the energy-loss spectra for soft and hard collisions are described by the following delta functions

$$\left.\frac{d\sigma_i}{dE}\right|_{\text{soft}} \propto N_i\ \delta(E - E_i), \tag{5.19}$$

and

$$\left.\frac{d\sigma_i}{dE}\right|_{\text{hard}} \propto N_i\ \delta(E - Q) \tag{5.20}$$

The main advantage of adopting an explicit model for the GOS is that it permits inelastic cross section calculations from first-principles. Thus, PENELOPE offers the capability of carrying out discrete simulation of inelastic collisions. Moreover, the particularly simple form of the Sternheimer–Liljequist GOS model yields analytic expression for all the physical quantities needed for mixed-CH simulation (e.g. hard inelastic cross section, restricted stopping power), including the soft-collision straggling parameter, Ω^2_{soft}, of equation (5.10). The latter enables PENELOPE to account for Gaussian straggling in soft inelastic collisions through equation (5.9), thus, setting it apart from other class II codes.

However, the collapse of inelastic cross sections to delta functions in the Sternheimer–Liljequist GOS model, see equations (5.19) and (5.20), has some important implications [28]. For example, equation (5.19) results in discrete energy values for the secondary electrons generated in soft collisions ($W = E_i - B_i$, with W being the kinetic energy of the secondary electron), that are unrealistic since they are not calculated according to the actual GOS of the material which has a continuous distribution. In addition, the hard collisions term of equation (5.20) is exactly equivalent to the Rutherford approximation where target electrons are free and at rest (exchange terms are added following the form of the Moller cross section formula). The Sternheimer–Liljequist GOS model used in PENELOPE yields collision stopping powers that are in good agreement with ICRU/NIST (available for electron energies above 1 keV) when the same *I*-value has been chosen for normalization of the GOS parameters. For liquid water and electron energies below a few hundred eV, the Sternheimer–Liljequist GOS model is known to overestimate the inelastic cross section (and stopping power) calculated from more elaborate models based on the dielectric response function which are used in some TS codes [28, 29].

The Geant4 code permits mixed CH simulation through its *low-energy* electromagnetic physics models which come in two flavors, namely, the 'Livermore' and the 'Penelope' models. The 'Penelope' models derive from a re-engineering of the PENELOPE code (version 2008). The 'Livermore' electron physics models are based on the EEDL (Evaluated Electron Data Library) and EADL (Evaluated Atomic Data Library) public data libraries which include information for the determination of cross sections and for the description of the final state of each physical interaction. Importantly, by taking into account the shell structure of atomic elements, they are able to account for binding effects and also simulate atomic de-excitation processes (such as fluorescence and Auger cascades). Depending on the production-cut, electron-impact ionization may be described by a continuous, discrete, or a mixed mode based on the Weizsacker–Williams model (as modified by Seltzer [30]). Specifically, for hard inelastic collisions, a binding-inclusive version of the Møller formula (equation (5.16)) is used

$$\left.\frac{d\sigma_i}{dE}\right|_{\text{hard}} = \frac{8\pi\, a_0^2 \mathrm{Ry}^2}{mc^2\beta^2} P_i N_i \left(\frac{1}{(W+B_i)^2} + \frac{1}{(T-W)^2} - \frac{1-b_0}{(W+B_i)(T-W)} + \frac{b_0}{T^2} + G_i\right), \tag{5.21}$$

where $E = W + B_i$ with W being the kinetic energy of the secondary electron liberated from a shell with binding energy B_i, $P_i = (\frac{T}{T + B_i + U_i})$ is the so-called 'focusing' (or accelerator) factor with U_i the average kinetic energy of the target electron at the ith shell, and G_i is a complicated function that results from averaging over an isotropic, hydrogenic distribution of orbital electron velocities. Note that the relation $W = E$ is assumed in the original Møller formula, equation (5.16), but not in equation (5.21). Therefore, equation (5.21) is expected to yield more realistic results at low incident energies than equation (5.16). For soft inelastic collisions a similar modification to the dipole part of the Weizsacker–Williams model is implemented

$$\left.\frac{d\sigma_i}{dE}\right|_{\text{soft}} = N_i\, I(W + B_i)\ \sigma_{\mathrm{PE}}(W + B_i), \tag{5.22}$$

with $\sigma_{PE}(W + B_i)$ the photoelectric cross section of the ith shell for an incident photon with energy $E = W + B_i$, and $I(W + B_i)$ is the virtual photon spectrum (which is given by a complicated expression that involves Bessel functions). Based on equations (5.21) and (5.22), Geant4 can simulate individual inelastic collisions in a discrete manner.

5.7 Role of condensed-history simulation in NRT

CH models are generally insensitive to materials structure and they have a simple material dependence. This greatly facilitates the application of class I and II codes to different transport media (they can practically handle any material composed of elements with $Z = 1 - 100$) and over a wide energy range (from keV to GeV energies). This is the underlying reason that makes these codes commonly referred to as *general-purpose* codes. Perhaps their most attractive feature in the context of NRT, is that a *single* code (of class I or II) can very efficiently simulate the transport of electrons (and photons) in both water and the high-Z atomic elements compromising the NPs. Many of these codes have become considerably user-friendly, can handle most geometries, and are publicly available, which further facilitates their application to emerging modalities (like NRT). On the other hand, one should be aware of the fact that the physics models used in class I and II codes have been developed for high-energy applications using physical approximations that require sufficiently large transport steps. As already discussed, this directly influences their spatial resolution. Furthermore, the physics models used in these codes do not account (or account only roughly) for binding effects in their ionization cross sections (while excitations are often neglected) which limits the accuracy with which the spectrum of secondary particles (mainly electrons but also photons) can be determined, which is a matter of high importance to NRT. Because of this deficiencies most class I or class II codes (e.g. MCNP, EGS4, FLUKA) terminate electron transport at 1 keV (or at 10 keV in older versions). The penetration range of 1 keV electrons in unit density water is some tens of nm which practically limits the dosimetric spatial resolution of these codes to hundreds of nm (depending on the required accuracy). Considering the additional limitations imposed by the step-size algorithms used in these codes, their overall spatial resolution is probably at the µm–mm level. In the context of NRT, this clearly renders class I and II codes unsuitable for calculating the microscopic DER, but makes them particularly effective for the macroscopic DER.

PENELOPE and Geant4 represent a special case of class II codes capable of simulating electron transport down to much lower energies. Specifically, PENELOPE permits discrete simulation down to 50 eV. Similarly, Geant4 permits discrete simulation of inelastic collisions down to the ionization potential of atomic elements. Therefore, these codes may be used (and have been used) for calculating the microscopic DER over sub-micron distances. However, the users of these codes should be aware that the discrete energy-loss models used in both codes pertain to *isolated* atoms. So, when these codes are applied to condensed-like media (like NPs or liquid water), their atomic cross sections are scaled (linearly) according to the mass density of the medium. This approximation is equivalent to the complete neglect of condensed-phase effects which are known to become important at sub-keV electron energies. Due to the above deficiencies, the often cited recommended tracking cut in PENELOPE is 100 eV (or higher) and in Geant4 (Livermore model) is 250 eV. Thus, simulation results by any of these two codes below a few hundred eV should be considered as semi-quantitative. The penetration range of a few hundred eV electrons in water is about ~10 nm which compromises the performance of these codes at the nanometer level.

It is noteworthy that recently some general-purpose Monte Carlo codes like MCNP (version 6) and PHITS (version 3.02) have extended their application range down to the nanoscale through the ad hoc implementation of TS models (along with their high-energy CH models).

5.8 Track-structure models

TS models aim to simulate all interactions (i.e. ionization, excitation, and elastic scattering) individually until the kinetic energy of the particles falls below the lowest excitation or ionization threshold of the material. Thus, in TS models $E_{prod} = T_{cut}$ with T_{cut} being in the eV scale (usually set at about 10 eV which is the ionization threshold in liquid water). Following Berger's classification, TS codes may be denoted as class III codes [31]. The principal advantage of TS models is that they provide a (near) complete description of the track, thus, offering a spatial resolution at the nanometer level (aside any quantum-mechanical uncertainties). On the other hand, such detail information is computer-intensive which makes the application of TS models at the clinical energy range impractical; with only few exceptions, TS models are commonly applied to electrons below a few hundred keV [10, 16].

TS models are conceptually simpler than CH models as they do not involve any 'artificial' parameters pertaining to the grouping of interactions which lead to step-size artifacts (i.e. the dependence of the results on the step-size). Moreover, within statistical uncertainties, the results of TS simulations are virtually exact, in the sense that they are identical to those that may be obtained from the exact solution of the transport equation with the same physics models. Although there is an obvious advantage of using TS models for calculating the microscopic DER, the transition from macroscopic (CH) to microscopic (TS) simulation is not always straightforward and requires much more detailed physics models than they are commonly available. For example, TS simulations require a large amount of input data in terms of integrated and differential cross sections for the individual collisions (elastic and inelastic). For the inelastic cross sections, in particular, they also require partial cross section corresponding to each ionization shell and excitation level. Unfortunately, many of these cross sections are not well-known, especially at low energies (<1 keV) where they become very sensitive to materials structure, composition, and density. It is therefore difficult to develop TS models that may be used reliably across the periodic table and at the different phases of matter (i.e. both in the gas and condensed-phase). As a result, TS codes are mostly specific-purpose codes and applicable to a single medium.

In the context of NRT, TS models must be available for at least two media, namely, in the NP itself and in the surrounding water medium. Note that NPs are not always composed of a single element, and water is not the only cellular target of interest at the nanoscale. So, eventually, TS models for different high-Z atoms and biological targets are needed in NRT. TS models are also particularly important if one aims to go beyond dosimetry and include radiobiological modeling which would require simulating also the chemical and biological stages of radiation action. Nevertheless, to a good approximation, TS models for just two-media (NP + water) may be adequate for many dosimetry studies (e.g. in calculating the microscopic DER). The main output of TS models is the cross sections for elastic and inelastic scattering, and the main differences between existing TS codes reside in these cross sections.

5.9 Track-structure models for water

The standard practice in NRT (and radiotherapy in general) is to report the DER in a water medium, since water represents on average ~70% (by weight) of living cells. Therefore, the availability of reliable interaction cross sections for water plays an important role. TS models for water have been used for over 40 years in micro-dosimetry and radiation biophysics, and more than a dozen TS codes have been reported in the literature [32], with the most widely known being NOREC (NIST—Oak Ridge Electron Code) [33] originally developed at the Oak Ridge National Laboratory (ORNL) and later improved at the National Institute of Standards and Technology (NIST), PARTRAC (Particle Track Code) [34] developed at the German Research Center for Environment and Health (GSF), and KURBUC (Kyushu University and Radiobiology Unit Code) [9], developed at UK's Medical Research Council and the Kyushu University in Japan (with important recent developments made at Karolinska Institute).

We can distinguish between two generations of TS models for water. In the **first generation**, TS models were based on water-vapor data which were (linearly) scaled to the density of the liquid phase (1 g cm^{-3}). The main motivation behind this so-called gas-phase approximation was the availability of *experimental* cross section data for water vapor. Data fitting has always been a popular approach for incorporating such data into the models. The general problem with data fitting is that almost always the data cover only a limited part of the parameter space, so there is a need for extrapolation and/or interpolation. For example, experimental cross section data are commonly obtained for only a small number of incident particle energies and, therefore, a method to extend them across the whole energy spectrum of interest must be adopted. To overcome this problem, theory-driven analytic representations of cross section data have been developed. It is generally accepted that experimental cross section data for water vapor have an uncertainty of about 10%–20%. Thus, an uncertainty margin of (at least) that level, also accompanies any theory- or data-driven parameterization.

Regarding the ionization cross section, which is the most important input, several models have been used in Monte Carlo codes. Perhaps the most known are the

Deutsch–Mark, Weizsacker–Williams, Kim–Rudd, and the Miller–Wilson–Manson models. The Deutsch–Mark model is based on Gryzinski's classical atomic collision formula but has the disadvantage that it is only applicable to the integrated ionization cross section. In contrast, the other three models (Weizsacker–Williams, Kim–Rudd, Miller–Wilson–Manson) permit calculation also of the differential ionization cross section which determines the energy distribution of secondary electrons. The starting point in all these models is the decomposition of the differential ionization cross section into a soft (distant) collision term and a hard (close) collision term as follows

$$\frac{d\sigma_i}{dE} = f_{\text{soft}} \frac{d\sigma_i}{dE}\bigg|_{\text{soft}} + f_{\text{hard}} \frac{d\sigma_i}{dE}\bigg|_{\text{hard}}, \tag{5.23}$$

where f_{soft} and f_{hard} represent (phenomenological) weighting factors that aim to produce the correct 'mixing' of soft and hard collisions. In principle, these weighting factors (f_{soft}, f_{hard}) are shell-specific, i.e. i-dependent. The exact description of $(d\sigma_i/dE)_{\text{soft}}$ and $(d\sigma_i/dE)_{\text{hard}}$ in equation (5.23) differs in the various models. In the Weizsacker–Williams model (as modified by Seltzer), it is assumed that $f_{\text{soft}} = f_{\text{hard}} = 1$ while $(d\sigma_i/dE)_{\text{soft}}$ is given by equation (5.22) and $(d\sigma_i/dE)_{\text{hard}}$ by equation (5.21). The Weizsacker–Williams model is used in the KURBUC*vap* code (the water-vapor version of the KURBUC code) [35] and also in the RETRACKS code [36]. In the Kim–Rudd model [37], on the other hand, the soft collision term is described by the leading term of Bethe's asymptotic expansion (the so-called dipole term), whereas the hard collision term by the Møller formula modified by the binary-encounter-approximation. The mixing coefficients f_{soft} and f_{hard} are not used explicitly, but they are built into the model (and obtained for each i) by requiring that the integrated ionization cross section and the stopping cross section agree asymptotically with the Bethe theory. The important outcome of the Weizsacker–Williams and Kim–Rudd models is that the secondary electron spectrum in ionization collisions can be calculated analytically, over a broad range of incident electron energies, through the T-dependence which is in-build to the $(d\sigma_i/dE)_{\text{soft}}$ and $(d\sigma_i/dE)_{\text{hard}}$ terms. Also, both models do not contain any fitted or adjustable parameters. Their main shortcoming is that the $(d\sigma_i/dE)_{\text{soft}}$ term requires as input the (ionization part of the) optical-oscillator-strength (OOS) (i.e. the GOS at $q = 0$). For most materials (including water), this information (which is not trivial) is most conveniently obtained from photoabsorption experiments taking advantage of the proportionality of the OOS to the photoelectric cross section, $\sigma_{\text{PE}}(E) \propto df(E, q = 0)/dE$. To bypass the problem of having to determine (by measurement or calculation) the OOS of each atomic or molecular shell, a simplified version of the Kim–Rudd model is available where the OOS is approximated by a simple analytic expression that corresponds to the ground state of hydrogen. In the literature, the original version of the Kim–Rudd model (with explicit knowledge of OOS) is known as the binary-encounter-dipole (BED) model, whereas its simplified version (with an approximate OOS) is referred to as the binary-encounter-Bethe (BEB) model. The BEB model is used in the latest version of the CPA100 code [38].

The inherent difficulty in calculating reliable mixing factors (f_{soft}, f_{hard}) has prompted the development of semi-empirical models. In the Miller–Wilson–Manson model [39] model one sets $f_{soft} = 1$ and determines $f_{hard} = f$ empirically through the expression:

$$f = \frac{\left(\frac{d\sigma_{\text{exp}}}{dE} - \frac{d\sigma_{\text{Bethe}}}{dE}\right)}{\left(\frac{d\sigma_{\text{BEA}}}{dE}\right)}. \tag{5.24}$$

The justification of equation (5.24) follows from Bethe's theory. According to this theory, at large incident energies T, the factor f can be considered independent of T. Then, from a set of experimental data of $(d\sigma/dE)_{\text{exp}}$ at certain T, equation (5.24) can be used to calculate f which may then be used at any other incident energy T. Although equation (5.24) has the advantage that the mixing factor f is deduced empirically, its main shortcoming is that the factor f cannot be considered independent of T for not too large T, thus, compromising the potential utility of the model at energies below ~1 keV. A form of the Miller–Wilson–Manson model is used in the MOCA code for water vapor (a precursor to PARTRAC). An empirical determination of f_{soft} and f_{hard} is also made in a model suggested by Rudd (which may be considered a precursor to the Kim–Rudd models). Rudd's electron model (there is also a version for heavy charged-particles) parameterizes the non-relativistic Møller formula (also called Mott inelastic cross section) after appropriate modifications so that it yields Bethe's asymptotic limit at high T. The empirical Rudd model is used in RETRACKS [36].

In summary, all the aforementioned models (Deutsch–Mark, Weizsacker–Williams, Kim–Rudd, Miller–Wilson–Manson) provide reliable analytic representations of the ionization cross section (integrated and/or differential) of atoms and molecules for intermediate- and high-energy electrons (above a few hundred eV). Their use in TS codes is often accompanied by data fitting at lower energies where the models are less reliable. Interestingly, the Kim–Rudd models (mostly the BED version) have shown to be reliable down to much lower energies, which have enhanced their popularity. It must be stressed that all the above models have been developed for atoms and molecules in the gas-phase.

The main criticism of the gas-phase approximation is that condensed-phase effects are generally non-linear, so density-scaled cross sections cannot reproduce faithfully electron transport in liquids or solids, especially at low energies. For example, the single-collision energy-loss spectrum changes drastically below 50 eV when water condenses from vapor to liquid (or solid), through the smearing and damping of discrete excitations and the emergence of collective (plasmon-like) excitations [9, 16]. These phase-effects directly influence the inelastic collisions of low-energy electrons (<100 eV). Perhaps less obvious is the fact that it also affects (to a smaller degree) higher energy electrons through their dipole interaction which is the origin of the different I-values in the stopping power of gaseous and liquid water. Therefore, the gas-phase approximation is less reliable (and its application must be discouraged) at the nanometer scale of condensed media where the interaction of low-energy electrons becomes critical.

The **second generation** of TS models for water employed interaction cross sections developed specifically for the liquid phase. In the absence of direct experimental cross section data, these TS models are mostly semi-theoretical. With respect to the calculation of inelastic cross sections the most established approach is based on the dielectric response function of the medium. The main advantage of this approach is that condensed-phase effects are built-in. The starting point of these calculations is the PWBA expression for the double differential cross section which in the non-relativistic limit (of most interest to TS models) reads [9, 16]:

$$\frac{d^2\sigma_{\text{PWBA}}}{dE\, dq} = \frac{1}{NZ}\frac{1}{\pi}\frac{1}{a_0 T}\frac{1}{q}\text{Im}\left[\frac{-1}{\varepsilon(E,\, q)}\right], \tag{5.25}$$

where $\varepsilon(E, q) = \varepsilon_1(E, q) + i\varepsilon_2(E, q)$ is the complex dielectric function and $\text{Im}[-1/\varepsilon(E, q)]$ the so-called energy loss function (ELF). The PWBA ignores exchange-correlation effects in e–e scattering. Thus, equation (5.25) describes the inelastic interaction between two opposite-spin electrons ($\sigma_{\text{PWBA}} \equiv \sigma_{\uparrow\downarrow}$). From equation (5.25) all quantities of interest related to inelastic scattering (e.g. integrated, single-differential, and stopping cross sections) can be calculated from appropriate integrations over q and/or E. Evidently, the practical use of equation (5.25) depends upon the availability of the dielectric function (or the ELF) over the entire range of E and q. The homogeneous electron gas is the only many-electron system where the dielectric function has been determined *analytically* under the random-phase approximation (RPA), yielding the celebrated Lindhard dielectric function. Unfortunately, calculating the dielectric function of real materials, such as liquids or amorphous solids, from first-principles is not feasible (even at the RPA level). At present, the development of semi-empirical dielectric functions that take advantage of experimental data at the optical limit ($q = 0$) and theory to extrapolate to finite momentum transfer ($q \neq 0$) seems to be the only viable approach. These so-called optical-data models of the dielectric function (or the ELF) have been quite successful in calculating reasonably accurate inelastic cross sections for sub-keV electrons in arbitrary solids and they are presently considered the state of the art [40].

Optical-data models are essentially formulated in terms of the Lindhard dielectric function of the homogeneous electron gas or its simplified plasmon-pole approximation. Extension to real materials is made by using a superposition of such functions to fit the available experimental data and treat the model parameters (transition energies, damping rates, oscillator strengths) as adjustable coefficients. The most popular optical-data models for calculating the ELF of an *arbitrary* solid are the Ritchie–Howie, Penn, and Ashley models. Yet another model is the MELF–GOS model. This model is recently receiving considerable attention owing to the improvements it offers over the earlier models by employing the Mermin dielectric function which allows lifetime broadening effects. For a review of the above models consult references [9, 16].

A problem with the above models is that their ELF cannot be directly partitioned to the various excitation and ionization channels, unless some 'outside' information (from experiments or *ab initio* calculations) is provided to the models. This partitioning is essential for simulating secondary electron cascade generation. Since the imaginary part of the dielectric function, $\varepsilon_2(E, q)$, describes single-electron excitations, the ELF is decomposed according to the expression

$$\mathrm{Im}\left[\frac{-1}{\varepsilon(E, q)}\right] = \sum_{k/n} \frac{\varepsilon_2^{(k/n)}(E, q)}{\varepsilon_1^2(E, q) + \varepsilon_2^2(E, q)}, \tag{5.26}$$

where the index k runs over all excitation levels and the index n runs over all ionization shells of liquid water. The denominator in equation (5.26), $|\varepsilon(E, q)|^2 = \varepsilon_1^2(E, q) + \varepsilon_2^2(E, q)$, represents the modifying effect of screening due to long-range polarization of the electronic subsystem of the medium. The real and imaginary parts of the dielectric function are not independent but they are related through the Kramers–Kronig (K–K) relations. The decomposition of ELF according to equation (5.26) permits the calculation of partial cross sections associated with the individual excitation levels (k) and ionization shells (n) by recasting equation (5.25) as follows

$$\frac{d^2\sigma_{\mathrm{PWBA}}^{(k/n)}}{dE\, dq} = \frac{1}{NZ}\frac{1}{\pi\, a_0 T}\frac{1}{q}\left\{\frac{\varepsilon_2^{(k/n)}(E, q)}{\varepsilon_1^2(E, q) + \varepsilon_2^2(E, q)}\right\}, \tag{5.27}$$

with

$$\frac{d^2\sigma_{\mathrm{PWBA}}}{dE\, dq} = \sum_{k}^{excit.} \frac{d^2\sigma_{\mathrm{PWBA}}^{(k)}}{dE\, dq} + \sum_{n}^{ioniz.} \frac{d^2\sigma_{\mathrm{PWBA}}^{(n)}}{dE\, dq}, \tag{5.28}$$

In principle equation (5.28) is all that is needed to perform discrete simulation of inelastic collisions. Its double integration (over q and E) allows us to sample the inelastic channel (ionization shell or excitation level), whereas its single integration (over q) allows us to sample the energy-loss and, for ionizations, the energy distribution of the ejected electrons.

In practice, for a model dielectric function to be useful, it must fulfill important sum rules and have a simple analytic form for arbitrary energy- and momentum-transfer. Currently, there are three major optical-data models of $\varepsilon(E, q)$ for liquid water that are suitable for use in TS models. The model developed by Ritchie and co-workers [41] at the Oak Ridge National Lab (ORNL); the model developed by Dingfelder and co-workers [42] at the German Research Center for Environment and Health (GSF), and the ECN model (Emfietzoglou–Cucinotta–Nikjoo) developed by Emfietzoglou and co-workers [43]. All the aforementioned models (ORNL, GSF, ECN) express the dielectric function of liquid water as a linear superposition of Drude-type functions (essentially equivalent to a gap-inclusive many-pole plasmon model)

$$\varepsilon(E, q) = 1 + \sum_{k/n} f_{k/n}(q) \frac{E_{\rm pl}^2}{E_{k/n}^2(q) - E^2 - iE\,\gamma_{k/n}(q)}, \tag{5.29}$$

where $E_{pl} = 4(\pi NZa_0^3)^{1/2}$ Ry is the nominal (volume or bulk) plasmon energy of the medium which depends upon its electron density. The models differ on the parameterization algorithm, the values of the Drude coefficients representing the strength ($f_{k/n}$), energy ($E_{k/n}$), and lifetime ($\hbar/\gamma_{k/n}$) of the individual transitions (k/n), and the extension to non-zero q through the dispersion relations $f_{k/n}(q)$, $E_{k/n}(q)$, and $\gamma_{k/n}(q)$. The optical limit of equation (5.29) mostly influences the inelastic cross section at high incident energies whereas its q-dependence is most important at low-medium energies. In total, five excitation levels (A^1B_1, B^1A_1, Ryd A+B, Ryd C+D, diffuse bands) and five outer-shell ionizations ($1b_1$, $3a_1$, $1b_2$, $2a_1$, and oxygen 1s) are considered in all three models (ORNL, GSF, ECN). The ORNL model also includes a plasmon excitation channel. The ORNL model is used in the NOREC code, the GSF model in the PARTRAC code, and the ECN model in the KURBUC*liq* code. The ORNL and GSF models use the same experimental optical data which cover a rather small portion of the excitation spectrum (up to 26 eV) of liquid water, neglect momentum-induced lifetime-broadening effects by setting $\gamma_{k/n}(q) = \gamma_{k/n}(0)$, and disperse the ionization energies by the impulse approximation $E_n(q) = E_n(0) + q^2/2m$. The ECN model is based on a more recent experimental data set which covers almost the entire excitation spectrum of the outer-shells of liquid water (up to ~150 eV) and extends to finite momentum transfer. An important feature of the ECN model is the inclusion, in a phenomenological manner, of exchange and correlation effects among the screening electrons, thus, going beyond RPA. This development, which introduces momentum-broadening and a departure from the impulse approximation, enables more accurate calculations of inelastic cross sections at sub-keV energies.

There are three main sources of uncertainty in optical-data models of the dielectric function [44]. The first concerns the source of optical data. In general, the available optical data span only a limited energy-loss range and different experimental techniques may exhibit sizeable discrepancies. Optical data are also not detailed enough, especially at small energy losses (0–20 eV) where the spectrum may be structure-rich [45–48]. The uncertainty in optical data is usually up to 20%–30%. This uncertainty mostly influences inelastic cross sections at high energies where forward scattering (where $q \approx 0$) dominates. A second source of uncertainty concerns the extrapolation of the optical data to finite momentum ($q \neq 0$). In general, this extrapolation is guided by the RPA dispersion relations of electron gas theory along with some known asymptotic limits. Such effects will mostly influence inelastic cross sections at low-medium energies where collisions with $q \neq 0$ (large-angle scattering) become dominant. The third source of uncertainty comes from the PWBA. This approximation neglects the exchange-correlation hole around the incident and struck electron which are important at low energies (below a few hundred eV). In TS simulations so far, only the exchange interaction between the incident and struck electron is considered in inelastic scattering. Calculations of inelastic cross sections that go beyond the two main approximations, namely, the RPA and PWBA, have been carried out recently by Emfietzoglou and co-workers [49, 50].

5.10 Track-structure codes for non-aqueous media

Monte Carlo models of keV electron scattering in solids are also of interest to materials analysis and characterization and, in particular, for interpreting and analyzing the signal from various experimental techniques used in the spectroscopy (e.g. electron energy-loss spectroscopy) and microscopy (e.g. scanning electron microscopy) of solids [51]. In these applications, the main interest is to quantify the fraction of primary electrons backscattered and/or transmitted, as well as the yield of secondary electron emission. The primary electron beam is commonly in the 10–100 keV energy range whereas the 'signal' electrons may have energies down to the eV scale. Thus, the tracking cut in these codes varies between 1–100 eV. The most common approach is to simulate elastic collisions in a discrete manner (i.e. using single-scattering cross sections) while calculating the energy-loss using a hybrid-CSDA scheme. The latter adopts a combination of continuous and discrete energy-loss models for the different inelastic channels by varying the production cut (in some ways resembling the mixed-CH models of inelastic collisions in class II codes).

A typical scheme is the following. The contribution of the outer-shells is calculated from a continuous energy-loss model through the following relation [52]

$$\left|\frac{dT}{dx}\right|_{\text{outer}} = \left|\frac{dT}{dx}\right|_{\text{Mod .Bethe}} - \left|\frac{dT}{dx}\right|_{\text{plasmon}} - \left|\frac{dT}{dx}\right|_{\text{inner}}, \tag{5.30}$$

where 'Mod. Bethe' denotes a modified Bethe formula. The use of the original Bethe stopping power formula in equation (5.30) is often avoided because it faces two fundamental problems, namely, it is not accurate for electrons below about 1–10 keV and it fails (becomes negative) for electron energies below $T < \frac{I}{1.166}$. So, it is fundamentally unsuited for electron transport down to the eV energy range of interest in these applications. Various modifications to the Bethe formula have been proposed (e.g. perhaps the most famous being the Joy–Luo empirical modification) and used successfully in equation (5.30). Alternatively, the outer-shell contribution in equation (5.30) is calculated directly within the PWBA using the dielectric function of the material

$$\left|\frac{dT}{dx}\right|_{\text{outer}} = \frac{1}{\pi\, a_0 T}\int E dE \int \frac{dq}{q} \text{Im}\left[\frac{-1}{\varepsilon(E,\, q)}\right], \tag{5.31}$$

where the q-integration is restricted to the single-electron continuum which extends over the interval $(q_c, q_{\max}]$ with $q_c = (2m)^{1/2}(E_F + E_{pl})^{1/2} - q_F$ (E_F the Fermi energy) being the critical momentum-transfer above which plasmons instantaneously decay (Landau damping) to single-electron excitations ($q > q_c$). The contribution of plasmon excitation is calculated from a discrete energy-loss model by sampling the single-differential inelastic cross section which is calculated within PWBA using the ELF approach

$$\left.\frac{d\sigma}{dE}\right|_{\text{plasmon}} = \frac{1}{NZ}\frac{1}{\pi\, a_0 T}\int \frac{dq}{q}\text{Im}\left[\frac{-1}{\varepsilon(E,\, q)}\right], \tag{5.32}$$

where the integration must now be restricted to the plasmon excitation range which extends over the interval $[q_{\min},\, q_c]$. The plasmon term in equation (5.30) is then given by

$$\left|\frac{dT}{dx}\right|_{\text{plasmon}} = NZ\int \frac{d\sigma_{\text{plasmon}}}{dE} E dE. \tag{5.33}$$

An important simplification is often made by assuming that plasmons are undamped (i.e. have infinite lifetime) and non-dispersive (i.e. are independent of q). Their inelastic mean free path (λ) is then given by the celebrated Quinn formula

$$\lambda_{pl}^{\text{Quinn}} = \frac{2a_0}{E_{pl}}T\left(\ln\frac{(P_{\text{F}}^2 + 2mE_{pl})^{1/2} - P_{\text{F}}}{P - (P^2 - 2mE_{pl})^{1/2}}\right)^{-1}, \tag{5.34}$$

with $P_{\text{F}} = (2mE_{\text{F}})^{1/2}$ and $P = (2mT)^{1/2}$. Under the above approximations, equation (5.33) simplifies to

$$\left|\frac{dT}{dx}\right|_{\text{plasmon}} = \frac{E_{pl}}{\lambda_{pl}^{\text{Quinn}}}. \tag{5.35}$$

Finally, the contribution of inner-shell ionizations is calculated from a discrete energy-loss model using single-scattering atomic ionization cross sections (e.g. the Gryzinski or Møller formula are often used)

$$\left.\frac{d\sigma}{dE}\right|_{\text{inner}} = \sum_{n}^{\text{ioniz}} \frac{d\sigma_n^{\text{atomic}}}{dE}, \tag{5.36}$$

with corresponding contribution to equation (5.30)

$$\left|\frac{dT}{dx}\right|_{\text{inner}} = \sum_n \left|\frac{dT}{dx}\right|_n = NZ\sum_n \int E\frac{d\sigma_n^{\text{ioniz}}}{dE}dE, \tag{5.37}$$

where the index n runs over those shells that are assumed to retain their atomic properties (e.g. the K, L, M shells). The contribution of each inner shell vanishes as the electron energy falls below the corresponding binding energy.

Although most of the Monte Carlo codes used in electron microscopy and spectroscopy (e.g. WinX [53], CASINO [54], MONSEL [55], NISTMonte [56]) cannot be strictly classified as TS codes, since they use both discrete and continuous energy-loss models, they have provided a great deal of validation of optical-data models of the dielectric function at sub-keV energies. An important development is the LEEPS (Low Energy Electron and Positron Simulation) code [31] developed at the University of Barcelona which employs TS models applicable down to 100 eV in a variety of solids based on inelastic cross sections from optical-data models. Inelastic cross sections are based on the PWBA (equation (5.25)) using an RPA dielectric function constructed from an optical-data model. Specifically, the LEEPS code adopts the Sternheimer–Liljequist GOS model (also used in PENELOPE) for the inner shells and a simple approximation to the Lindhard model for the outer-shells. In that sense, LEEPS may be considered as a more accurate low-energy extension of PENELOPE.

5.11 The case of TRAX and Geant4-DNA

The TRAX code [57] and the Geant4-DNA [58–60] low-energy package of Geant4 represent two codes of particular interest to NRT since they offer TS models for both water and (high-Z) NPs. With respect to NPs, TRAX uses the Kim-Rudd model for calculating ionization cross sections for each atomic shell with parameters pertaining to isolated atoms (gas-phase approximation). Solid-state effects are considered using the Quinn formula for bulk plasmon excitation (which neglects both plasmon damping and dispersion). For water, excitation and ionization cross sections in TRAX are based on parameterization of experimental data using the first-order term of Bethe's asymptotic expansion, $\sigma_{\mathrm{exc/ioniz}}(T) \propto AT^{-1}\ln(T/B)$ with A, B being empirical coefficients. Below a few hundred eV (where the Bethe asymptote is invalid) the experimental data are used directly. The energy deposition in inelastic collisions is set equal to the average excitation energy and the average binding energy which are also parameterized as a function of incident energy T using simple polynomials. The single-differential ionization cross section (or secondary electron spectrum) is assumed to follow the simple relation $d\sigma_{\mathrm{ioniz}}/dW \propto [1 + (W/C)^2]^{-1}$ with C being an empirical coefficient.

In the Geant4-DNA package several TS models are available for electron interactions. For gold NPs a relativistic form of BEB, called relativistic-binary-encounter-Bethe–Vriens (RBEBV) model along with the Quinn model for plasmon excitations have been implemented [61, 62]. More recently, the ELF approach was used to establish inelastic cross sections using the plasmon-pole approximation for the dielectric function based on optical data for solid gold [63]. For water the Geant4-DNA package includes three alternative TS models (which correspond to different cross sections for elastic and inelastic scattering), namely, the default model, the model developed at the University of Ioannina (hereafter the 'Ioannina' model), and the CPA100 model. The default model covers the electron incident energy range from a few eV to 1 MeV. Excitation and ionization cross sections (both integrated and differential) are calculated numerically within the PWBA using the dielectric function of equation (5.29) following the parameterization of [29]. Below a few hundred eV corrections to the PWBA are applied. For the K-shell (of the oxygen atom) total and differential cross sections for electron-impact ionization are calculated analytically from the binary-encounter-approximation-with-exchange model (BEAX) using atomic parameters. The Ioannina model [64, 65] is restricted to the low-energy range from 10 eV to 10 keV. It is based on the same general form of the dielectric function with the default model, but uses an improved algorithm for the partitioning of the ELF to the different excitation levels and ionization shells. The modified ELF of the Ioannina model yields improved low-energy inelastic cross sections. Finally, the CPA100 model [38] corresponds to a re-engineering of the CPA100 code initially developed by Terrissol and co-workers in the '80s (covering the 11 eV–250 keV energy range). It includes excitation cross sections calculated from the optical-data model of the dielectric function by Dingfelder and co-workers [42] and ionization cross sections calculated using a relativistic extension of the BEB model.

5.12 Surface effects

In limited media, when the electrons move towards the surface region (or interface between two different media), the probability of surface excitations gradually dominates over that of bulk excitations. Surface excitations take place at a small region near the surface (both from outside and inside the material) that typically extends up to a few nm. The probability of surface excitations is known to increase with decreasing distance from the surface, target thickness, and particle energy; thus, making them particularly relevant to low-energy electron interactions with nanostructures (including NPs). However, owing to the coupling between bulk and surface excitation modes that are orthogonal, the increased contribution of surface excitations to inelastic scattering in the near-surface region results in a reduction of the corresponding bulk contribution (the so-called Begrenzungs effect) [66]. This near-cancellation effect has sometimes been used as a justification for assuming a spatially-independent inelastic cross section (equal to the asymptotic bulk value) in limited media. In NRT, the presence of surface excitations has (at least) two obvious implications. First, outgoing electrons may excite surface modes even when outside the material. Thus, there is an additional energy-loss channel (associated with the NP) for electrons moving in the water medium in close vicinity to NP. Second, in metallic systems, surface excitations are associated with surface plasmons which exhibit a clear shift towards lower energy losses as compared to the bulk (or volume) plasmon. In planar (semi-infinite) geometries this shift is roughly by a factor of $\frac{1}{\sqrt{2}}$ [67]. Since plasmons are mainly decaying via single-electron excitations, the presence of surface plasmons further enhances the release of very low-energy electrons (typically below 10–20 eV) which, in turn, may significantly increase the energy deposition in the surrounding water medium within the first few nm from the NP.

To a first approximation, the energy-loss to surface excitations can be conveniently treated within the dielectric approach (described above), by taking advantage of the relation between the *surface* ELF (which describes the spectrum of surface excitations in planar geometries) and the *bulk* dielectric function of the medium, i.e. $ELF_{surface} = \mathrm{Im}[\frac{-1}{\varepsilon_{bulk}(E, q = 0) + 1}]$. For practical calculations, the above definition is often extended to $q \neq 0$ [68]. Thus, through the concept of the surface ELF, direct usage of optical-data models of the bulk material can be made, which facilitates the calculation of inelastic cross sections to surface excitation modes within the PWBA by an expression similar to equation (5.25). Other approximations specific to spherical geometries (relevant to NPs) have also been developed to make the calculations tractable [69].

5.13 Role of TS models in NRT

The main advantage of TS models compared to CH models is their high spatial resolution. Neglecting the possibility of coherent scattering effects at very low energies [70], TS models permit the simulation of electron transport collision-by-collision down to the eV scale with a resolution of the order of atomic (or molecular) dimensions. TS models are therefore ideally suited for calculating the microscopic dose enhancement and should be preferred over CH models when a spatial resolution down to 1–10 nm is sought for.

However, one should be aware of the limitations of such models. For example, TS models are generally considered to have an overall higher uncertainty compared to CH models. Within the validity range of the PWBA (for electrons above a few hundred eV) optical-data models of the dielectric function, when carefully implemented, may offer inelastic cross sections which, for liquid water in particular, are probably correct to within ~10%. At lower energies, especially below 50–100 eV, a larger uncertainty is expected (which is hard to quantify). Another issue of particular relevance to NRT is that TS models have a rather complex material dependence and, therefore, they are medium-specific. Moreover, since their application range extends down to very low energies, TS models are very sensitive to the phase of the medium (i.e. gas versus liquid/solid). All the above make the development of reliable TS models for different media a very time consuming effort. TRAX and Geant4 (via its Geant4-DNA extension) are two codes that offer TS models down to the eV scale in both water and NPs, which makes them very attractive for NRT. However, with the exception of the Geant4-DNA package, the physics models used in both TRAX and Geant4 pertain to isolated atoms and molecules (gas-phase approximation) which may compromise their performance at low electron energies and at the nanometer level.

5.14 Monte Carlo codes in NRT

In table 5.1 we present an overview of Monte Carlo models and codes that are available for electron transport (the list of codes is not exhaustive). Table 5.2

Table 5.1. Overview of Monte Carlo models and codes for electron transport (the list of codes is not exhaustive).

Monte Carlo model classification	Main physics input	Codes	Medium
CSDA	Stopping power; Elastic scattering cross sections	WinX, CASINO, MONSEL, NISTMonte	Elemental solids
Class I condensed-history	Energy-loss straggling function; Multiple elastic scattering theory	ETRAN, ITS, MCNP	All elements (and compounds)
Class II condensed-history	Restricted stopping power; δ-ray ionization cross section; Multiple elastic scattering theory	EGS, PENELOPE, Geant4, FLUKA, PHITS	All elements (and compounds)
Track structure	Interaction cross sections (elastic, excitation, ionization)	NOREC, PARTRAC, KURBUC, RE/RITRACKS, Geant4-DNA, TRAX, PHITS3.02	Water
		Geant4-DNA, RE/RITRACKS, TRAX, LEEPS	Selected media (including high-Z NP)
		MCNP6	All elements

summarizes the published work on Monte Carlo (nano/micro/macro) dosimetry for NRT using gold (Au) NPs, which are by far the most studied NP. The search is based on the SCOPUS database (as of August 14, 2017) using the keywords gold, nanoparticle, and Monte Carlo. For each of these papers, we have separately listed the Monte Carlo code used for radiation transport simulations in the AuNP and the surrounding biological medium (often approximated as liquid water). The frequency of each different Monte Carlo code (CH or TS) is depicted in figure 5.1. The Geant4 simulation toolkit has clearly been the most used Monte Carlo code for both AuNPs and water. The MCNP code comes second, followed by EGS and PENELOPE. From the roughly 30 papers that use Geant4 for their simulations, a small number (<5) have used it through the GATE or TOPAS software. Interestingly, only a relatively small numbers of studies (~10) have used a TS code, with Geant4-DNA being by far the most frequently used.

Table 5.2. Summary of published work on Monte Carlo codes for (nano/micro/macro) dosimetry in NRT using AuNPs. Search based on the SCOPUS database (as of August 14, 2017) using the keywords gold, nanoparticle, and Monte Carlo. For each paper we have separately listed the Monte Carlo code used for radiation transport simulations in the AuNP and the surrounding water medium.

Year	1st author	AuNP	WATER	Primary beam
2004	Schulte [71]	Geant4	Geant4	Proton
2005	Cho [72]	EGS and MCNP	EGS and MCNP	Photons
2009	Zhang [73]	Geant4	Geant4	Photons
2009	Cho [74]	EGS and MCNP	EGS and MCNP	Photons
2009	Montenegro [75]	Geant4	Geant4	Photons
2010	Cho [76]	MCNP	MCNP	Photons
2010	Van den Heuvel [77]	MCNP	MCNP	Photons
2010	Marques [78]	PENELOPE	PENELOPE	Photons
2010	Jones [79]	EGS	NOREC	Photons
2011	Leung [80]	Geant4	Geant4	Photons
2011	Lechtman [81]	PENELOPE and MCNP	PENELOPE and MCNP	Photons
2011	McMahon [82]	Geant4	Geant4-DNA	Photons
2011	McMahon [83]	Geant4	Geant4-DNA	Photons
2012	Mousavie [84]	MCNP	MCNP	Photons
2012	Chow [85]	Geant4	NOREC	Photons
2012	Toossi [86]	MCNP	MCNP	Photons
2012	Chow [87]	Geant4	Geant4	Electrons
2013	Ghorbani [88]	MCNP	MCNP	Photons
2013	Khadem-Abolfazli [89]	MCNP		Photons
2013	Tsiamas [90]	EGS and Geant4	Geant4	Photons
2013	Detappe [91]		EGS	Photons
2013	Mesbahi [92]	MCNP	MCNP	Photons
2013	Lechtman [93]	PENELOPE	PENELOPE	Photons
2013	Garnica-Garza [94]	PENELOPE	PENELOPE	Photons
2013	Douglass [95]	Geant4	Geant4-DNA	Photons
2013	Amato [96]	Geant4	Geant4	Photons
2013	Cai [97]	MCNP	MCNP	Photons
2013	Zygmanski [98]	Geant4	Geant4	Photons
2013	Amato [99]	Geant4	Geant4	Photons
2014	Li [100]	EGS and PENELOPE	EGS and PENELOPE and Geant4-DNA	Photons
2014	Ezzati [101]	MCNP	MCNP	Photons
2014	Tsiamas [102]	EGS	EGS	Photons
2014	Walzlein [57]	TRAX	TRAX	Protons, electrons
2014	Reynoso [103]	EGS and MCNP	EGS and MCNP	Photons
2014	Jeynes [104]	Geant4	Geant4	Protons
2014	Lin [105]	Geant4 (TOPAS)	Geant4-DNA (TOPAS)	Photons, protons
2015	Khosravi [106]	MCNP	MCNP	Photons

2015	Khosravi [107]	MCNP	MCNP	Photons
2015	Kakade [108]	EGS	EGS	Photons
2015	Asadi [109]	MCNP	MCNP	Photons
2015	Kirkby [110]	PENELOPE	PENELOPE	Photons
2015	Azorin-Vega [111]		PENELOPE	Electrons
2015	Shin [112]	Geant4	Geant4	Alpha
2015	Xie [113]	PARTRAC	PARTRAC	Photons
2015	Chow [114]	Geant4	NOREC	Photons
2015	Hao [115]		EGS	Photons
2015	Lin [116]	Geant4 (TOPAS)	Geant4 (TOPAS)	Protons, photons
2015	Zabihzadeh [117]	MCNP	MCNP	Photons
2015	Rakowski [118]	Geant4	Geant4	Photons
2015	Martinez-Rovira [119]	Geant4 (GATE)	Geant4-DNA (GATE)	Protons
2015	Spirou [120]	Geant4 (GATE)	Geant4 (GATE)	Photons
2015	Khadem-Abolfazli [121]	MCNP	MCNP	Photons
2016	Paro [122]	EGS	EGS	Photons
2016	Berbeco [123]		EGS	Photons
2016	Le Loirec [124]	PENELOPE	PENELOPE	Photons
2016	McNamara [125]	Geant4	Geant4	Photons
2016	McMahon [126]	Geant4	Geant4-DNA	Photons
2016	McQuaid [127]	Geant4	Geant4	Photons
2016	Koger [128]	PENELOPE	PENELOPE	Photons
2016	Dou [129]	EGS	EGS	Photons
2016	Cho [130]	Geant4 (TOPAS)	Geant4-DNA (TOPAS)	Protons
2016	Retif [131]	Geant4 (GATE)	Geant4 (GATE)	Photons
2016	Tran [132]	Geant4	Geant4-DNA	Protons
2016	Chow [133]	Geant4	Geant4	Photons, electrons
2016	Asadi [134]	MCNP	MCNP	Photons
2016	Yook [135]	MCNP	MCNP	Electrons
2016	Cho [136]	Geant4 (TOPAS)	Geant4 (TOPAS)	Protons, photons
2016	Belamri [137]	Geant4	Geant4	Protons
2016	Kwon [138]	Geant4	Geant4	Protons
2016	McKinnon [139]	Geant4	Geant4-DNA	Protons
2016	Koger [140]	PENELOPE	PENELOPE	Photons
2017	Martinov [141]	EGS	EGS	Photons
2017	Brivio [142]	MCNP	MCNP	Photons
2017	Byrne [143]	Geant4	Geant4	Photons
2017	Rezaei [144]	MCNP	MCNP	Photons
2017	Hwang [145]	MCNP	MCNP	Photons

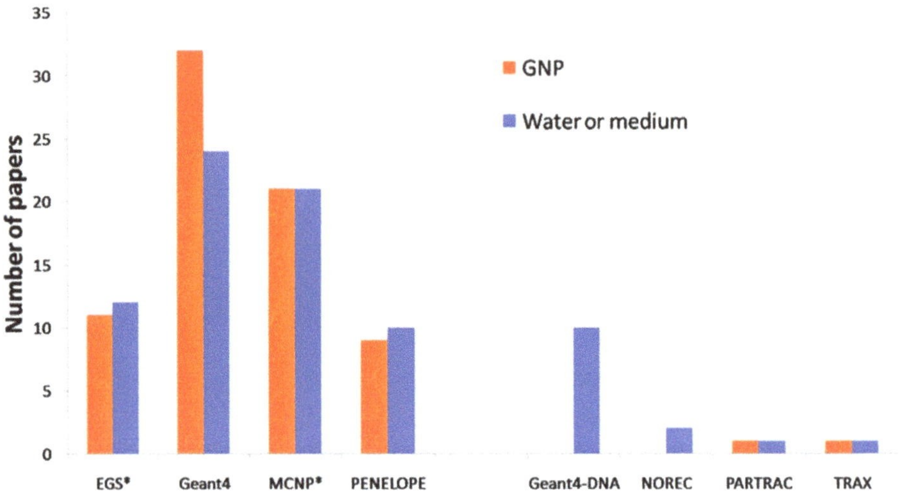

Figure 5.1. Number of papers using a particular Monte Carlo code for electron transport simulation in gold nanoparticles (GNP) (orange bar) and in the surrounding water medium (blue bar) as obtained from our search in the SCOPUS database (as of August 14, 2017) which is summarized in table 5.1. A small number of papers (<5) that use Geant4 through the GATE or TOPAS software are counted under Geant4. (*) Under EGS and MCNP we include all their different versions (e.g. EGSnrc is counted under EGS).

References

[1] Ngwa W, Kumar R, Sridhar S, Korideck H, Zygmanski P, Cormack R A, Berbeco R and Makrigiorgos G M 2014 Targeted radiotherapy with gold nanoparticles: current status and future perspectives *Nanomedicine* **9** 1063–82

[2] Zygmanski P and Sajo E 2016 Nanoscale radiation transport and clinical beam modeling for gold nanoparticle dose enhanced radiotherapy (GNPT) using X-rays *Br. J. Radiol.* **89** 20150200

[3] Jain S, Hirst D G and O'Sullivan J M 2012 Gold nanoparticles as novel agents for cancer therapy *Br. J. Radiol.* **85** 101–13

[4] Haume K, Rosa S, Grellet S, Śmiałek M A, Butterworth K T, Solov'yov A V, Prise K M, Golding J and Mason N J 2016 Gold nanoparticles for cancer radiotherapy: a review *Cancer Nanotechnol.* **7** 8

[5] Schuemann J, Berbeco R, Chithrani D B, Cho S H, Kumar R, McMahon S J, Sridhar S and Krishnan S 2016 Roadmap to clinical use of gold nanoparticles for radiation sensitization *Int. J. Radiat. Oncol. Biol. Phys.* **94** 189–205

[6] Retif P, Pinel S, Toussaint M, Frochot C, Chouikrat R, Bastogne T and Barberi-Heyob M 2015 Nanoparticles for radiation therapy enhancement: the key parameters *Theranostics* **5** 1030–45

[7] Detappe A *et al* 2016 Key clinical beam parameters for nanoparticle-mediated radiation dose amplification *Sci. Rep.* **6** 34040

[8] Chetty I J *et al* 2007 Report of the AAPM Task Group No. 105: Issues associated with clinical implementation of Monte Carlo-based photon and electron external beam treatment planning *Med. Phys.* **34** 4818–53

[9] Nikjoo H, Emfietzoglou D, Liamsuwan T, Taleei R, Liljequist D and Uehara S 2016 Radiation track, DNA damage and response—a review *Rep. Prog. Phys.* **79** 116601
[10] Salvat F and Fernández-Varea J M 2009 Overview of physical interaction models for photon and electron transport used in Monte Carlo codes *Metrologia* **46** S112
[11] Nikjoo H, Taleei R, Liamsuwan T, Liljequist D and Emfietzoglou D 2016 Perspectives in radiation biophysics: From radiation track structure simulation to mechanistic models of DNA damage and repair *Radiat. Phys. Chem.* **128** 3–10
[12] Kawrakow I and Bielajew A F 1998 On the condensed history technique for electron transport *Nucl. Instrum. Methods Phys. Res., Sect.* B **142** 253–80
[13] Berger M J 1963 Monte Carlo calculation of the penetration and diffusion of fast charged particles *Methods Comput. Phys.* **1** 135–215
[14] Seltzer S M 1991 Electron-photon Monte Carlo calculations: The ETRAN code *Int. J. Radiat. Appl. Instrum. Part* A **42** 917–41
[15] Goorley J T *et al* 2013 *Initial MCNP6 Release Overview - MCNP6 version 1.0, United States*
[16] Nikjoo H, Uehara S and Emfietzoglou D 2012 *Interaction of Radiation with Matter* (Boca Raton, FL: CRC Press)
[17] Berger M J, Coursey J, Zucker M and Chang J 1998 Stopping-power and range tables for electrons, protons, and helium ions *ICRU Report 49* (Gaithersburg, MD: NIST Physics Laboratory)
[18] Llovet X, Powell C J, Salvat F and Jablonski A 2014 Cross sections for inner-shell ionization by electron impact *J. Phys. Chem. Ref. Data* **43** 013102
[19] Nahum A E 1999 Condensed-history Monte-Carlo simulation for charged particles: what can it do for us? *Radiat. Environ. Biophys.* **38** 163–73
[20] Nelson W R, Hirayama H and Rogers D W 1985 EGS4 code system *Stanford Linear Accelerator Center, Menlo Park, CA (USA)*
[21] Kawrakow I, Mainegra-Hing E, Rogers D W O, Tessier F and Walters B R B 2017 The EGSnrc code system: Monte Carlo simulation of electron and photon transport *NRCC Report PIRS-701*
[22] Agostinelli S *et al* 2003 G4—a simulation toolkit *Nucl. Instrum. Methods Phys. Res., Sect.* A **506** 250–303
[23] Allison J *et al* 2006 Geant4 developments and applications *IEEE Trans. Nucl. Sci.* **53** 270–8
[24] Allison J *et al* 2016 Recent developments in Geant4 *Nucl. Instrum. Methods Phys. Res., Sect.* A **835** 186–225
[25] Salvat F, Fernández-Varea J M and Sempau J 2009 PENELOPE-2008: A code system for Monte Carlo simulation of electron and photon transport, in: OECD-NEA (Ed.) the Workshop Proc. June, OECD-NEA, Issy-les-Moulineaux, France
[26] Ferrari A, Sala P R and Fasso A 2005 *J. Ranft, FLUKA: A multi-particle transport code (Program version 2005)*
[27] Liljequist D 1985 Simple generalized oscillator strength density model applied to the simulation of keV electron-energy-loss distributions *J. Appl. Phys.* **57** 657–65
[28] Fernández-Varea J M, González-Muñoz G, Galassi M E, Wiklund K, Lind B K, Ahnesjö A and Tilly N 2012 Limitations (and merits) of PENELOPE as a track-structure code *Int. J. Radiat. Biol.* **88** 66–70
[29] Emfietzoglou D 2003 Inelastic cross-sections for electron transport in liquid water: a comparison of dielectric models *Radiat. Phys. Chem.* **66** 373–85

[30] Seltzer S M 1988 Cross sections for bremsstrahlung production and electron-impact ionization *Monte Carlo Transport of Electrons and Photons* ed T M Jenkins, W R Nelson and A Rindi (Boston, MA: Springer) pp 81–114

[31] Fernández-Varea J M 1998 Monte Carlo simulation of the inelastic scattering of electrons and positrons using optical-data models *Radiat. Phys. Chem.* **53** 235–45

[32] Nikjoo H, Uehara S, Emfietzoglou D and Cucinotta F 2006 Track-structure codes in radiation research *Radiat. Meas.* **41** 1052–74

[33] Semenenko V A, Turner J E and Borak T B 2003 NOREC, a Monte Carlo code for simulating electron tracks in liquid water *Radiat. Environ. Biophys.* **42** 213–7

[34] Friedland W, Dingfelder M, Kundrát P and Jacob P 2011 Track structures, DNA targets and radiation effects in the biophysical Monte Carlo simulation code PARTRAC *Mutat. Res.* **711** 28–40

[35] Uehara S, Nikjoo H and Goodhead D T 1993 Cross-sections for water vapour for the Monte Carlo electron track structure code from 10 eV to the MeV region *Phys. Med. Biol.* **38** 1841–58

[36] Plante I and Cucinotta F A 2009 Cross sections for the interactions of 1 eV–100 MeV electrons in liquid water and application to Monte-Carlo simulation of HZE radiation tracks *New J. Phys.* **11** 063047

[37] Kim Y-K and Rudd M E 1994 Binary-encounter-dipole model for electron-impact ionization *Phys. Rev.* A **50** 3954–67

[38] Bordage M C, Bordes J, Edel S, Terrissol M, Franceries X, Bardiès M, Lampe N and Incerti S 2016 Implementation of new physics models for low energy electrons in liquid water in Geant4-DNA *Phys. Med.* **32** 1833–40

[39] Miller J, Wilson W and Manson S 1985 Secondary electron spectra: a semi-empirical model *Radiat. Prot. Dosim.* **13** 27–30

[40] Emfietzoglou D, Kyriakou I, Abril I, Garcia-Molina R and Nikjoo H 2012 Inelastic scattering of low-energy electrons in liquid water computed from optical-data models of the Bethe surface *Int. J. Radiat. Biol.* **88** 22–8

[41] Ritchie R H, Hamm R N, Turner J E, Wright H A and Bolch W E 1991 Radiation interactions and energy transport in the condensed phase *Physical and Chemical Mechanisms in Molecular Radiation Biology* ed W A Glass and M N Varma (Boston, MA: Springer) pp 99–135

[42] Dingfelder M, Hantke D, Inokuti M and Paretzke H G 1999 Electron inelastic-scattering cross sections in liquid water *Radiat. Phys. Chem.* **53** 1–18

[43] Emfietzoglou D, Cucinotta F A and Nikjoo H 2005 A complete dielectric response model for liquid water: a solution of the Bethe Ridge problem *Radiat. Res.* **164** 202–11

[44] Emfietzoglou D, Kyriakou I, Garcia-Molina R and Abril I 2017 Inelastic mean free path of low-energy electrons in condensed media: beyond the standard models *Surf. Interface Anal.* **49** 4–10

[45] Chantler C T and Bourke J D 2014 Electron inelastic mean free path theory and density functional theory resolving discrepancies for low-energy electrons in copper *J. Phys. Chem.* A **118** 909–14

[46] Heller J M, Hamm R N, Birkhoff R D and Painter L R 1974 Collective oscillation in liquid water *J. Chem. Phys.* **60** 3483–6

[47] Hayashi H, Watanabe N, Udagawa Y and Kao C-C 2000 The complete optical spectrum of liquid water measured by inelastic x-ray scattering *Proc. Natl Acad. Sci.* **97** 6264–6

[48] Hayashi H and Hiraoka N 2015 Accurate measurements of dielectric and optical functions of liquid water and liquid benzene in the VUV region (1–100 eV) using small-angle inelastic x-ray scattering *J. Phys. Chem.* B **119** 5609–23
[49] Emfietzoglou D, Kyriakou I, Garcia-Molina R and Abril I 2013 The effect of static many-body local-field corrections to inelastic electron scattering in condensed media *J. Appl. Phys.* **114** 144907
[50] Emfietzoglou D, Kyriakou I, Garcia-Molina R, Abril I and Nikjoo H 2013 Inelastic cross sections for low-energy electrons in liquid water: exchange and correlation effects *Radiat. Res.* **180** 499–513
[51] Dapor M 2014 *Transport of Energetic Electrons in SolidsSpringer Tracts in Modern Physics* vol 257 (Berlin: Springer) p 81
[52] Shimizu R and Ze-Jun D 1992 Monte Carlo modelling of electron-solid interactions *Rep. Prog. Phys.* **55** 487–531
[53] Gauvin R, Lifshin E, Demers H, Horny P and Campbell H 2005 Win x-ray: A new Monte Carlo program that computes x-ray spectra obtained with a scanning electron microscope *Microsc. Microanal.* **12** 49–64
[54] Hovington P, Drouin D and Gauvin R 1997 CASINO: A new Monte Carlo code in C language for electron beam interaction —part I: Description of the program *Scanning* **19** 1–14
[55] Lowney J R 1996 Monte Carlo simulation of scanning electron microscope signals for lithographic metrology *Scanning* **18** 301–6
[56] Ritchie N W M 2005 A new Monte Carlo application for complex sample geometries *Surf. Interface Anal.* **37** 1006–11
[57] Wälzlein C, Scifoni E, Krämer M and Durante M 2014 Simulations of dose enhancement for heavy atom nanoparticles irradiated by protons *Phys. Med. Biol.* **59** 1441–58
[58] Incerti S *et al* 2010 The Geant4-DNA project *Int. J. Model. Simul. Sci. Comput.* **01** 157–78
[59] Bernal M A *et al* 2015 Track structure modeling in liquid water: a review of the Geant4-DNA very low energy extension of the Geant4 Monte Carlo simulation toolkit *Phys. Med.* **31** 861–74
[60] Incerti S *et al* 2018 Geant4-DNA example applications for track structure simulations in liquid water: a report from the Geant4-DNA project *Med. Phys.* **45** 722–39
[61] Sakata D *et al* 2016 An implementation of discrete electron transport models for gold in the Geant4 simulation toolkit *J. Appl. Phys.* **120** 244901
[62] Sakata D *et al* 2018 Geant4-DNA for track-structure simulations for gold nanoparticles: the importance of electron discrete models in nanometer volumes *Med. Phys.* **45** 2230–42
[63] Sakata D, Kyriakou I, Tran H N, Bordage M C, Rosenfeld A, Ivanchenko V, Incert S, Emfietzoglou D and Guatelli S 2019 Electron track structure simulations in a gold nanoparticle using Geant4-DNA *Phys. Med.* **63** 98–104
[64] Kyriakou I, Incerti S and Francis Z 2015 Technical note: improvements in GEANT4 energy-loss model and the effect on low-energy electron transport in liquid water *Med. Phys.* **42** 3870–6
[65] Kyriakou I, Šefl M, Nourry V and Incerti S 2016 The impact of new Geant4-DNA cross section models on electron track structure simulations in liquid water *J. Appl. Phys.* **119** 194902
[66] Salvat-Pujol F and Werner W S M 2013 Surface excitations in electron spectroscopy. Part I: dielectric formalism and Monte Carlo algorithm *Surf. Interface Anal* **45** 873–94
[67] Ritchie R H 1957 Plasma losses by fast electrons in thin films *Phys. Rev.* **106** 874–81

[68] Kyriakou I, Emfietzoglou D, Garcia-Molina R, Abril I and Kostarelos K 2011 Simple model of bulk and surface excitation effects to inelastic scattering in low-energy electron beam irradiation of multi-walled carbon nanotubes *J. Appl. Phys.* **110** 054304
[69] Verkhovtsev A, McKinnon S, de Vera P, Surdutovich E, Guatelli S, Korol A V, Rosenfeld A and Solov'yov A V 2015 Comparative analysis of the secondary electron yield from carbon nanoparticles and pure water medium *Eur. Phys. J.* D **69** 116
[70] Thomson R M and Kawrakow I 2011 On the Monte Carlo simulation of electron transport in the sub-1 keV energy range *Med. Phys.* **38** 4531–4
[71] Schulte R, Bashkirov V, Li T, Liang Z, Sadrozinski H F W and Williams D C 2004 Nanoparticle-enhanced proton computed tomography: a Monte Carlo simulation study *2nd IEEE Int. Symp. on Biomedical Imaging: Macro to Nano* 1354–6
[72] Cho S H 2005 Estimation of tumour dose enhancement due to gold nanoparticles during typical radiation treatments: a preliminary Monte Carlo study *Phys. Med. Biol.* **50** N163–73
[73] Zhang S X, Gao J, Buchholz T A, Wang Z, Salehpour M R, Drezek R A and Yu T-K 2009 Quantifying tumor-selective radiation dose enhancements using gold nanoparticles: a Monte Carlo simulation study *Biomed. Microdevices* **11** 925–33
[74] Cho S H, Jones B L and Krishnan S 2009 The dosimetric feasibility of gold nanoparticle-aided radiation therapy (GNRT) via brachytherapy using low-energy gamma-/x-ray sources *Phys. Med. Biol.* **54** 4889–905
[75] Montenegro M, Nahar S N, Pradhan A K, Huang K and Yu Y 2009 Monte Carlo simulations and atomic calculations for auger processes in biomedical nanotheranostics *J. Phys. Chem.* A **113** 12364–9
[76] Cho S, Jeong J H, Kim C H and Yoon M 2010 Monte Carlo simulation study on dose enhancement by gold nanoparticles in brachytherapy *J. Korean Phys. Soc.* **56** 1754–8
[77] Van den Heuvel F, Locquet J-P and Nuyts S 2010 Beam energy considerations for gold nano-particle enhanced radiation treatment *Phys. Med. Biol.* **55** 4509–20
[78] Marques T, Schwarcke M, Garrido C, Zucolot V, Baffa O and Nicolucci P 2010 Gel dosimetry analysis of gold nanoparticle application in kilovoltage radiation therapy *J. Phys. Conf. Ser.* **250** 012084
[79] Jones B L, Krishnan S and Cho S H 2010 Estimation of microscopic dose enhancement factor around gold nanoparticles by Monte Carlo calculations *Med. Phys.* **37** 3809–16
[80] Leung M K K, Chow J C L, Chithrani B D, Lee M J G, Oms B and Jaffray D A 2011 Irradiation of gold nanoparticles by x-rays: Monte Carlo simulation of dose enhancements and the spatial properties of the secondary electrons production *Med. Phys.* **38** 624–31
[81] Lechtman E, Chattopadhyay N, Cai Z, Mashouf S, Reilly R and Pignol J P 2011 Implications on clinical scenario of gold nanoparticle radiosensitization in regards to photon energy, nanoparticle size, concentration and location *Phys. Med. Biol.* **56** 4631–47
[82] McMahon S J *et al* 2011 Biological consequences of nanoscale energy deposition near irradiated heavy atom nanoparticles *Sci. Rep.* **1** 18
[83] McMahon S J *et al* 2011 Nanodosimetric effects of gold nanoparticles in megavoltage radiation therapy *Radiother. Oncol.* **100** 412–6
[84] Mousavie Anijdan S H, Shirazi A, Mahdavi S R, Ezzati A, Mofid B, Khoei S and Zarrinfard M A 2012 Megavoltage dose enhancement of gold nanoparticles for different geometric set-ups: Measurements and Monte Carlo simulation *Iran. J. Radiat. Res.* **10** 183–6

[85] Chow J C L, Leung M K K, Fahey S, Chithrani D B and Jaffray D A 2012 Monte Carlo simulation on low-energy electrons from gold nanoparticle in radiotherapy *J. Phys. Conf. Ser.* **341** 012012

[86] Bahreyni Toossi M T, Ghorbani M, Mehrpouyan M, Akbari F, Sobhkhiz Sabet L and Soleimani Meigooni A 2012 A Monte Carlo study on tissue dose enhancement in brachytherapy: a comparison between gadolinium and gold nanoparticles *Australas. Phys. Eng. Sci. Med.* **35** 177–85

[87] Chow J C L, Leung M K K and Jaffray D A 2012 Monte Carlo simulation on a gold nanoparticle irradiated by electron beams *Phys. Med. Biol.* **57** 3323–31

[88] Ghorbani M, Bakhshabadi M, Golshan A and Knaup C 2013 Dose enhancement by various nanoparticles in prostate brachytherapy *Australas. Phys. Eng. Sci. Med.* **36** 431–40

[89] Khadem-Abolfazli M, Mahdavi M, Mahdavi S R M and Ataei G 2013 Dose enhancement effect of gold nanoparticles on MAGICA polymer gel in mega voltage radiation therapy *Int. J. Radiat. Res.* **11** 55–61

[90] Tsiamas P *et al* 2013 Impact of beam quality on megavoltage radiotherapy treatment techniques utilizing gold nanoparticles for dose enhancement *Phys. Med. Biol.* **58** 451–64

[91] Detappe A, Tsiamas P, Ngwa W, Zygmanski P, Makrigiorgos M and Berbeco R 2013 The effect of flattening filter free delivery on endothelial dose enhancement with gold nanoparticles *Med. Phys.* **29** e1–e46

[92] Mesbahi A, Jamali F and Garehaghaji N 2013 Effect of photon beam energy, gold nanoparticle size and concentration on the dose enhancement in radiation therapy *Bioimpacts* **3** 29–35

[93] Lechtman E, Mashouf S, Chattopadhyay N, Keller B M, Lai P, Cai Z, Reilly R M and Pignol J P 2013 A Monte Carlo-based model of gold nanoparticle radiosensitization accounting for increased radiobiological effectiveness *Phys. Med. Biol.* **58** 3075–87

[94] Garnica-Garza H M 2013 Microdosimetry of x-ray-irradiated gold nanoparticles *Radiat. Prot. Dosim.* **155** 59–63

[95] Douglass M, Bezak E and Penfold S 2013 Monte Carlo investigation of the increased radiation deposition due to gold nanoparticles using kilovoltage and megavoltage photons in a 3D randomized cell model *Med. Phys.* **40** 0717101–9

[96] Amato E, Italiano A, Leotta S, Pergolizzi S and Torrisi L 2013 Monte Carlo study of the dose enhancement effect of gold nanoparticles during x-ray therapies and evaluation of the anti-angiogenic effect on tumour capillary vessels *J. X-Ray Sci. Technol.* **21** 237–47

[97] Cai Z, Pignol J-P, Chattopadhyay N, Kwon Y L, Lechtman E and Reilly R M 2013 Investigation of the effects of cell model and subcellular location of gold nanoparticles on nuclear dose enhancement factors using Monte Carlo simulation *Med. Phys.* **40** 1141011–8

[98] Zygmanski P, Liu B, Tsiamas P, Cifter F, Petersheim M, Hesser J and Sajo E 2013 Dependence of Monte Carlo microdosimetric computations on the simulation geometry of gold nanoparticles *Phys. Med. Biol.* **58** 7961–77

[99] Amato E, Italiano A and Pergolizzi S 2013 Gold nanoparticles as a sensitising agent in external beam radiotherapy and brachytherapy: A feasibility study through Monte Carlo simulation *Int. J. Nanotechnol.* **10** 1045–54

[100] Li W B, Müllner M, Greiter M B, Bissardon C, Xie W Z, Schlatll H, Oeh U, Li J L and Hoeschen C 2014 Monte Carlo simulations of dose enhancement around gold nanoparticles used as x-ray imaging contrast agents and radiosensitizers *Proc. SPIE* 90331K

[101] Ezzati A O, Mahdavi S R and Anijdan H M 2014 Size effects of gold and iron nanoparticles on radiation dose enhancement in brachytherapy and teletherapy: a Monte Carlo study *Iran. J. Med. Phys.* **11** 253–9
[102] Tsiamas P, Mishra P, Cifter F, Berbeco R I, Marcus K, Sajo E and Zygmanski P 2014 Low-Z linac targets for low-MV gold nanoparticle radiation therapy *Med. Phys.* **41** 021701
[103] Reynoso F J, Manohar N, Krishnan S and Cho S H 2014 Design of an Yb-169 source optimized for gold nanoparticle-aided radiation therapy *Med. Phys.* **41** 1017091–9
[104] Jeynes J C G, Merchant M J, Spindler A, Wera A C and Kirkby K J 2014 Investigation of gold nanoparticle radiosensitization mechanisms using a free radical scavenger and protons of different energies *Phys. Med. Biol.* **59** 6431–44
[105] Lin Y, McMahon S J, Scarpelli M, Paganetti H and Schuemann J 2014 Comparing gold nano-particle enhanced radiotherapy with protons, megavoltage photons and kilovoltage photons: a Monte Carlo simulation *Phys. Med. Biol.* **59** 7675–89
[106] Khosravi H, Hashemi B, Mahdavi S R and Hejazi P 2015 Effect of gold nanoparticles on prostate dose distribution under Ir-192 internal and 18 MV external radiotherapy procedures using gel dosimetry and monte carlo method *J. Biomed. Phys. Eng.* **5** 3–14
[107] Khosravi H, Hashemi B, Mahdavi S R and Hejazi P 2015 Target dose enhancement factor alterations related to interaction between the photon beam energy and gold nanoparticles' size in external radiotherapy: using Monte Carlo method *Koomesh* **17** 255–61
[108] Kakade N and Sharma S 2015 Dose enhancement in gold nanoparticle-aided radiotherapy for the therapeutic photon beams using Monte Carlo technique *J. Cancer Res. Ther.* **11** 94–7
[109] Asadi S, Vaez-zadeh M, Masoudi S F, Rahmani F, Knaup C and Meigooni A S 2015 Gold nanoparticle-based brachytherapy enhancement in choroidal melanoma using a full Monte Carlo model of the human eye *J. Appl. Clin. Med. Phys.* **16** 344–57
[110] Kirkby C and Ghasroddashti E 2015 Targeting mitochondria in cancer cells using gold nanoparticle-enhanced radiotherapy: a Monte Carlo study *Med. Phys.* **42** 1119–28
[111] Azorín-Vega E P, Zambrano-Ramírez O D, Rojas-Calderón E L, Ocampo-García B E and Ferro-Flores G 2015 Tumoral fibrosis effect on the radiation absorbed dose of 177Lu–Tyr3-octreotate and 177Lu–Tyr3-octreotate conjugated to gold nanoparticles *Appl. Radiat. Isot.* **100** 96–100
[112] Shin J I *et al* 2015 Simulation study of dose enhancement in a cell due to nearby carbon and oxygen in particle radiotherapy *J. Korean Phys. Soc.* **67** 209–17
[113] Xie W Z, Friedland W, Li W B, Li C Y, Oeh U, Qiu R, Li J L and Hoeschen C 2015 Simulation on the molecular radiosensitization effect of gold nanoparticles in cells irradiated by x-rays *Phys. Med. Biol.* **60** 6195–213
[114] Chow J C L 2015 Characteristics of secondary electrons from irradiated gold nanoparticle in radiotherapy *Handbook of Nanoparticles* ed M Aliofkhazraei (Cham: Springer) pp 1–18
[115] Hao Y, Altundal Y, Moreau M, Sajo E, Kumar R and Ngwa W 2015 Potential for enhancing external beam radiotherapy for lung cancer using high-Z nanoparticles administered via inhalation *Phys. Med. Biol.* **60** 7035–44
[116] Lin Y, Paganetti H, McMahon S J and Schuemann J 2015 Gold nanoparticle induced vasculature damage in radiotherapy: comparing protons, megavoltage photons, and kilovoltage photons *Med. Phys.* **42** 5890–902
[117] Zabihzadeh M and Arefian S 2015 Tumor dose enhancement by nanoparticles during high dose rate 192 Ir brachytherapy *J. Cancer Res. Ther.* **11** 752–9

[118] Rakowski J T, Laha S S, Snyder M G, Buczek M G, Tucker M A, Liu F, Mao G, Hillman Y and Lawes G 2015 Measurement of gold nanofilm dose enhancement using unlaminated radiochromic film *Med. Phys.* **42** 5937–44

[119] Martínez-Rovira I and Prezado Y 2015 Evaluation of the local dose enhancement in the combination of proton therapy and nanoparticles *Med. Phys.* **42** 6703–10

[120] Spirou S V, Makris D and Loudos G Does the setup of Monte Carlo simulations influence the calculated properties and effect of gold nanoparticles in radiation therapy? *Phys. Med.: Eur. J. Med. Phys.* **31** 817–21

[121] Khadem Abolfazli M, Mahdavi S R and Ataei G 2015 Studying effects of gold nanoparticle on dose enhancement in megavoltage radiation *J. Biomed. Phys. Eng.* **5** 185–90

[122] Paro A D, Hossain M, Webster T J and Su M 2016 Monte Carlo and analytic simulations in nanoparticle-enhanced radiation therapy *Int. J. Nanomed.* **11** 4735–41

[123] Berbeco R I, Detappe A, Tsiamas P, Parsons D, Yewondwossen M and Robar J 2016 Low Z target switching to increase tumor endothelial cell dose enhancement during gold nanoparticle-aided radiation therapy *Med. Phys.* **43** 436–42

[124] Le Loirec C, Chambellan D and Tisseur D 2016 Image-guided treatment using an x-ray therapy unit and gold nanoparticles: test of concept *Radiat. Prot. Dosim.* **169** 331–5

[125] McNamara A L, Kam W W Y, Scales N, McMahon S J, Bennett J W, Byrne H L, Schuemann J, Paganetti H, Banati R and Kuncic Z 2016 Dose enhancement effects to the nucleus and mitochondria from gold nanoparticles in the cytosol *Phys. Med. Biol.* **61** 5993–6010

[126] McMahon S J, Paganetti H and Prise K M 2016 Optimising element choice for nanoparticle radiosensitisers *Nanoscale* **8** 581–9

[127] McQuaid H N *et al* 2016 Imaging and radiation effects of gold nanoparticles in tumour cells**6** 19442

[128] Koger B and Kirkby C 2016 A method for converting dose-to-medium to dose-to-tissue in Monte Carlo studies of gold nanoparticle-enhanced radiotherapy *Phys. Med. Biol.* **61** 2014

[129] Dou Y *et al* 2016 Size-tuning ionization to optimize gold nanoparticles for simultaneous enhanced CT imaging and radiotherapy *ACS Nano* **10** 2536–48

[130] Cho J, Gonzalez-Lepera C, Manohar N, Kerr M, Krishnan S and Cho S H 2016 Quantitative investigation of physical factors contributing to gold nanoparticle-mediated proton dose enhancement *Phys. Med. Biol.* **61** 2562–81

[131] Retif P, Bastogne T and Barberi-Heyob M 2016 Robustness analysis of a Geant4-GATE simulator for nanoradiosensitizers characterization *IEEE Trans. Nanobiosci.* **15** 209–17

[132] Tran H N *et al* 2016 Geant4 Monte Carlo simulation of absorbed dose and radiolysis yields enhancement from a gold nanoparticle under MeV proton irradiation *Nucl. Instrum. Methods Phys. Res., Sect.* B **373** 126–39

[133] Chow J C L 2016 Photon and electron interactions with gold nanoparticles: A Monte Carlo study on gold nanoparticle-enhanced radiotherapy *Nanobiomaterials in Medical Imaging: Applications of Nanobiomaterials* (Amsterdam: Elsevier) 45–70

[134] Asadi S, Vaez-zadeh M, Vahidian M, Marghchouei M and Masoudi S F 2016 Ocular brachytherapy dosimetry for 103Pd and 125I in the presence of gold nanoparticles: a Monte Carlo study *J. Appl. Clin. Med. Phys.* **17** 90–9

[135] Yook S, Cai Z, Lu Y, Winnik M A, Pignol J-P and Reilly R M 2016 Intratumorally injected 177Lu-labeled gold nanoparticles: gold nanoseed brachytherapy with application for neoadjuvant treatment of locally advanced breast cancer *J. Nucl. Med.* **57** 936–42

[136] Cho J, Wang M, Gonzalez-Lepera C, Mawlawi O and Cho S H 2016 Development of bimetallic (Zn@Au) nanoparticles as potential PET-imageable radiosensitizers *Med. Phys.* **43** 4775–88

[137] Belamri C, Dib A S A and Belbachir A H 2016 Monte Carlo simulation of proton therapy using bio-nanomaterials *J. Radiother. Pract.* **15** 290–5

[138] Kwon J, Sutherland K, Hashimoto T, Shirato H and Date H 2016 Spatial distributions of dose enhancement around a gold nanoparticle at several depths of proton Bragg peak *Nucl. Instrum. Methods Phys. Res., Sect.* B **384** 113–20

[139] McKinnon S, Guatelli S, Incerti S, Ivanchenko V, Konstantinov K, Corde S, Lerch M, Tehei M and Rosenfeld A 2016 Local dose enhancement of proton therapy by ceramic oxide nanoparticles investigated with Geant4 simulations *Phys. Med.: Eur. J. Med. Phys.* **32** 1584–93

[140] Koger B and Kirkby C 2016 Optimization of photon beam energies in gold nanoparticle enhanced arc radiation therapy using Monte Carlo methods *Phys. Med. Biol.* **61** 8839–53

[141] Martinov M P and Thomson R M 2017 Heterogeneous multiscale Monte Carlo simulations for gold nanoparticle radiosensitization *Med. Phys.* **44** 644–53

[142] Brivio D, Nguyen P L, Sajo E, Ngwa W and Zygmanski P 2017 A Monte Carlo study of I-125 prostate brachytherapy with gold nanoparticles: dose enhancement with simultaneous rectal dose sparing via radiation shielding *Phys. Med. Biol.* **62** 1935–48

[143] Byrne H L, Gholami Y and Kuncic Z 2017 Impact of fluorescence emission from gold atoms on surrounding biological tissue—implications for nanoparticle radio-enhancement *Phys. Med. Biol.* **62** 3097–110

[144] Rezaei H, Zabihzadeh M, Ghorbani M, Goli Ahmadabad F and Mostaghimi H 2017 Evaluation of dose enhancement in presence of gold nanoparticles in eye brachytherapy by 103Pd source *Australas. Phys. Eng. Sci. Med.* **40** 545–53

[145] Hwang C, Kim J M and Kim J 2017 Influence of concentration, nanoparticle size, beam energy, and material on dose enhancement in radiation therapy *J. Radiat. Res.* **58** 405–11

IOP Publishing

Nanoparticle Enhanced Radiation Therapy
Principles, methods and applications
Erno Sajo and Piotr Zygmanski

Chapter 6

Nanoparticle-aided radiation therapy: challenges of treatment planning

C Kirkby and B Koger

6.1 Introduction

Nanoparticle-aided radiation therapy (NPRT) offers the potential to engineer solutions to some of the common constraints in conventional radiation therapy (RT) that otherwise limit its effectiveness as a treatment for various cancers. The major factors that currently limit the efficacy of RT lie at its intersection with disease biology and chemistry. These factors include: (i) identifying the precise location of the disease (tumor), (ii) limitations in tracking the disease location in real-time, (iii) the need to limit dose to normal organs-at-risk while still achieving local control of the tumor, (iv) the inability to differentiate between tumor cells and normal ones in scenarios where a target volume contains both, and (v) the inability to target tumor cells exclusively in a mixed scenario. While this list is not exhaustive, nanoparticles (in the form of nano-spheres, rods, cages, and other nano-scale structures) hold a great deal of promise to make headway against these limiting problems [1, 2].

In this chapter, we are primarily concerned with the challenges of planning RT treatments in scenarios where NPs are administered to the patient prior to radiation therapy treatments so as to act as radiosensitizing[1] agents. As with any RT treatment planning, the ultimate goal is to plan the best possible treatment based on an accurate prediction of clinical outcome for the individual patient, a plan which is derived from information about patient anatomy and physiology, largely from CT, MRI and PET images. *Clinical outcome* is broadly defined here, incorporating local tumor control, suppression of systemic disease, symptom relief, as well as

[1] The term *radiosensitizing* here is broadly defined. In this chapter we focus on the radiation dose enhancement properties of NPs composed of high atomic number (high-Z) elements. Strictly speaking, a radiosensitizing agent is one which alters the biochemical response to a given radiation dose. Toward the end of the chapter, however, we review the evidence for NP-induced biological effects, which may also play an important role in NPRT.

doi:10.1088/978-0-7503-2396-3ch6

limiting the normal tissue toxicities. It should be noted that even in the absence of any radiosensitizing agents, accurate predictions of clinical outcome for any given treatment plan are not without challenges [3–6].

The function of any therapeutic radiosensitizing agent is to amplify the desired end effect from a given dose of ionizing radiation. In principle, NPs can be engineered to accumulate preferentially in a specific target volume, i.e. a tumor and the microscopic disease surrounding it, based on its physiological properties. For example, since microvasculature structure in tumors tends to have larger pores than in normal tissue and since tumors tend to have poor lymphatic drainage, NPs can passively accumulate in the tumor interstitium, in a phenomenon known as the enhanced permeability and retention (EPR) effect [7, 8]. More active targeting options are also available such as conjugating NPs with glucose to target tumors via metabolic pathways [9, 10] or with oligonucleotides, peptides, antibodies or lipids [11], to take advantage of other inherent processes and ultimately lead to the accumulation of NPs in targeted cells.

Because of this ability to preferentially collect at the disease site, there is tremendous interest in using NPs for both diagnostic and therapeutic purposes. Radiologically, the use of NPs with high atomic numbers (high Z) can make them serve as effective contrast agents in x-ray-based *in vivo* imaging modalities [12]. In this respect they open up avenues for exploring the first two factors identified above that limit the efficacy of conventional RT, potentially enabling advances in disease detection, diagnosis, monitoring of its progression or regression or even tracking tumor position in real time during RT. Further, the larger interaction cross section of high-Z NPs relative to that of soft tissue can increase the absorbed dose near the NPs (generally within a few hundred nm of the NP surface). If dose near the NPs increases and the NPs are localized within a tumor, higher doses of therapeutic radiation to a tumor may be achieved while still keeping the dose to organs at risk to an acceptable level, thus enabling a means to address the third limiting factor defined above. Additionally, because the energy deposition around high-Z NPs tends to be highly localized, NPRT may offer the potential to target cancer at cellular or sub-cellular scales.

The focus in this chapter is to examine the specific challenges to planning RT treatments when NPs accumulate in a target volume and that target volume is irradiated in an attempt to generate a specific effect (generally the sterilization of all clonogenic cancer cells). These challenges are numerous, but they can be broken into two distinct categories: establishing accurate, meaningful dosimetry, and from that predicting biological effects.

Accurate and meaningful dosimetry needs to be established both in terms of computed and measureable quantities. Photon radiation interacts more readily with high-Z NPs than soft tissue, and such interactions can release more energy into the surrounding biological media in a highly localized manner. A similar effect is seen with protons and heavy ions, but this chapter will focus on photon-based NPRT scenarios. Accurate and meaningful dosimetry requires an understanding of the energy deposition process in the presence of high-Z NPs at both the more traditional macroscopic scales (i.e. from tens of centimeters down to millimeters), as well as at the microscopic scale (i.e. down to nanometers). For NPRT treatment planning such dosimetry computations will need to be fast and ideally come without massive increases in computing power. Further, they will ultimately require rigorous experimental validation within a well-defined commissioning process.

The second distinct challenge is translating from dosimetry into the meaningful prediction of biological effect. Clinical experience in radiation oncology is intimately related to accurate and precise dosimetry (determination of physical dose or ionizing energy deposited in the tissue). In traditional RT, the relationship between dosimetry and biological effect is relatively well characterized at the macroscopic scale. Treatment planning generally focuses on physical dose, and detailed models of biological effect are usually an optional part of treatment planning. However, when dose is enhanced in a heterogeneous manner on microscopic scales, as it is with high-*Z* NPs, the resulting enhancement of biological effect can become a complex function dependent on specific details of the irradiation scenario. NP physical characteristics (such as composition, size, shape, and coating), their macroscopic concentration, degree of cellular uptake and relative locations within each cell, as well as cell-specific properties that result in heterogeneous distributions of NPs (at nano-, micro- or macro-scales) all impact the way in which physical dose can be translated into a biological effect. In the context of NPRT, there is a greater need for the direct incorporation of biological effect models in order to translate from the complex patterns of dose enhancement into effects that can be optimized.

6.2 Nature of energy absorption near high-*Z* NPs

Before delving into the specific challenges to NPRT, we will first review photon interactions with high-*Z* NPs and the subsequent dispersion of energy into the surrounding media. This will highlight how the majority of energy to a medium added as a result of an interaction inside an NP is actually deposited within a few hundred nm of the NP, which leads directly into some of the challenges with dosimetry and modelling biological effect in the presence of such NPs.

High-*Z* NPs present a larger interaction cross section to x-rays than to soft tissue, particularly in the kilovoltage energy range. In external beam radiotherapy, x-rays interact with soft tissue primarily via Compton (incoherent) scattering. They can also interact through the pair production process for energies above 1.022 MeV, and through the photo-electric effect at very low energies (e.g. brachytherapy sources below 50 keV). Since Compton scattering is the dominant process in soft tissues between approximately 50 keV to 20 MeV, the probability of interaction tends to scale directly with the relative electron density of the medium. At lower energies or in media with higher effective atomic numbers, however, the photoelectric effect becomes the dominant mode of interaction.

The mass photoelectric coefficient, τ/ρ, is proportional to an exponential power, m, of Z the atomic number, or Z_{eff}, the effective atomic number of a compound medium. The value of m is approximately 3, (~4 above the K-edge). τ/ρ also scales inversely with the cube of photon energy, i.e.

$$\frac{\tau}{\rho} \propto \frac{Z^m}{(h\nu)^3}. \tag{6.1}$$

Hence at keV energies, photons interact much more readily with high-Z materials than low-Z materials. In figure 6.1, we have plotted the total mass attenuation coefficient for some common materials used for NPs—gold ($Z = 79$), silver ($Z = 47$), and hafnium oxide ($Z_{\text{eff}} \sim 63$)—compared to soft tissue ($Z_{\text{eff}} \sim 7$), as well as the ratio of cross-sections for each material to that of water as a function of incident photon energy. Clearly, these coefficients can differ from that of soft tissue by up to two

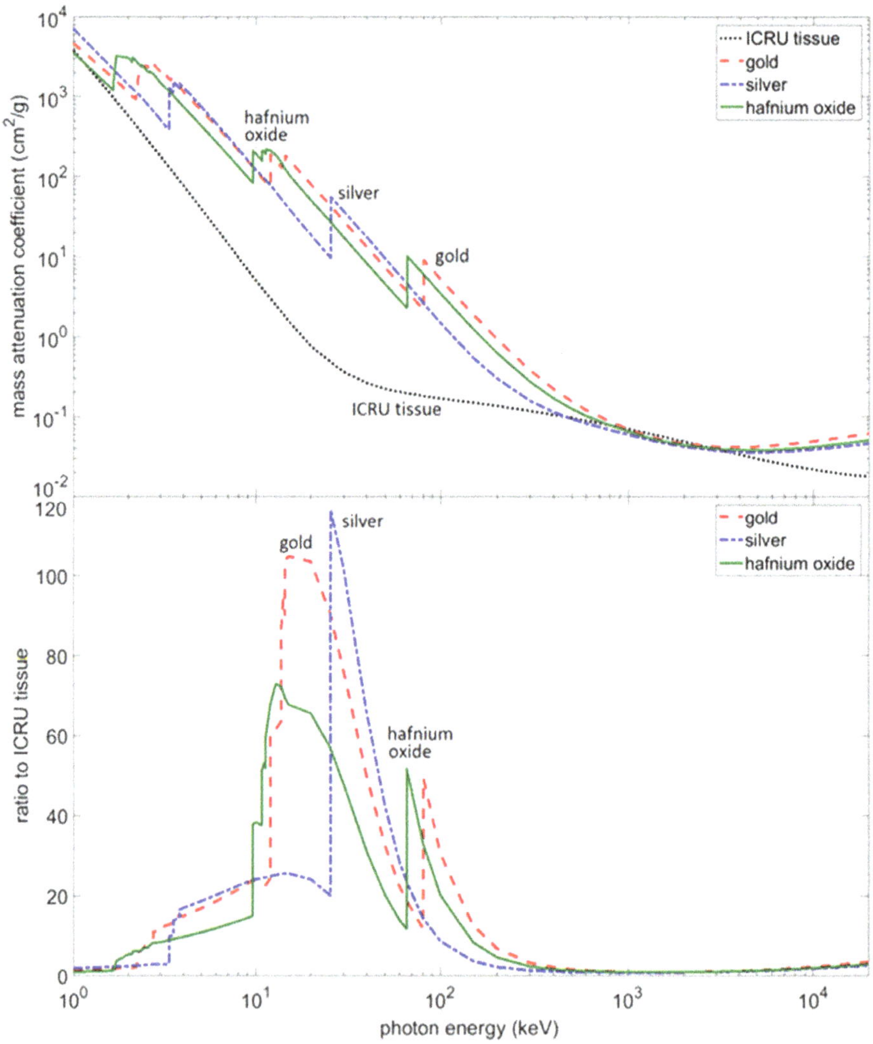

Figure 6.1. The mass attenuation coefficients for some common materials used in high-Z NPs (top), and the ratio for each high-Z material relative to soft tissue. Data are taken from the XCOM database [13]. The ratio can change by two orders of magnitude.

orders of magnitude (in the case of gold and silver), meaning that at certain energies, photons will interact in the high-Z material much more frequently than with tissue. In principle, if high-Z NPs collect at a specific location within an otherwise low-Z medium, many more interactions will occur in each NP on irradiation, releasing more ionizing electrons into the medium and thereby enhancing dose and subsequent radiation effects.

This suggests that the ratio of mass energy absorption coefficients relative to soft tissue is a predictor of dose enhancement, and it can be in terms of spatially averaged dose, but there is more to the story.

It is important to bear in mind that NP dose enhancement is largely a stochastic process on very small scales. Even under conditions of high photon beam exposures and low photon energies, photon interactions within any given high-Z NP can be rare, simply because of their small size. For example, McMahon *et al* reported that a 20 nm gold NP exposed to 100 keV x-rays would experience only 0.001 photon interactions per Gy deposited in the surrounding water volume [14]. That said, once a photon interacts within an NP, a cascade of events can be triggered that will ultimately lead to a statistically predictable pattern of energy deposition in the surrounding medium that is larger than what would otherwise occur in the absence of the NP. And these patterns will likely superimpose on each other, since even though the number ionizations per NP is small, the number of NPs in or near a given cell can range from the hundreds to tens of thousands [15–17], thus exposing a given cell to a Poisson probability distribution of extra ionization events.

An ionization photon interaction in a high-Z NP will generally create a Compton or photo-electron, often accompanied by multiple short-ranged Auger electrons. These will have sufficient energy to leave the immediate site of the interaction, potentially escape from the NP, and produce subsequent ionizations along a track within the medium surrounding it. Ionizations in the medium generate highly reactive radical species, which can then go on to interact with and potentially damage biologically sensitive structures such as the DNA (in addition to any direct damage done by ionizations within the sensitive structures themselves). Still, it is important to bear in mind that the majority of these interactions occur only within a few hundred nanometers of the NP in which the initial interaction took place.

The physical quantity *absorbed dose* is used as an effective quantity for conventional treatment planning (i.e. without nanoparticles) for several reasons. It can be measured on macroscopic scales with high degrees of precision and accuracy, it can be calculated consistently and reliably through heterogeneous volumes, and it can be monitored and controlled leading to reliable accumulation during radiation treatments. Additionally, it has long-established relationships with a variety of biological end points such as cell survival, tumor control probability and normal tissue complication probability.

Generally speaking, absorbed dose is a measure of the energy absorbed within a finite mass, making it a quantity that is well defined only on relatively macroscopic scales (i.e. much larger than typical cell dimensions), and for relatively high exposure levels. As mentioned, on small scales the energy from ionizing radiation is imparted into a medium along charged-particle tracks. In scenarios where a target (e.g. a cell nucleus, DNA macromolecule, mitochondrion, etc) is sufficiently small, very few charged-particle tracks may pass through it for a given exposure level. In these cases, the energy absorbed by the target volume can vary drastically between similar targets, making the absorbed energy a stochastic quantity [18, 19]. Therefore, it becomes necessary to describe energy deposition in terms of well-parameterized probability distribution rather than a single quantity, bringing dose deposition into the realm of microdosimetry. The stochastic analog of absorbed dose is *specific energy*, or $z = d\varepsilon/dm$ where $d\varepsilon$ is the energy deposited from a single interaction or track through a given small volume and dm is the mass associated with that volume. It bears noting that in much of the literature on NP dose enhancement, the term *dose* is sometimes used informally for this quantity.

Despite the stochastic nature of photon interactions with an NP, once a photon does interact, the patterns of energy deposition in the vicinity of the irradiated high-Z NP are predictable. When a photon interacts, it generates low-energy electrons. Though individual paths followed by electrons that escape high-Z NPs can be tortuous, their ranges are determined by their initial energy. A plot of electron range in water as a function of the initial kinetic energy of the electron is given in figure 6.2, showing a comparison of results from the literature. There is some discrepancy between sources, as definitions of 'range' can vary in the literature, and uncertainties in the charged particle transport process can become somewhat large at lower energies (below 1 keV), even for sophisticated track-structure Monte Carlo codes [20, 21]. For energies below 1 keV, quantum mechanical uncertainty can also become significant [22]. Details aside, based on figure 6.2, it is clear that the initial kinetic energies of any electrons that escape a high-Z NP, dictate the spatial distribution of the energy they impart into the media surrounding the NP.

To illustrate this effect, we investigate the case of an isolated 25 nm radius spherical gold NP (GNP) in a water medium exposed to monoenergetic photons. Results from Monte Carlo simulations of this scenario are shown in figures 6.3 and 6.4. Other NPs will follow similar trends, though the numerical values will differ.

The dosimetric implications of emissions from photon interactions in NPs can be surmised from figure 6.3. The dose per photon incident on the NP was scored in concentric spherical shells around the GNP[2]. We also included a plot of the dose with the irradiated volume defined as water (blue broken curve) for incident photons of 40 keV. To provide some context for the curves, at 10 keV, the probability of a directly incident photon interacting with the NP is roughly 7.4×10^{-3}. At 1 MeV, this probability is about 3.5×10^{-6}. The photon fluence required to deliver 2 Gy (in the absence of any high-Z NPs) from a 6 MV, 10×10 cm^2 field at a depth of 10 cm, translates to just more than 6 photons passing through the volume occupied by the 25 nm radius GNP. The fluence would be greater for lower energy spectra. In a clinical scenario, the doses presented in figure 6.3 would be superimposed on a

---

[2] Notes on the simulation details:

- Dose from primary beam photon interactions in the surrounding media is not superimposed on these doses.
- Although the dose is binned with radial symmetry, emissions are not necessarily isotropic [29].

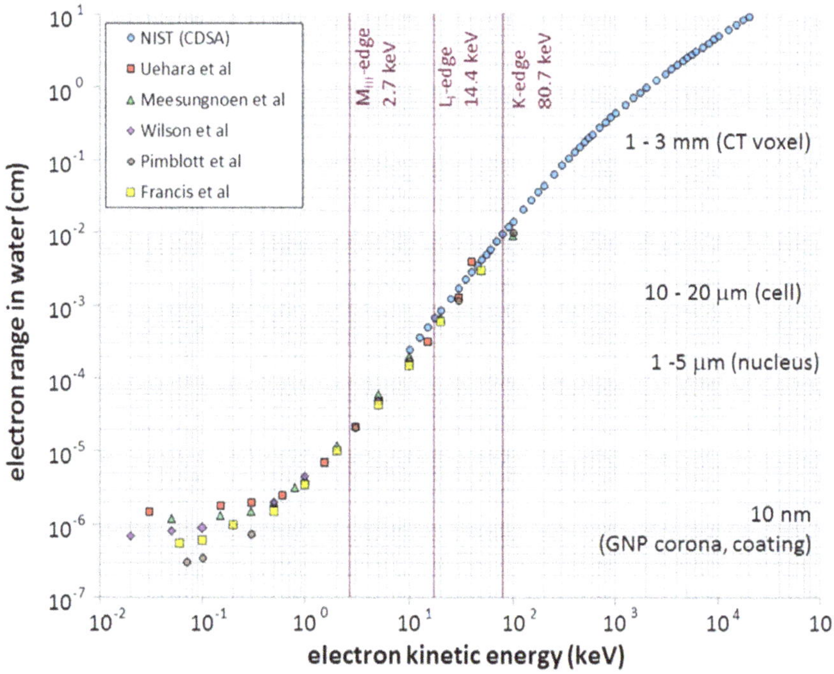

Figure 6.2. A plot of electron ranges in water as a function of kinetic energy is shown as taken from several sources. The NIST continuous slowing down approximation (CSDA) data (blue circles) [23] are shown down to 10 keV. Also shown are electron penetration ranges from Uehara *et al* (red squares) [24], Meesungnoen *et al* (green triangles) [25], Wilson *et al* (purple diamonds) [26], Pimblott *et al* (grey circles) [27], and Francis *et al* (yellow squares) [28]. We have also superimposed violet lines on the data to show the approximate energies of K, L_I, and M_{III} edges, and pointed out the approximate dimensions of common objects of interest on the right for context. Electron ranges are reasonably consistent down to approximately 1 keV. The variation at lower energies reflects the uncertainties in the various methods of calculating electron range as well as differences in the approach.

background of dose that would result from radiation interacting in the surrounding medium, which was not modelled here.

Interactions in the GNPs give rise to a spectrum of photo-electrons, Auger electrons, characteristic x-rays and to a lesser extent Compton electrons [29, 30]. In most cases these will escape the GNP and go on to interact with the surrounding media. The dose surrounding the GNP in figure 6.3 falls off roughly as a power law relation with an exponent between about −1.9 and −2.5, out to the maximum range of the emitted photoelectrons. More subtle structure to each curve results from the emissions of much lower energy Auger electrons. When the photo-electron range is exceeded, the dose drops sharply over some orders of magnitude and then resumes with a tail due to emitted characteristic x-rays.

Figure 6.4 zooms in on the first 5000 nm surrounding the GNP. The 10 keV incident photon case (red dashed line) shows a substantial drop in dose per ionisation beyond about 2000 nm as the highest energy electrons that can be emitted from such interactions reach the end of their range. The tail beyond 3000 nm is due

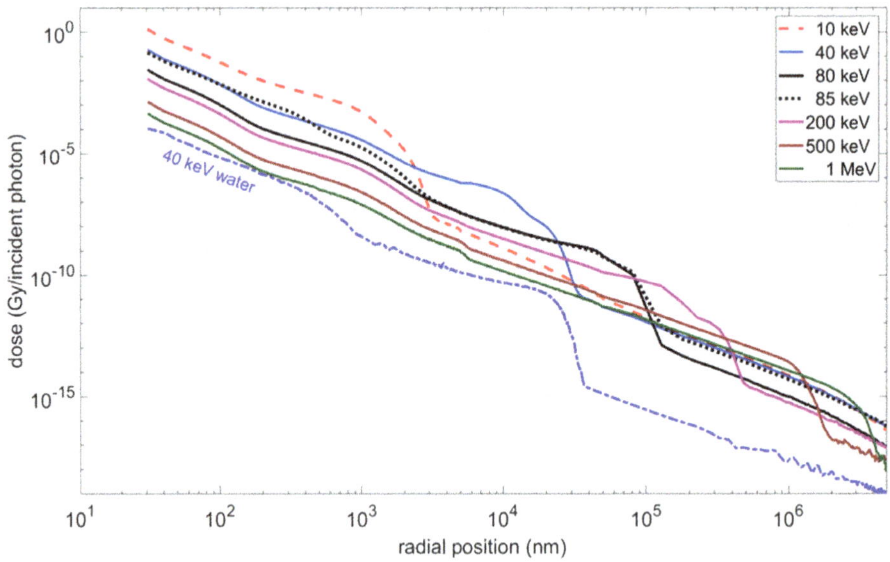

Figure 6.3. Monte Carlo predicted dose as a function of distance from a 25 nm radius GNP, normalized per photon incident on the GNP, shown for incident photons of selected energies. Each curve is characterized by a roughly inverse square falloff out to the approximate range of the emitted electrons (see figure 6.2) after which the curve drops sharply a few orders of magnitude and then continues on into a tail due to dose spreading out from the emission of fluorescent x-rays. Also shown is a similar curve for 40 keV photons incident on an equivalent volume of water (dashed blue).

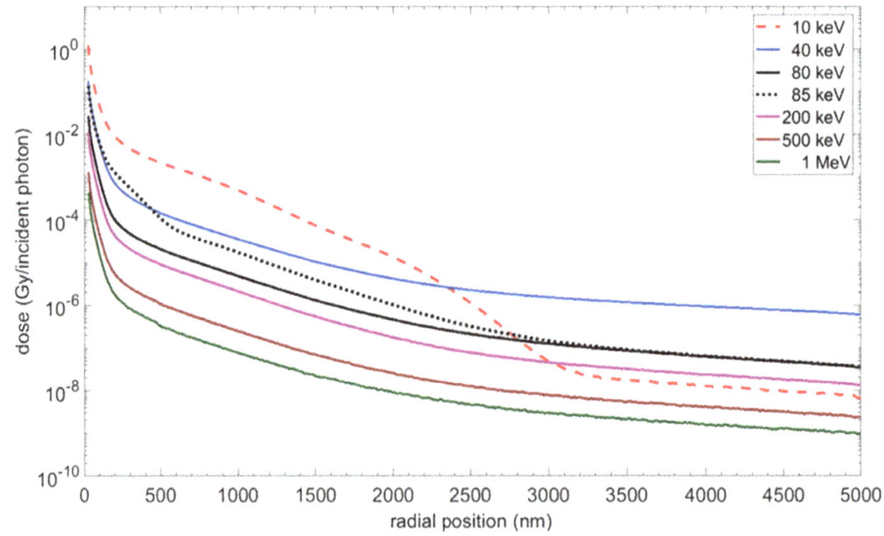

Figure 6.4. A closer look at the energy deposition patterns presented in figure 6.3, over the first 5000 nm plotted on a log-linear scale.

to characteristic x-rays emitted from the GNP. The 85 keV incident photon case (black dashed line) shows a characteristic bulge between 200 nm and 600 nm. This is because the 85 keV photons are just above the 80.7 keV K-edge of gold. After overcoming the binding energy, the emitted photo-electrons from K-shell interactions have only 4.3 keV of kinetic energy and therefore have a range of only a few hundred nm. Dose deposited beyond this point is due solely to interactions with the L-shell and higher.

The implications of this pattern of energy release into the surrounding medium are far-reaching. When a photon interaction within a high-Z NP occurs, a substantial amount of energy may be released into the surrounding medium, but the majority of that energy is deposited within a few hundred nm of the NP. Because of this highly localized pattern of dose deposition, the specific location of each NP relative to any sensitive structures within the cell can play a critical role in determining an individual cell's response when it is irradiated in the presence of high-Z NPs. This high localization of dose suggests that the overall pattern of energy deposition within a cell can be quite heterogeneous, especially at low incident photon energies. Sophisticated models that can account for the dose heterogeneity, the stochastic nature of the ionization events, and the stochastic arrangements of GNPs within cells may be required to accurately predict cellular response [2].

High-Z NPs are often coated with different materials or macromolecules for more active targeting of cancer cells or for controlling their pharmacokinetic properties such a biological half-life. A common coating such as polyethylene glycol (PEG) typically has a thickness of 5–30 nm [31, 32]. Figure 6.3 suggests that over a distance of 30 nm from the surface of otherwise bare GNPs the dose per ionization can drop by an order of magnitude in water-equivalent media. Hence, if such a coating remains intact at the time of irradiation, it can absorb a substantial amount of the total energy that escapes the high-Z NP. This has the potential to mitigate any desired enhancement effect [31, 33].

Another major implication from these curves is that while at larger distances dose enhancement is small, it can accumulate to clinically significant levels when many NPs are present. Figure 6.3 suggests that doses of 7.7×10^{-8} Gy/incident photon to 4.9×10^{-4} Gy/incident photon occur at 10 μm from each GNP. While this may not seem significant at first, it is not unreasonable to observe uptakes of 10^4 GNPs per cell [15, 34, 35]. And for typical irradiation scenarios there are multiple photons incident on any given NP. Even though not all incident photons will necessarily interact, there is potential for small, stochastic contributions to accumulate into a significant increase in dose on cell-to-cell scales or greater, i.e. the macroscopic scale.

The accumulation of high-Z NPs can have other dosimetric consequences as well. High-Z NPs commonly tend to collect in clusters within cells, rather than disperse homogeneously. This is partially because of the endocytosis process of NP uptake where the NPs are encapsulated into a vacuole as they are transported into a cell [36, 37]. When tightly clustered, substantial portions of the energy released by each high-Z NP may be absorbed by the neighbouring high-Z NPs [38]. When this energy is cross-absorbed by gold, the dose enhancement effect is again mitigated.

From a macroscopic point of view (on the order of mm), the large-scale uptake of high-*Z* NPs in a tumor or other irradiated tissue can change its attenuation properties. Because the depth of radiation penetration is a function of energy, this implies a complex trade-off relationship between the spectrum of incident photons, the concentration of high-*Z* NPs and the depth of the target volume in a patient [39, 40].

As we consider the challenges of treatment planning in the context of NPRT, we shall build on the concepts developed here.

6.3 Uptake and dispersion prediction of NPs

Accurate treatment planning in radiation therapy requires an accurate estimation of absorbed dose within both the directly targeted volume and any organs-at-risk. According to the International Atomic Energy Agency, 'all forms of radiotherapy should be applied as accurately as reasonably achievable (AAARA), technical and biological factors being taken into account [41].' In NPRT, high-*Z* NPs will modify the absorbed dose in the irradiated volume, as discussed in the previous section: high amounts of energy will be deposited in a stochastic manner over sub-cellular distances, and small amounts of energy will have the potential to accumulate and lead to non-stochastic dose enhancements on larger scales. Collectively, the presence of high-*Z* NPs can lead to an overall sensitization enhancement effect.

But how accurately can the sensitization effect be predicted?

While the overall NPRT sensitization effect may not derive *entirely* from the radiation dosimetry, accurate dosimetry in the presence of high-*Z* NPs is at least a major variable that needs to be addressed for effective treatment planning. Accurate dosimetry relies on an accurate understanding of the spatial-temporal distribution of the high-*Z* NPs at both the macroscopic and microscopic scales. Thus, the next major challenge to effective NPRT treatment planning is predicting this distribution, at least in a statistical sense, based on information that can be gathered from multi-scale and multi-modality imaging studies.

6.4 Nanoparticle distribution within tissues and organs

On the macroscopic scale, it is important to understand which tissues and organs the NPs can be expected to accumulate in and the timescales involved. NPs tend to collect most prominently in the liver and spleen with smaller amounts collecting in other organs [42]. The specific pharmacokinetic behavior of NPs is dictated by a number of properties including: size, shape, coating, surface charge, and conjugate materials when applied for active targeting.

Size plays a critical role in the fate of NPs *in vivo*, particularly when administered through intravenous injection. *Passive targeting* of NPs to tumors takes advantage the EPR phenomenon [7, 8]. The pores in normal, healthy blood vessels are typically up to about 5–12 nm in size [43], while the blood vessel diameter ranges between 3–20 μm with a peak around 3–5 μm and the density is in the range of 10^2–10^3 mm^{-2}. Due to the rapid growth that occurs in solid tumors and the associated angiogenesis, tumor blood vessels tend to be larger with diameters in the range of 5–50 μm, peaking at 10–20 μm, and have larger pores, up to several hundred nm [44]. The difference in pore sizes allows NPs with sizes between these limits to move easily into the tumor interstitium, but less easily into that of healthy tissues, leading to a preferential uptake within tumors over healthy tissues. Still, some accumulation in healthy tissue does occur. NPs with dimensions smaller than about 6 nm tend to be cleared rapidly by the kidneys [45, 46]. NPs with dimensions greater than 100 nm tend to be taken up by macrophages and eliminated or accumulate in the healthy liver or spleen [45].

Size can also play a role in the distribution of NPs within different organs, as well as biological half-life (the time it takes a given concentration of NPs to be reduced to half its initial value within a given organ or tissue) [42, 47]. The half-life of GNPs in the blood administered intravenously tends to decrease with increasing GNP size in the 20 nm to 100 nm range with half-lives ranging from 0.4 h to 51.1 h (with additional dependence on coating) [48]. Size can also dictate movement of NPs within a tumor—an environment that is generally heterogeneous in properties such as pH, pO_2 or vascular density. Large particles tend not to travel far from blood vessels. Smaller particles penetrate further, but are more transient [49].

With respect to NP shape, the literature suggests advantages of for non-spherical shapes in terms of improved circulation time, and target tissue binding, but disadvantages in terms of cellular uptake [36, 45]. NP charge has also been shown to influence uptake with positively charged NPs being associated with a higher uptake in nonphagocytic cells and phagocytic cells preferentially taking up negatively charged NPs [50]. Even clustering NPs together in aggregates has been shown to result in differential uptakes between cells lines [51].

Blood circulation time, and therefore tumor uptake, can also be increased by coating the surface of NPs with a material such as polyethylene glycol (PEG), which may act to shield the NP's surface charge and provide a hydrophilic surface [45, 48]. However, this same property may inhibit internalization of the NPs into cells [45]. The addition of more active targeting agents such as antibodies or peptides to the NPs has been more recently explored as a strategy to increase accumulation in tumors, [2, 49, 52] and while this has generally improved uptake, there is yet to be an optimal strategy defined [52].

6.5 Determination of NP concentrations on the macroscopic scale

In the context of planning external beam radiotherapy using CT-images, modern treatment planning systems (Monte Carlo or grid-based linear Boltzmann equation solving algorithms) simulating megavoltage photon beams can achieve dose calculation uncertainties on the order of 2%–3% or better even in heterogeneous media [53, 54]. Conventional treatment planning relies on a voxelized CT image data set, from which the information relevant to the radiation transport calculations (i.e. relative electron density and effective atomic number, Z_{eff}) can be extracted. It also relies on the assumption that tissues are homogeneous over 1–3 mm distance scales, a condition that will no longer be satisfied in NPRT. Adding high-Z NPs to tissue changes its attenuation properties as a medium, which is precisely what enables the exciting work being done with high-Z NPs as contrast-enhancing agents in x-ray imaging scenarios [55–59]. So how well can NP concentration in tissue be resolved with current, conventional tools?

In principle, the average concentration of NPs in a given CT scan voxel can be derived from the calibrated HU number associated with that voxel. Early work scanning known concentrations of GNPs suggests a linear relation between HU and concentration up to a saturation threshold at approximately 500 mM (which is likely well beyond any practical uptake concentration in an NPRT scenario) [60]. The slope of this relation is approximately 5 ± 1 HU mM^{-1}, with subtle dependencies on the imaging spectrum and GNP size [60, 61]. Conceptually, if a patient could be imaged prior to any NP administration and later at some time t after NPs have been administered, and if the images are registered, differences in HU values for a given voxel could be attributed to the accumulation of NPs.

For a typical CT simulator used for radiotherapy treatment planning, it is reasonable to expect the uncertainty of the HU value for a given voxel to be within ± 20 HU compared to the true value [41]. Tolerances for water or water-equivalent media can certainly be tighter, but they often apply to mean values measured over many voxels of the same material [62], hence an uncertainty for any given voxel of 20 HU is not unreasonable. Given the slope of 5 ± 1 HU mM^{-1}, such an uncertainty would mean that the concentration could be determined to within only 4 mM or about 0.8 mg g^{-1} for GNPs using conventional CT simulation techniques. More specialized techniques such as K-edge spectral CT may reduce this detection threshold to a theoretical minimum of approximately 0.2 mg g^{-1}, though a more realistic limit may be around 0.5 mg g^{-1} [63].

This does beg the question of what NP concentration resolution is necessary for effective NPRT treatment planning. The answer to that depends on what concentrations of NPs are both safe for administration and generate the desired radiosensitization effect.

Initial Monte Carlo calculations suggested that GNP concentrations on the order of several mg g^{-1} were necessary to double the dose otherwise delivered in the absence of GNPs [29, 35, 64]. For such cases, conventional CT simulation may have been sufficient. However experimental measurements of radiosensitization have demonstrated substantial increases in biological effect when cells containing concentrations of GNPs below 1 mg g^{-1} were irradiated [65]. This implies that effective treatment planning may require the ability to resolve finer concentrations. Alternative approaches to quantifying NP uptake are under development. Optical imaging, surface enhanced Raman scattering, and photoacoustic imaging have been shown to detect GNPs down to μg g^{-1} concentrations [2], but they are not without their own limitations in terms of penetration depth. X-ray fluorescence CT has the potential to detect such low concentrations with the ability to penetrate deep into a patient, but current experimental apparatus requires extreme collimation, which may make routine patient scanning impractical [66–68]. Other options include SPECT, which could detect NPs labelled with gamma-emitting nuclides, but suffer from practical resolution limits, or MRI, which may be capable of detecting low NP concentrations, but will required the use of very-high (7 T) magnetic fields [2], which are still largely under experimental development and not in routine clinical use.

6.6 Cellular internalization

Regardless of modality, the ability to determine NP concentration *in vivo* is likely to be limited in spatial resolution to volumes on the order of 1 mm^3, which will contain roughly 10^5–10^7 cells. While information about macroscopic NP distribution may be available, questions of microscopic distribution would not be answered by *in vivo* imaging. Are the NPs confined to microvasculature or extra-cellular fluid, or are they internalized into cells? If so, to what degree—how many NPs enter into a given cell? Within each cell, where are the NPs located relative to sensitive structures such as the DNA? Are the NPs confined within vacuoles, or do they disperse through the cytoplasm? Do they penetrate the nucleus? And what about cell-to-cell heterogeneity of the distributions? Given the highly localized nature of dose deposition near high-Z NPs, as discussed above, the answers to such questions are likely to play a significant role in determining biological response.

Of course answering such questions for all cells in a given patient is impractical. At the microscopic scale, NP spatial distributions and cellular uptake must be inferred on a statistical basis via models of pharmacokinetic behavior.

6.7 Dosimetry in the presence of NPs

Some of the key advantages of NPRT on a macroscopic scale can be seen in an example of an arc-therapy treatment using GNPs shown in figure 6.5. In the centre of the brain, a model tumor volume is delineated with a thick black line. In figure 6.5(a) the tumor volume is assumed to have a uniform GNP uptake of 15 mg g^{-1} and is irradiated with a 200 kVp photon source. A conventional 6 MV treatment is shown in figure 6.5(b) for comparison. Profiles along the left-right direction through isocenter are shown in figure 6.5(c).

In the NPRT case, the region of high dose (for example the 95% isodose line) is determined by the *intersection* of the arc therapy irradiated volume and the presence of the GNPs (in high concentration). In contrast, the high dose region in conventional treatments is determined entirely by the arc therapy irradiated volume. The lower energy photon spectra in the NPRT case results in a much sharper penumbra outside of the tumor volume. This is both because of the sharper percentage depth dose curve at 200 kVp compared to that from a 6 MV beam and the limited range of electrons generated in the GNP interactions. This means that in theory, if high-Z NPs can be engineered to accumulate in a solid tumor, and not just in the gross tumor volume but in the microscopic extensions of the disease that may not be resolved through imaging, the prescribed dose can be delivered to those volumes. Normal tissues with an absence of high-Z NPs will receive substantially less dose, even when they are directly irradiated.

It is of course important to underscore that figure 6.5 presents an idealized case, with attention only to dosimetry at the macroscopic (~mm) scale. Though GNP uptake of 15 mg g^{-1} has been reported in animal models in the literature [69], toxicity and rapid elimination issues may present challenges to achieving such concentrations in humans [70]. Obtaining uniform uptake of high-Z NPs in a clinically relevant volume, while restricting uptake in surrounding tissues to

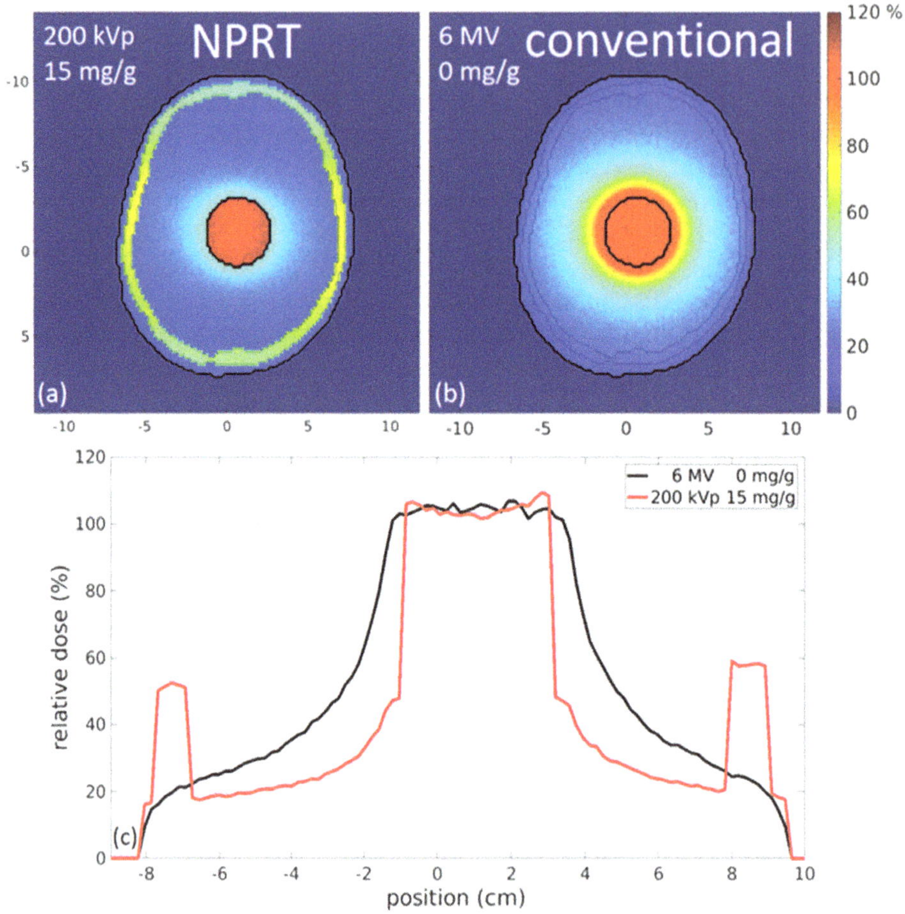

Figure 6.5. Example dose distributions from Monte Carlo simulations of arc therapy treatments for a brain with a spherical tumor (radius 2 cm). (a) A 200 kVp photon source with a uniform distribution of GNPs at 15 mg g^{-1} within the tumor volume. (b) A 6 MV source without GNPs in the same target volume. Bone is outlined in thin black lines. Distances are in cm. (c) Dose profiles along the left–right axis through isocentre demonstrate the dose differences on the macroscopic scale.

inconsequential levels, is a substantial challenge. Further, dosimetry over the macroscopic scale is only part of the picture. As previously discussed, energy deposition around high-Z NPs is highly heterogeneous and stochastic on sub-cellular scales.

Effective planning of NPRT will require dosimetry that is: (i) accurate in biological media modified by the presence of high-Z NPs, incorporating that into conventional radiation transport calculations on macroscopic scales, and (ii) meaningful at the microscopic scale, incorporating the expected high levels of dose heterogeneity. This is known as the two-stage or multi-scale problem [1].

There are a number of different possible approaches to the multi-scale problem, each with advantages and disadvantages. The first set of approaches are more conventional, where the dosimetry is considered only on the macroscopic (mm) scale. As in figure 6.5, doses are calculated in voxels and dose enhancement only comes into play when NP uptake is large enough to enhance the mean dose through a given voxel. In these approaches, additional sensitization enhancement effects would need to be inferred from clinical experience, similar to approaches used with radiosensitizing drugs. In the second set of approaches, more detailed calculations performed at the sub-cellular scale and based on pharmacokinetic models of NP uptake and detailed Monte Carlo simulations can be used to estimate sensitisation enhancement on a statistical basis.

6.8 NPRT dosimetry on the macroscopic scale

In conventional external beam radiation therapy, as shown in figure 6.5, the medium through which radiation is transported (i.e. the patient) is generally broken into cubic voxels of approximately 1–3 mm in size. The content of each voxel is determined from CT simulation. Relative electron densities or mass densities are mapped from HU values using quasi-linear mapping techniques based on phantom measurements [62]. Effective atomic numbers (Z_{eff}) are determined in a similar way using step-functions, with most voxels within the patient defaulting to soft tissue ($Z_{\text{eff}} \sim 7.4$). For a given beam configuration or modulated delivery the dose to each voxel is determined using either convolution-superposition algorithms, numerical algorithms for directly solving the linear Boltzmann equation, or Monte Carlo methods.

When a volume in a patient (e.g. a tumor) acquires a large concentration (several mg g^{-1}) of high-Z NPs, the presence of the NPs will give rise to unique challenges to calculating the mean dose within each voxel. The presence of high-Z NPs may alter the radiation transport through each voxel. Figure 6.6 illustrates the approximate magnitude of this concern with an example plotting the relative difference in attenuation through a soft tissue medium as the GNP content (GC) in the medium is increased, i.e.

$$f_{\text{att}}(\text{GC}) = \frac{e^{-\mu_{\text{soft tissue}} \cdot x} - e^{-\mu_{\text{GNP}}(\text{GC}) \cdot x}}{e^{-\mu_{\text{soft tissue}} \cdot x}}, \tag{6.2}$$

where $\mu_{\text{GNP}}(GC)$ is the linear attenuation coefficient, averaged over the relevant photon spectrum, and weighted by the indicated gold content, GC in terms of milligram of gold per gram of soft tissue, x = 1 cm, and $\mu_{\text{soft tissue}}$ is the linear attenuation coefficient in soft tissue with no GNPs present. Figure 6.6 shows that differences in attenuation of 1% cm^{-1} manifest between gold content of about 0.4 mg g^{-1} (80 kVp) and 6 mg g^{-1} (6 MV). Therefore, for concentrations of high-Z NPs in this ballpark, it becomes necessary to account for the NP content in the tissue at the time of irradiation, even if one plans to completely infer sensitization enhancement on a protocol basis. This also implies the potential for high-Z NP shielding effects that may reduce otherwise anticipated dose enhancement effects and alter dosimetry to downstream tissues [39, 71].

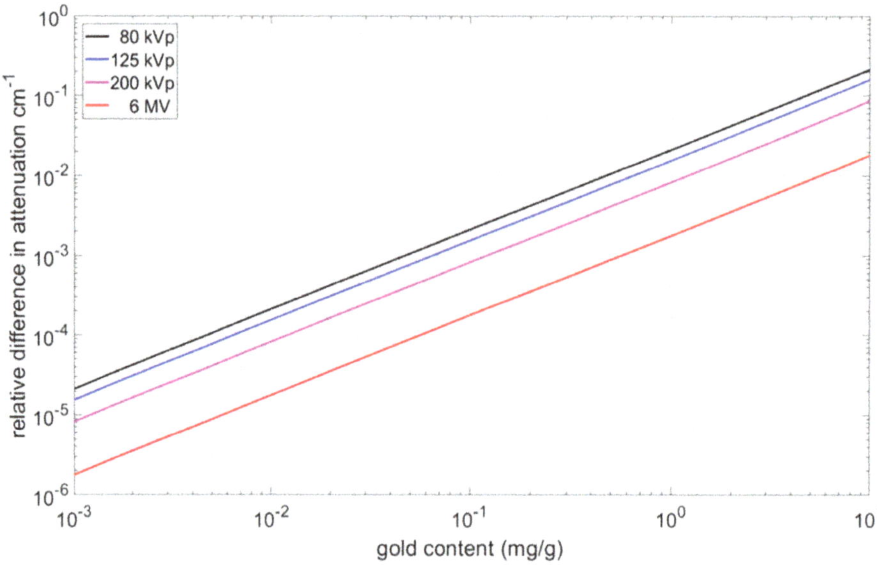

Figure 6.6. The relative difference in linear attenuation through a path length of 1 cm (equation (6.2)) is plotted as a function of GNP content in a soft tissue medium for different photon spectra, demonstrating that, particularly at higher concentrations, high-*Z* NP content in tissue at the time of irradiation is a non-negligible aspect of radiation transport.

A further challenge is the assignment of Z_{eff} to voxels from CT data. For conventional megavoltage external beam therapies without high-*Z* NPs, it is generally sufficient to assume that most voxels are roughly equivalent to soft tissue and scale them by relative electron density. Accurate tissue models are a concern in brachytherapy treatment planning with differences in tissue composition translating into dose discrepancies on the order of 10% in some cases [72, 73], particularly because of the low photon energies involved. In many NPRT scenarios (involving kilovoltage energies and higher Z_{eff}), the photoelectric effects will play a larger role, which will require accurate mapping of Z_{eff} from a CT image set. In figure 6.7, the relative difference in mass energy-absorption coefficients is plotted for different photon spectra as a function of GNP content, i.e.

$$f_{\text{en}}(\text{GC}) = \frac{\left.\frac{\mu_{en}}{\rho}\right|_{\text{GNP(GC)}} - \left.\frac{\mu_{en}}{\rho}\right|_{\text{soft tissue}}}{\left.\frac{\mu_{en}}{\rho}\right|_{\text{soft tissue}}}, \tag{6.3}$$

where $\mu_{\text{EN}}/\rho|_{\text{GNP(GC)}}$ is the mass energy-absorption coefficient averaged over the given spectra for a given concentration of GNPs (*GC*) and the subscript 'soft tissue' denotes an absence of GNPs. Since absorbed dose is generally proportional to this quantity, it serves as a good approximation to the error expected when a voxel of incorrect Z_{eff} is used. As shown, for the GNP example, a 2% error in voxel dose can occur with gold content of about 0.06 mg g^{-1} (80 kVp) and just over 1 mg g^{-1}

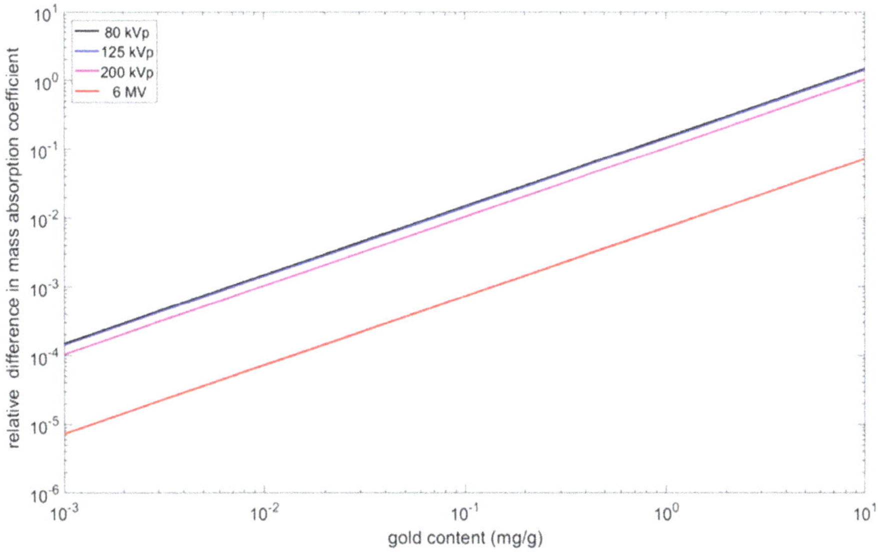

Figure 6.7. The difference in mass absorption coefficients of media with GNPs relative to soft tissue alone is plotted as a function of GNP content. This demonstrates the approximate magnitude of voxel dose errors when a volume is incorrectly assigned Z_{eff} for soft tissue when it in fact has high-Z NP content.

(6 MV). Even with a sophisticated dose calculation algorithm, the GIGO (garbage in garbage out) principle still applies. So strategies will need to be developed to identify voxels where high-Z NPs will accumulate at the time of treatment such that the approximate NP content can be determined and the appropriate Z_{eff} assigned.

The concentration of high-Z NPs will also change with time, presenting yet another challenge for effective NPRT dosimetry. As already discussed, biological half-lives of NPs have a complex dependence on the properties of the tissues or organs they are taken up by as well as the NP physical properties themselves, resulting in half-lives that can vary from minutes to days [48]. If the high-Z NP concentration changes appreciably between the time of simulation imaging and treatment delivery, such changes will need to be accounted for. It may be possible to monitor large concentration changes with imaging equipment such as on-board cone-beam CT systems, but it is more likely that uptake and elimination will have to rely on models of NP pharmacokinetic behaviour.

In conventional external beam radiation therapy, dose from daily imaging protocols is not typically incorporated into the treatment plan. Dose from typical kilovoltage CBCT systems will tend to fall in the range of 0.2–3 cGy depending on the image site and protocol/technique applied [74], and therefore generally less than 2% of a 200 cGy fraction. But with high-Z NPs acting to enhance dose at the lower energies used by imaging systems, daily imaging dose will increase and may need to be incorporated into the treatment plan. This may present an additional challenge because often more than a single study is required to accurately set up a patient, and multiple images may be necessary to track the uptake and elimination of the high-Z NPs in time.

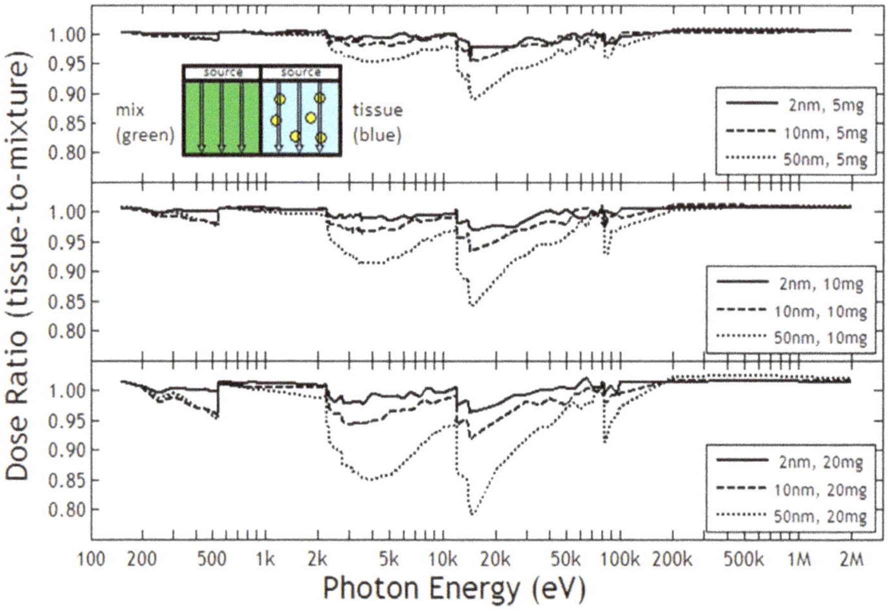

Figure 6.8. The ratio of dose directly deposited in tissue when GNPs are explicitly modelled in a simulation to that in a gold–tissue mixture (see inset) as a function of photon energy as shown for a variety of GNP diameters (given in nm in the legend) and concentrations (given in mg Au/g tissue in the legend) [75]. Copyright 2016 IOP Publishing Ltd. Adapted with permission. All rights reserved.

When dose is scored on a macroscopic scale as in figure 6.5, the entire dose to a voxel containing high-*Z* NPs is not biologically relevant. On the microscopic scale, some of that energy remains within the NPs and will not have any effect on the surrounding biological medium. One study used Monte Carlo simulations to calculate the ratio of dose directly to tissue in a ~micrometer-sized volume where the NPs were explicitly modelled and the dose to the tissue exclusively could be isolated (D_{tis}), to that where the volume was modelled as a uniform 'mixture' material which would include dose to both tissue and gold seen as a single medium (D_{mix}), i.e. *Dose Ratio* = D_{tis}/D_{mix}. These results, shown in figure 6.8, demonstrate the approximate magnitude of this effect as a function of energy (more pronounced near K and L edges), gold concentration (becomes more substantial with more GNPs), and NP diameter (larger diameters absorb more electrons internally) [75]. In extreme cases it can be a 20% effect, though for smaller NPs, kilovoltage energy spectra that can realistically penetrate a phantom, and lower GNP concentrations the effect is fairly small.

Perhaps the most significant challenge to NPRT in terms of macroscopic level radiation transport is that of determining an appropriate radiation source (specifically in terms of energy spectrum) to achieve desired dose enhancement effects. Based on equation (6.1), lower photon energies result in a higher interaction cross section in high-*Z* NPs. However, lower energy photon beams also attenuate more when traversing tissue. This leads to an energy optimization problem, the solution of which will depend on the depth and dimensions of a given target volume relative to a radiation source [39, 40]. An effective treatment plan will need not only account for any dose enhancement in isolation, but relative to the dose delivered elsewhere in the plan to the organs at risk, as with any other radiation therapy treatment planning scenario. A plan that effectively doubles the mean tumor dose but brings the skin dose beyond an acceptable level for toxicities would not be viable. An example of this can be seen in figure 6.5. Bone from the patient skull is contoured with thin black lines. The 200 kVp spectrum that provides a reasonable balance between GNP dose enhancement and penetration also increases the dose to bone from about 20% to almost 60% of the prescription dose.

There are out-of-field effects and general sensitivities to the source spectrum to consider as well. The spectrum from a given therapeutic source is not uniform across a field. Given the sensitivity of high-Z NP dose enhancement to the energy of the photons incident on the NPs, it becomes clear that detailed, accurate source models, more so than in conventional radiation therapy, are necessary for accurate dosimetry. As an example, IMRT fields can have a substantial amount of dose delivered via out-of-field phantom scatter, which will have a different spectrum (lower mean energy) than that of the primary beam, which can alter the expected dose enhancement [76]. Secondly, since the NP uptake will not be perfectly targeted in practice, peripheral tissues and organs at risk are also likely to contain some NPs. Moving out of the primary field, the mean energy of a 6 MV beam can drop from ~1.5 MeV to 0.36 MeV over only a few centimeters [77]. Since the out-of-field spectrum is of lower energy than that in-field, there is a risk of any peripheral NPs enhancing the out-of-field dose and delivering unnecessary dose to healthy tissues [78].

Also underlining the importance of an accurate spectrum model for dose calculations is sensitivity enhancement observed when cells loaded with high-Z NPs are irradiated with megavoltage beams [79, 80]. The mean energy of these beams might suggest minimal dose enhancement on the macroscopic scale. When the simulation performed in figure 6.5(b) is repeated with a volume containing the 15 mg g^{-1} GNP mixture, the calculated dose is relatively similar to that without the NPs. But in general these spectra are not without a low energy component. Some groups have looked at techniques such as modifying target materials and removing flattening filters as a means of increasing dose enhancement or increasing the low energy portions of megavoltage spectra [81, 82]. However, to really understand and effectively predict the dose enhancement effects, it becomes necessary to turn to more detailed models that incorporate the microscopic picture.

6.9 NPRT dosimetry on the microscopic scale

The challenges to accurate dosimetry outlined in the previous section are not insurmountable. However, when the scope of the problem is limited to the macroscopic picture, even with accurate dosimetry, it may still be of limited value for predicting therapeutic effects and planning treatments. Let us define clinically relevant levels of dose enhancement to be 5% or greater when calculated on the macroscopic scale. Achieving these levels of enhancement requires relatively high concentrations of high-Z NPs (several mg g^{-1} for GNPs) and low energy, kilovoltage photon spectra. Yet, there is plenty of *in vitro* experimental evidence demonstrating that the enhancement of biological effects, such as cell survival, can occur using megavoltage sources and lower NP concentrations [16, 80, 83–88]. This suggests that there is more detail to the story of nanoparticle dosimetry than dose enhancement on the macroscopic scale.

In this section we consider the details on a much smaller scale. The energy deposition patterns shown in figures 6.3 and 6.4 suggest that the vast majority of excess energy deposited in a medium containing high-Z NPs will be deposited within a few hundred nm of each NP. In turn, this implies that the location of each NP relative to sensitive structures within a given cell may play a very important role in the cell's overall response. Determining the pattern of energy deposition on the microscopic scale, at least in a statistical sense, can then be used to inform models of biological response [14, 89–91].

One approach to generating maps of expected dose values on such small scales is a point kernel technique [38, 92]. Figure 6.9 presents a hypothetical scenario. The same brain patient depicted in figure 6.5, with a volume containing a known quantity of GNPs outlined in black, is irradiated. For simplicity, we have only drawn a single incident beam angle. However, now we are interested in the energy deposition pattern to an arbitrary microscopic volume within the patient, rather than macroscopic volumes. These microscopic volumes are roughly the size of a cell or cellular organelle, small enough that the high-Z NPs can be considered explicitly. In principle, if the fluence differential in energy through a voxel and the local arrangement of high-Z NPs are known or can be predicted on a statistical basis, we should be able to calculate the expected dose at any given point in that volume.

To establish a framework for determining dose on the microscopic scale we consider the dose to a very small volume dV, centered at some position $\bar{x} = (x, y, z)$ as shown on the right-hand side of figure 6.9. Under irradiation, this volume will

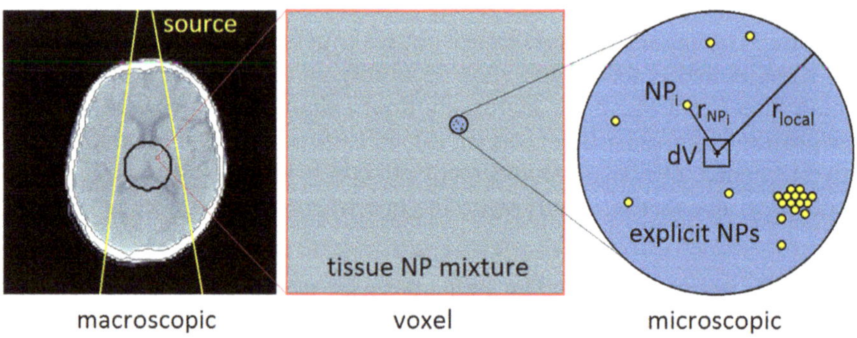

Figure 6.9. A hypothetical scenario where a phantom containing high-Z NPs is irradiated. The left side shows the macroscopic picture where the radiation travels through a voxelized geometry. Each voxel (~mm) in the phantom is taken as a homogeneous mixture of soft tissue and high-Z NPs determined by the mean uptake within the voxel. On the right we zoom in to the microscopic scale where NPs are defined explicitly. Within the tissue NP mixture a local volume can be defined by a distance r_{local} (~10 μm). Inside of r_{local} the NPs can be considered explicitly. Outside of this, they may be treated as mixture material with an effective atomic number and density resulting from a bulk aggregate of the medium and NPs together.

absorb dose from electrons generated by photon interactions in the surrounding high-Z NPs as well as the surrounding medium. Dose contributions from each high-Z NP, NP_i, will depend on their positions relative to the sensitive volume, i.e. $\bar{r}_{NP_i} = (\bar{x} - \bar{x}_{NP_i})$. The steep dose gradients around any given NP will mean that for those NPs closest to dV, even small changes in their relative positions will result in large differences in expected dose. As the distance from the NP to dV increases, this sensitivity diminishes to the point where dose contributions from distant particles really only depend on the bulk density or become negligible.

To distinguish these scales, and for purposes of computational efficiency, we define a 'local volume' (shown as a blue circle in figure 6.9, center and right) with a radius of r_{local}. Typically, r_{local} would be on the order of about ten microns (see figure 6.10). Beyond this distance, different random distributions of NPs with the same bulk density show very little variance between random particle placements. Inside the volume defined by r_{local}, NPs can be considered explicitly. The total dose to dV, $D(\bar{x})$, is then a combination of dose arising from interactions in the surrounding 'non-local' medium (including both NPs and soft tissue) and carried in by electrons if they have sufficient range, interactions in the local medium, and interactions in each local NP.

The macroscopic voxel dose in the absence of any local NPs can be defined as $D_{mac}(\bar{x})$. This value can be calculated by a conventional treatment planning system. It represents contributions from photon interactions in the surrounding tissue medium. For higher average NP concentrations the voxel dose can change as shown in the previous section, adding some dose to dV from higher energy, longer range, electrons. Under such circumstances one may be able to use cavity theory to extract the dose to tissue from the dose calculated in media containing an NP-tissue mixture from beyond r_{local}. To this value, contributions from individual NPs in the

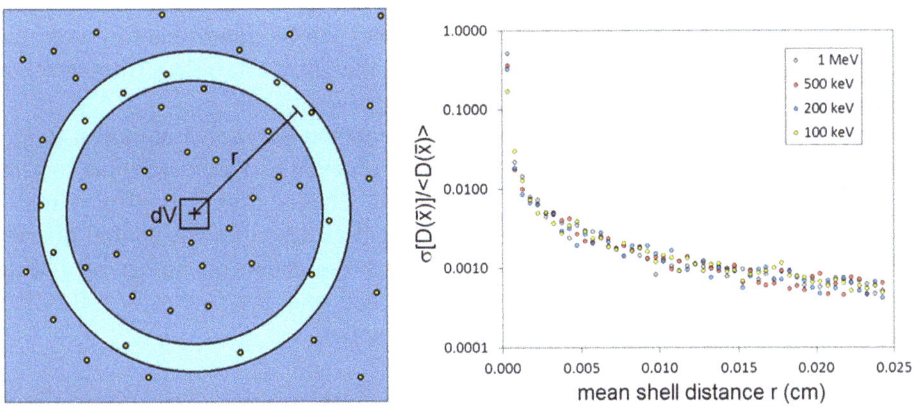

Figure 6.10. For a random distribution of GNPs at a bulk mass ratio of 1 mg g^{-1}, the dose, $D(\bar{x})$, to a small volume dV can be calculated for a series of concentric shells (depicted on the left side). Over multiple cases, the relative standard deviation in possible doses contributed from each shell falls rapidly with distance from dV (right side). At approximately 10 μm the relative standard deviation in dose drops below 1% for a broad range of incident energies. The specific geometrical configuration of GNPs strongly influences dose inside this distance. Therefore, we define r_{local} at approximately 10 μm.

local volume (or possibly clusters of NPs depending on the details of the calculation) can then be added,

$$D(\bar{x}) = D_{\mathrm{mac}}(\bar{x}) + \sum_{i=1}^{N_{\mathrm{NP}}}[D_{\mathrm{NP}_i}(\bar{x}) - D_{\mathrm{tisNP}_i}(\bar{x})]. \tag{6.4}$$

Such a summation requires a detailed knowledge of the local distribution of NPs at the time of irradiation. The term $D_{\mathrm{NP}_i}(\bar{x})$ is the dose at $\bar{x}$ resulting from the ith NP (or NP cluster) located at a position $\bar{x}_{\mathrm{NP}_i}$ within $\mathrm{r}_{\mathrm{local}}$. For completeness we subtract the term $D_{\mathrm{tisNP}_i}(\bar{x})$, which would be the dose contribution to dV from an equivalent volume of tissue the NP has displaced (this term tends only to be relevant for higher energy cases where the mass attenuation coefficients of the NP material and tissue are similar). In cases where many NPs are packed very close together, equation (6.4) may over-estimate dose contributions because the NPs themselves can absorb electrons generated in neighbouring NPs [38]. To generate values or lookup tables to determine $D_{\mathrm{NP}_i}(\bar{x})$ we typically turn to Monte Carlo simulations that score dose as a function of radial distance from the NP, r, per incident photon fluence of a given energy on the NP, $\frac{D\mathrm{NP}(E,r)}{\Phi\mathrm{NP}(E)}$, such as those presented in figures 6.3 and 6.4. Then

$$D_{\mathrm{NP}_i}(\bar{x}) = K\int_0^{E_{max}} \Phi_{\mathrm{NP}}(E,\, \bar{x}_{\mathrm{NP}_i})\frac{D_{NP}(E,\, r_{\mathrm{NP}_i})}{\Phi_{\mathrm{NP}}(E)}dE. \tag{6.5}$$

Here $\Phi_{\mathrm{NP}}(E,\, \bar{x}_{\mathrm{NP}_i})$ is the photon fluence, differential in energy, at energy E, incident on the ith NP, and the integration is performed over the full photon spectrum. In most cases the photon fluence across a small cavity defined by r_{local} will be uniform and not vary from NP to NP. The term K is a constant to maintain the same normalization scheme as that used for $D_{\mathrm{mac}}(\bar{x})$, such as dose per monitor unit.

An expectation value for the dose (or specific energy) deposited over a sensitive volume of interest (e.g. the cell nucleus, DNA, etc) can be determined by averaging $D(\bar{x})$ over that volume. Equations (6.4) and (6.5) therefore establish a framework for detailed dosimetry in the presence of high-Z NPs.

Obviously it would be too computationally intensive to solve equation (6.4) in detail for all possible NP distributions in a patient, even if it were possible to know the precise location of each NP within. This underscores the importance of establishing an accurate probability distribution that describes the spatial distribution, clustering and local density of NPs within the cells and media of a target volume. This will likely be established with detailed imaging studies of NP cellular uptake and accurate models of NP pharmacokinetics.

6.10 Challenges to modelling biological response

While dose can certainly be enhanced by NPs, the next major challenge with respect to treatment planning in NPRT is translating from the resulting dose distribution into a reliable prediction of clinical response. Ultimately, clinicians interested in using NPs as radiation sensitizers must have the confidence to know what combination of NP type, conjugates, concentration, delivery method, beam type, energy and exposure level will combine to produce a desired clinical effect.

Typically in response to radiation exposure, cell survival is expressed in terms of a surviving fraction. From this, quantities such as tumor control probability or normal tissue complication probability may be calculated and clinical response may be inferred. For sparsely ionizing radiation (e.g. x-rays), the surviving fraction can be related to the mean dose absorbed over a relatively large volume (containing many cells) by a linear quadratic relation [3, 4]. This approach simplifies a relatively complex biological process into something that can be expressed by only a few adjustable parameters. But as we've shown, high-Z NPs can generate highly heterogeneous dose distributions and amplify the stochastic nature of tracks running through target volumes, which can make predictions of biological response based on mean doses calculated over larger volumes problematic.

6.11 Further evidence for an NP-induced biological effect

The indirect mechanism of radiation-induced cell kill results from charged particle tracks inducing reactive oxygen species as well as reactive nitrogen species that can interact chemically with and generate lesions on macromolecules such as DNA. In one report, experimental measurements of the yield of hydroxyl radicals produced in aqueous solutions were not explained by dose alone, but could be explained with the addition of a catalytic-like reaction at the water–NP interface [93]. This suggests that in some cases NPs can enhance this indirect mechanism of cell kill.

NPs also have the potential to alter typical progression through the cell cycle, leading to an increase in the number of cells in the G2 and M phases [9, 94–97]. Cells in these phases tend to exhibit a higher sensitivity to a given dose of radiation. Hence, some NPs may indirectly make a population of proliferating cancer cells more sensitive on average simply by causing them to spend more time in the radiosensitive phases.

Another of the 'Rs' dictating cellular response to radiation is *repair*. Not all DNA damage has lethal consequences for a cell. Lesions, even double strand breaks, can be repaired, enabling a damaged cell to survive. NPs have also demonstrated the potential to interfere with the mechanics of DNA repair. Experiments showing the same degree of DNA damage initially had higher degrees of residual damage when NPs were present [80, 98, 99]. Not only does this suggest that the timeline following radiation exposure in the presence of NPs is important, but that models of DNA repair, once damage has been done may not hold to any benchmarks established in the absence of NPs.

The DNA is not the only sensitive structure within a cell. Other organelles such as mitochondria are known to play a role in cell proliferation, metabolism, and in triggering apoptotic response. GNPs have been shown to induce changes in mitochondrial membrane polarization and oxidation, which infers potential changes to overall radiosensitization [98]. In fact it may even be possible to use NPs to specifically target mitochondria [92].

Details of the specific mechanisms that determine the sensitivity enhancement aside, there is a need to translate from the set of possible heterogeneous dose distributions at the microscopic scale into predictions of biological, and ultimately treatment, response.

One proposal for translating the heterogeneous distributions of specific energy that result from the presence of high-Z NPs is a local effect model or LEM [14, 89, 91]. The LEM was initially proposed as a means of determining surviving fractions for high LET radiations [100–102]. McMahon *et al* proposed that this model could be applied to scenarios where high-Z NPs generate heterogeneous dose distributions when interacting with sparsely ionizing radiation (i.e. x-rays), and demonstrated success in modeling the surviving fraction for MDA-231 cells as a function of dose for 1.9 nm diameter GNPs [14]. In principle, rather than determining overall response from the mean expected dose through a given cell, the model attempts to calculate the probability of survival based on the dose to each point in the cell and integrates that over the volume to determine the probability of survival. One of the limitations of the model is that it does not account for the fact that certain sub-cellular volumes may play a more important role than others in governing overall survival when the cell is exposed to a heterogeneous distribution of specific energy.

Lechtman *et al* proposed a modification to the LEM model, which they referred to as a GNP radiosensitization predictive model [90]. After randomly distributing GNPs through model cell volumes, they used Monte Carlo-based track structure simulations to generate detailed specific energy distribution patterns through the cell nuclei. They then applied a modified probability density function over that volume to estimate the number of lethal lesions. This model was able to generate predictions of sensitivity enhancement for GNP-exposed PC-3 cells consistent with experimental results.

In addition to cellular response, it is also worth considering physiological response and patterns of cell kill. NPs introduced into the bloodstream can accumulate not just in the tumor itself, but in the microvasculature supporting it. The accumulation of GNPs in tumor microvasculature can potentially be harnessed as an anti-angiogenesis or anti-vascular therapy to prevent tumor growth [103, 104]. This of course has complex implications in that disruptions to the vasculature may create a hypoxic, radio-resistant tumor [105, 106] or disrupt the pharmacokinetics expected to deliver the NPs to their targets over the course of an extended NPRT treatment.

6.12 Conclusions and a look forward

Effective treatment planning for NPRT is going to be extremely challenging. As shown in this chapter, the dose enhancing properties of high-Z NPs are likely to generate a more effective form of radiotherapy when the pharmacokinetics of the NPs result in their preferential accumulation within a tumor. In a best case scenario this offers the potential to conform the radiation therapy dose distribution and lines of iso-effect to the physiology of the disease and dramatically reduce dose to peripheral organs at risk, reducing toxicities that would otherwise result from conventional approaches to treatment. But the challenges are numerous.

Accurate treatment planning will require: (i) accurate estimates of high-Z NP concentrations at macroscopic (voxel-to-voxel) scales, which are limited by conventional technologies, (ii) accurate calculations of the dose distribution on at least the macroscopic scale, (iii) the ability to extend the dosimetry into the microscopic (sub-cellular) scale, which in turn requires accurate models of the heterogeneous cellular uptake and sub-cellular distribution of NPs, and (iv) techniques to translate from dose and sub-cellular energy deposition patterns to biological effects, including effects the NPs may have on cellular response to radiation.

NPRT is likely to evolve with advances in these various challenges informing a 'top-down' experimental clinical trial approach where different combinations of NPs with different properties and conjugates are combined with radiation in an informed and well-designed manner, where clinical protocols will evolve from successful clinical outcomes.

References

[1] Zygmanski P and Sajo E 2016 Nanoscale radiation transport and clinical beam modeling for gold nanoparticle dose enhanced radiotherapy (GNPT) using x-rays *Br. J. Radiol.* **89** 20150200

[2] Schuemann J, Berbeco R, Chithrani D B, Cho S H, Kumar R, McMahon S J, Sridhar S and Krishnan S 2016 Roadmap to clinical use of gold nanoparticles for radiation sensitization *Int. J. Radiat. Oncol. Biol. Phys.* **94** 189–205

[3] Dale R G and Jones B 2007 *Radiobiological Modelling in Radiation Oncology* (London: The British Institute of Radiology)

[4] Joiner M and van der Kogel A 2009 *Basic Clinical Radiobiology* (London: Hodder Arnold)

[5] Supiot S, Lisbona A, Paris F, Azria D and Fenoglietto P 2010 ['Dose-painting': myth or reality?] *Cancer Radiother.* **14** 554–62

[6] Grau C, Overgaard J, Hoyer M, Tanderup K, Lindegaard J C and Muren L P 2015 Biology-guided adaptive radiotherapy (BiGART) is progressing towards clinical reality *Acta Oncol.* **54** 1245–50

[7] Maeda H, Fang J, Inutsuka T and Kitamoto Y 2003 Vascular permeability enhancement in solid tumor: various factors, mechanisms involved and its implications *Int. Immunopharmacol.* **3** 319–28

[8] Steichen S D, Caldorera-Moore M and Peppas N A 2013 A review of current nanoparticle and targeting moieties for the delivery of cancer therapeutics *Eur. J. Pharm. Sci.* **48** 416–27

[9] Geng F, Song K, Xing J Z, Yuan C, Yan S, Yang Q, Chen J and Kong B 2011 Thio-glucose bound gold nanoparticles enhance radio-cytotoxic targeting of ovarian cancer *Nanotechnology* **22** 285101

[10] Kong T, Zeng J, Wang X, Yang X, Yang J, McQuarrie S, McEwan A, Roa W, Chen J and Xing J Z 2008 Enhancement of radiation cytotoxicity in breast-cancer cells by localized attachment of gold nanoparticles *Small* **4** 1537–43

[11] Giljohann D A, Seferos D S, Daniel W L, Massich M D, Patel P C and Mirkin C A 2010 Gold nanoparticles for biology and medicine *Angew. Chem. Int. Ed. Engl.* **49** 3280–94

[12] Hahn M A, Singh A K, Sharma P, Brown S C and Moudgil B M 2011 Nanoparticles as contrast agents for in-vivo bioimaging: current status and future perspectives *Anal. Bioanal. Chem.* **399** 3–27

[13] Berger M J, Hubbell J H, Seltzer S M, Chang J, Coursey J S, Skukmar R, Zucker D S and Olsen K 2010 *XCOM: Photon Cross Sections Database NBSIR 87-3597* (Gaithersburg, MD: National Institute of Science and Technology, Physical Measurement Laboratory, Radiation Physics Division)

[14] McMahon S J *et al* 2011 Biological consequences of nanoscale energy deposition near irradiated heavy atom nanoparticles *Sci. Rep.* **1** 18

[15] Chithrani B D, Ghazani A A and Chan W C 2006 Determining the size and shape dependence of gold nanoparticle uptake into mammalian cells *Nano Lett.* **6** 662–8

[16] Chithrani D B, Jelveh S, Jalali F, van Prooijen M, Allen C, Bristow R G, Hill R P and Jaffray D A 2010 Gold nanoparticles as radiation sensitizers in cancer therapy *Radiat. Res.* **173** 719–28

[17] Chithrani D B, Dunne M, Stewart J, Allen C and Jaffray D A 2009 Cellular uptake and transport of gold nanoparticles incorporated in a liposomal carrier *Nanomedicine* **6** 161–9

[18] Menzel H-G *et al* 2011 Report 86: Quantification and reporting of low-dose and other heterogeneous exposures *J. ICRU* **11** 1–77

[19] ICRU 1983 *ICRU Report 36: Microdosimetry* (Bethesda, MD: International Commission on Radiation Units and Measurements)

[20] Nikjoo H and Lindborg L 2010 RBE of low energy electrons and photons *Phys. Med. Biol.* **55** R65–R109

[21] Fernandez-Varea J M, Gonzalez-Munoz G, Galassi M E, Wiklund K, Lind B K, Ahnesjo A and Tilly N 2012 Limitations (and merits) of PENELOPE as a track-structure code *Int. J. Radiat. Biol.* **88** 66–70

[22] Thomson R M and Kawrakow I 2011 On the Monte Carlo simulation of electron transport in the sub-1 keV energy range *Med. Phys.* **38** 4531–4

[23] Berger M J, Coursey J S, Zucker M A and Chang J 2005 *ESTAR, PSTAR, and ASTAR: Computer Programs for Calculating Stopping-Power and Range Tables for Electrons, Protons, and Helium Ions (version 1.2.3)* (Gaithersburg, MD: National Institute of Standards and Technology) Available: http://physics.nist.gov/Star [2017, Sept. 15]

[24] Uehara S, Nikjoo H and Goodhead D T 1999 Comparison and assessment of electron cross sections for Monte Carlo track structure codes *Radiat. Res.* **152** 202–13

[25] Meesungnoen J, Jay-Gerin J P, Filali-Mouhim A and Mankhetkorn S 2002 Low-energy electron penetration range in liquid water *Radiat. Res.* **158** 657–60

[26] Wilson W E, Miller J H, Lynch D J, Lewis R R and Batdorf M 2004 Analysis of low-energy electron track structure in liquid water *Radiat. Res.* **161** 591–6

[27] Pimblott S M and Siebbeles L D A 2002 Energy loss by non-relativistic electrons and positrons in liquid water *Nucl. Instrum. Methods Phys. Res.* B **194** 237–50

[28] Francis Z, Incerti S, Capra R, Mascialino B, Montarou G, Stepan V and Villagrasa C 2011 Molecular scale track structure simulations in liquid water using the Geant4-DNA Monte-Carlo processes *Appl. Radiat. Isot.* **69** 220–6

[29] Lechtman E, Chattopadhyay N, Cai Z, Mashouf S, Reilly R and Pignol J P 2011 Implications on clinical scenario of gold nanoparticle radiosensitization in regards to photon energy, nanoparticle size, concentration and location *Phys. Med. Biol.* **56** 4631–47

[30] Gadoue S M, Toomeh D, Zygmanski P and Sajo E 2017 Angular dose anisotropy around gold nanoparticles exposed to x-rays *Nanomedicine* **13** 1653–61

[31] Spaas C *et al* 2016 Dependence of gold nanoparticle radiosensitization on functionalizing layer thickness *Radiat. Res.* **185** 384–92

[32] Wang C-H *et al* 2008 Optimizing the size and surface properties of polyetheylene glycol (PEG)-gold nanoparticles by intense x-ray irradiation *J. Phys. D: Appl. Phys.* **41** 195301

[33] Koger B and Kirkby C 2017 Dosimetric effects of polyethylene glycol surface coatings on gold nanoparticle radiosensitization *Phys. Med. Biol.* **62** 8455–69

[34] Lechtman E and Pignol J P 2017 Interplay between the gold nanoparticle sub-cellular localization, size, and the photon energy for radiosensitization *Sci. Rep.* **7** 13268

[35] Cho E C, Zhang Q and Xia Y 2011 The effect of sedimentation and diffusion on cellular uptake of gold nanoparticles *Nat. Nanotechnol.* **6** 385–91

[36] Chithrani B D and Chan W C 2007 Elucidating the mechanism of cellular uptake and removal of protein-coated gold nanoparticles of different sizes and shapes *Nano Lett.* **7** 1542–50

[37] Alkilany A M and Murphy C J 2010 Toxicity and cellular uptake of gold nanoparticles: what we have learned so far? *J. Nanopart. Res.* **12** 2313–33

[38] Kirkby C, Koger B, Suchowerska N and McKenzie D R 2017 Dosimetric consequences of gold nanoparticle clustering during photon irradiation *Med. Phys.* **44** 6560–9

[39] Koger B and Kirkby C 2016 Optimization of photon beam energies in gold nanoparticle enhanced arc radiation therapy using Monte Carlo methods *Phys. Med. Biol.* **61** 8839–53

[40] McMahon S J, Mendenhall M H, Jain S and Currell F 2008 Radiotherapy in the presence of contrast agents: a general figure of merit and its application to gold nanoparticles *Phys. Med. Biol.* **53** 5635–51

[41] van der Merwe D, Van Dyk J, Healy B, Zubizarreta E, Izewska J, Mijnheer B and Meghzifene A 2017 Accuracy requirements and uncertainties in radiotherapy: a report of the International Atomic Energy Agency *Acta Oncol.* **56** 1–6

[42] Hirn S *et al* 2011 Particle size-dependent and surface charge-dependent biodistribution of gold nanoparticles after intravenous administration *Eur. J. Pharm. Biopharm.* **77** 407–16

[43] Sarin H 2010 Physiologic upper limits of pore size of different blood capillary types and another perspective on the dual pore theory of microvascular permeability *J. Angiogenes. Res.* **2** 14

[44] Unezaki S, Maruyama K, Hosoda J I, Nagae I, Koyanagi Y, Nakata M, Ishida O, Iwatsuru M and Tsuchiya S 1996 Direct measurement of the extravasation of polyethylglycol-coated liposomes into solid tumor tissue by *in vivo* fluorescence microscopy *Int. J. Pharm.* **144** 11–7

[45] Duan X and Li Y 2013 Physicochemical characteristics of nanoparticles affect circulation, biodistribution, cellular internalization, and trafficking *Small* **9** 1521–32

[46] Choi H S, Liu W, Misra P, Tanaka E, Zimmer J P, Itty Ipe B, Bawendi M G and Frangioni J V 2007 Renal clearance of quantum dots *Nat. Biotechnol.* **25** 1165–70

[47] Huang K *et al* 2012 Size-dependent localization and penetration of ultrasmall gold nanoparticles in cancer cells, multicellular spheroids, and tumors *in vivo ACS Nano* **6** 4483–93

[48] Perrault S D, Walkey C, Jennings T, Fischer H C and Chan W C 2009 Mediating tumor targeting efficiency of nanoparticles through design *Nano Lett.* **9** 1909–15

[49] Albanese A, Tang P S and Chan W C 2012 The effect of nanoparticle size, shape, and surface chemistry on biological systems *Annu. Rev. Biomed. Eng.* **14** 1–16
[50] Frohlich E 2012 The role of surface charge in cellular uptake and cytotoxicity of medical nanoparticles *Int. J. Nanomed.* **7** 5577–91
[51] Albanese A and Chan W C 2011 Effect of gold nanoparticle aggregation on cell uptake and toxicity *ACS Nano* **5** 5478–89
[52] Bazak R, Houri M, El Achy S, Kamel S and Refaat T 2015 Cancer active targeting by nanoparticles: a comprehensive review of literature *J. Cancer Res. Clin. Oncol.* **141** 769–84
[53] Chetty I J *et al* 2007 Report of the AAPM Task Group No. 105: Issues associated with clinical implementation of Monte Carlo-based photon and electron external beam treatment planning *Med. Phys.* **34** 4818–53
[54] Hoffmann L, Jorgensen M B, Muren L P and Petersen J B 2012 Clinical validation of the Acuros XB photon dose calculation algorithm, a grid-based Boltzmann equation solver *Acta Oncol.* **51** 376–85
[55] Popovtzer R, Agrawal A, Kotov N A, Popovtzer A, Balter J, Carey T E and Kopelman R 2008 Targeted gold nanoparticles enable molecular CT imaging of cancer *Nano Lett.* **8** 4593–6
[56] Reuveni T, Motiei M, Romman Z, Popovtzer A and Popovtzer R 2011 Targeted gold nanoparticles enable molecular CT imaging of cancer: an *in vivo* study *Int. J. Nanomed.* **6** 2859–64
[57] Curry T, Kopelman R, Shilo M and Popovtzer R 2014 Multifunctional theranostic gold nanoparticles for targeted CT imaging and photothermal therapy *Contrast Media Mol. Imaging* **9** 53–61
[58] Meir R, Motiei M and Popovtzer R 2014 Gold nanoparticles for *in vivo* cell tracking *Nanomedicine* **9** 2059–69
[59] Hainfeld J F, Slatkin D N, Focella T M and Smilowitz H M 2006 Gold nanoparticles: a new x-ray contrast agent *Br. J. Radiol.* **79** 248–53
[60] Galper M W, Saung M T, Fuster V, Roessl E, Thran A, Proksa R, Fayad Z A and Cormode D P 2012 Effect of computed tomography scanning parameters on gold nanoparticle and iodine contrast *Invest. Radiol.* **47** 475–81
[61] Xu C, Tung G A and Sun S 2008 Size and concentration effect of gold nanoparticles on x-ray attenuation as measured on computed tomography *Chem. Mater.* **20** 4167–9
[62] Mutic S, Palta J R, Butker E K, Das I J, Huq M S, Loo L N, Salter B J, McCollough C H and Van Dyk J 2003 Quality assurance for computed-tomography simulators and the computed-tomography-simulation process: report of the AAPM Radiation Therapy Committee Task Group No. 66 *Med. Phys.* **30** 2762–92
[63] Alivov Y, Baturin P, Le H Q, Ducote J and Molloi S 2014 Optimization of K-edge imaging for vulnerable plaques using gold nanoparticles and energy resolved photon counting detectors: a simulation study *Phys. Med. Biol.* **59** 135–52
[64] Cai Z, Pignol J P, Chattopadhyay N, Kwon Y L, Lechtman E and Reilly R M 2013 Investigation of the effects of cell model and subcellular location of gold nanoparticles on nuclear dose enhancement factors using Monte Carlo simulation *Med. Phys.* **40** 114101
[65] Butterworth K T, McMahon S J, Taggart L E and Prise K M 2013 Radiosensitization by gold nanopartiles: effective at megavoltage energies and potential role of oxidative stress *Transl. Cancer Res.* **2** 269–79

[66] Cheong S K, Jones B L, Siddiqi A K, Liu F, Manohar N and Cho S H 2010 X-ray fluorescence computed tomography (XFCT) imaging of gold nanoparticle-loaded objects using 110 kVp x-rays *Phys. Med. Biol.* **55** 647–62
[67] Jones B L, Manohar N, Reynoso F, Karellas A and Cho S H 2012 Experimental demonstration of benchtop x-ray fluorescence computed tomography (XFCT) of gold nanoparticle-loaded objects using lead- and tin-filtered polychromatic cone-beams *Phys. Med. Biol.* **57** N457–67
[68] Manohar N, Reynoso F J and Cho S H 2013 Experimental demonstration of direct L-shell x-ray fluorescence imaging of gold nanoparticles using a benchtop x-ray source *Med. Phys.* **40** 080702
[69] Hainfeld J F, Smilowitz H M, O'Connor M J, Dilmanian F A and Slatkin D N 2013 Gold nanoparticle imaging and radiotherapy of brain tumors in mice *Nanomedicine* **8** 1601–9
[70] Khlebtsov N and Dykman L 2011 Biodistribution and toxicity of engineered gold nanoparticles: a review of *in vitro* and *in vivo* studies *Chem. Soc. Rev.* **40** 1647–71
[71] Martinov M P and Thomson R M 2017 Heterogeneous multiscale Monte Carlo simulations for gold nanoparticle radiosensitization *Med. Phys.* **44** 644–53
[72] Landry G, Reniers B, Murrer L, Lutgens L, Gurp E B, Pignol J P, Keller B, Beaulieu L and Verhaegen F 2010 Sensitivity of low energy brachytherapy Monte Carlo dose calculations to uncertainties in human tissue composition *Med. Phys.* **37** 5188–98
[73] Afsharpour H, Pignol J P, Keller B, Carrier J F, Reniers B, Verhaegen F and Beaulieu L 2010 Influence of breast composition and interseed attenuation in dose calculations for post-implant assessment of permanent breast 103Pd seed implant *Phys. Med. Biol.* **55** 4547–61
[74] Hioki K, Araki F, Ohno T, Nakaguchi Y and Tomiyama Y 2014 Absorbed dose measurements for kV-cone beam computed tomography in image-guided radiation therapy *Phys. Med. Biol.* **59** 7297–313
[75] Koger B and Kirkby C 2016 A method for converting dose-to-medium to dose-to-tissue in Monte Carlo studies of gold nanoparticle-enhanced radiotherapy *Phys. Med. Biol.* **61** 2014–24
[76] Tsiamas P *et al* 2013 Impact of beam quality on megavoltage radiotherapy treatment techniques utilizing gold nanoparticles for dose enhancement *Phys. Med. Biol.* **58** 451–64
[77] Kry S F, Titt U, Ponisch F, Followill D, Vassiliev O N, White R A, Mohan R and Salehpour M 2006 A Monte Carlo model for calculating out-of-field dose from a varian 6 MV beam *Med. Phys.* **33** 4405–13
[78] Brivio D, Zygmanski P, Arnoldussen M, Hanlon J, Chell E, Sajo E, Makrigiorgos G M and Ngwa W 2015 Kilovoltage radiosurgery with gold nanoparticles for neovascular age-related macular degeneration (AMD): a Monte Carlo evaluation *Phys. Med. Biol.* **60** 9203–13
[79] Jain S, Hirst D G and O'Sullivan J M 2012 Gold nanoparticles as novel agents for cancer therapy *Br. J. Radiol.* **85** 101–13
[80] Jain S *et al* 2011 Cell-specific radiosensitization by gold nanoparticles at megavoltage radiation energies *Int. J. Radiat. Oncol. Biol. Phys.* **79** 531–9
[81] Berbeco R I, Detappe A, Tsiamas P, Parsons D, Yewondwossen M and Robar J 2016 Low Z target switching to increase tumor endothelial cell dose enhancement during gold nanoparticle-aided radiation therapy *Med. Phys.* **43** 436
[82] Tsiamas P, Mishra P, Cifter F, Berbeco R I, Marcus K, Sajo E and Zygmanski P 2014 Low-Z linac targets for low-MV gold nanoparticle radiation therapy *Med. Phys.* **41** 021701
[83] Enferadi M, Fu S Y, Hong J H, Tung C J, Chao T C, Wey S P, Chiu C H, Wang C C and Sadeghi M 2018 Radiosensitization of ultrasmall GNP-PEG-cRGDfK in ALTS1C1

exposed to therapeutic protons and kilovoltage and megavoltage photons *Int. J. Radiat. Biol.* **94** 124–36

[84] Liu C J *et al* 2008 Enhanced x-ray irradiation-induced cancer cell damage by gold nanoparticles treated by a new synthesis method of polyethylene glycol modification *Nanotechnology* **19** 295104

[85] Rezaee Z, Yadollahpour A, Bayati V and Negad Dehbashi F 2017 Gold nanoparticles and electroporation impose both separate and synergistic radiosensitizing effects in HT-29 tumor cells: an *in vitro* study *Int J Nanomed.* **12** 1431–9

[86] Rahman W N 2010 Gold nanoparticles: novel radiobiological dose enhancement studies for radiation therapy, synchrotron based microbeam and stereotactic radiotherapy *PhD Thesis* Royal Melbourne Institute of Technology (RMIT University), Melbourne, Victoria, Australia

[87] Ma N, Wu F G, Zhang X, Jiang Y W, Jia H R, Wang H Y, Li Y H, Liu P, Gu N and Chen Z 2017 Shape-dependent radiosensitization effect of gold nanostructures in cancer radiotherapy: comparison of gold nanoparticles, nanospikes, and nanorods *ACS Appl. Mater. Interfaces* **9** 13037–48

[88] Liu C J *et al* 2010 Enhancement of cell radiation sensitivity by pegylated gold nanoparticles *Phys. Med. Biol.* **55** 931–45

[89] Brown J M C and Currell F J 2017 A local effect model-based interpolation framework for experimental nanoparticle radiosensitisation data *Cancer Nanotechnol.* **8** 1

[90] Lechtman E, Mashouf S, Chattopadhyay N, Keller B M, Lai P, Cai Z, Reilly R M and Pignol J P 2013 A Monte Carlo-based model of gold nanoparticle radiosensitization accounting for increased radiobiological effectiveness *Phys. Med. Biol.* **58** 3075–87

[91] McMahon S J *et al* 2011 Nanodosimetric effects of gold nanoparticles in megavoltage radiation therapy *Radiother. Oncol.* **100** 412–6

[92] Kirkby C and Ghasroddashti E 2015 Targeting mitochondria in cancer cells using gold nanoparticle-enhanced radiotherapy: a Monte Carlo study *Med. Phys.* **42** 1119–28

[93] Sicard-Roselli C, Brun E, Gilles M, Baldacchino G, Kelsey C, McQuaid H, Polin C, Wardlow N and Currell F 2014 A new mechanism for hydroxyl radical production in irradiated nanoparticle solutions *Small* **10** 3338–46

[94] Roa W *et al* 2009 Gold nanoparticle sensitize radiotherapy of prostate cancer cells by regulation of the cell cycle *Nanotechnology* **20** 375101

[95] Wang C, Jiang Y, Li X and Hu L 2015 Thioglucose-bound gold nanoparticles increase the radiosensitivity of a triple-negative breast cancer cell line (MDA-MB-231) *Breast Cancer* **22** 413–20

[96] Wang C, Li X, Wang Y, Liu Z, Fu L and Hu L 2013 Enhancement of radiation effect and increase of apoptosis in lung cancer cells by thio-glucose-bound gold nanoparticles at megavoltage radiation energies *J. Nanopart. Res.* **15** 1642

[97] Zhu C D, Zheng Q, Wang L X, Xu H F, Tong J L, Zhang Q A, Wan Y and Wu J Q 2015 Synthesis of novel galactose functionalized gold nanoparticles and its radiosensitizing mechanism *J. Nanobiotechnol.* **13** 67

[98] Taggart L E, McMahon S J, Currell F, Prise K M and Butterworth K T 2014 The role of mitochondrial function in gold nanoparticle mediated radiosensitisation *Cancer Nanotechnol.* **5** 5

[99] Cui L, Tse K, Zahedi P, Harding S M, Zafarana G, Jaffray D A, Bristow R G and Allen C 2014 Hypoxia and cellular localization influence the radiosensitizing effect of gold nanoparticles (AuNPs) in breast cancer cells *Radiat. Res.* **182** 475–88
[100] Scholz M and Kraft G 1994 Calculation of heavy ion inactivation probability based on track structure, x-ray sensitivity and target size *Radiat. Prot. Dosim.* **52** 29–33
[101] Scholz M and Kraft G 2004 The physical and radiobiological basis of the local effect model: a response to the commentary by R. Katz *Radiat. Res.* **161** 612–20
[102] Scholz M and Kraft G 1996 Track structure and the calculation of biological effects of heavy charged particles *Adv. Space Res.* **18** 5–14
[103] Berbeco R I, Ngwa W and Makrigiorgos G M 2011 Localized dose enhancement to tumor blood vessel endothelial cells via megavoltage x-rays and targeted gold nanoparticles: new potential for external beam radiotherapy *Int. J. Radiat. Oncol. Biol. Phys.* **81** 270–6
[104] Detappe A, Tsiamas P, Ngwa W, Zygmanski P, Makrigiorgos M and Berbeco R 2013 The effect of flattening filter free delivery on endothelial dose enhancement with gold nanoparticles *Med. Phys.* **40** 031706
[105] Ghasroddashti E, Kirkby C and Morrison H 2012 PD-0401: modelling tumour vasculature and radiation response using a simulated annealing approach *Radiother. Oncol.* **99** S160–1
[106] Kirkby C and Ghasroddashti E 2011 SU-E-T-08: A pO_2-based vascular tumour model for iterative radiobiological modelling *Med. Phys.* **38** 3487

Chapter 7

Nanoparticle enhanced radiotherapy: quality assurance perspective

Piotr Zygmanski, Davide Brivio and Erno Sajo

7.1 General

Nanoparticle enhanced radiotherapy (NPRT) uses high-Z nanoparticles (NPs) to enhance energy deposition at the cellular and/or molecular levels. NPRT is one of the emerging radiotherapy modalities with dozens of papers published each year, yet systematic treatment of the subject from the quality assurance (QA) perspective has not been attempted so far [1–3]. The production and use of radiation in medical imaging and treatment of cancer is a multifaceted enterprise requiring quality assurance (QA) and quality control (QC) [4–10]. Maintaining high QA standards is essential in designing and performing research, reporting findings, as well as in clinical implementations of new techniques or application of routine treatments.

Quality assurance of medical procedures, equipment and software is carried out in order to guarantee that the application of radiation is according to the prescription and it is safe, accurate and effective. The introduction of NPs into therapy and imaging naturally increases the demands for keeping high QA standards, and calls for the development of new or additional QA methodologies and metrics of quality that address issues that are specific to high-Z (HZ) NPs. Since currently nanoparticle-based medical procedures are in the preclinical research stage or in the experimental clinical stage, QA methods are not yet established and QA guidelines have not been developed. In the following, we adopt a radiotherapy (RT) perspective on quality assurance for NPRT.

Radiotherapy involves a chain of activities starting with delineation of tumor using MRI, PET and CT images, and planning the treatment in the CT space, which is directly suitable for dose calculations. In the treatment planning stage, dose is computed by converting patient CT data to electron densities of tissue. Next, treatment fields are optimized, including proper beam arrangement and spatio-dynamic modulation of flux of each field. This process is facilitated by commercial

doi:10.1088/978-0-7503-2396-3ch7

software, referred to as treatment planning system (TPS). During the commissioning stage of TPS, its dose calculation and optimization algorithms have to be tested and validated against experimental data prior to their intended uses. The accuracy of TPS systems depends on multiple factors and it is not homogeneous across multidimensional parameter space (spatial coordinates, depth, field size, energy, position with respect to field edges, type of heterogeneity, proximity to surface, time, etc). Before each radiotherapy treatment, the tumor has to be localized and targeted with radiation at 1 mm spatial accuracy and about 1%–5% absolute dose accuracy in the high-dose regions. In low-dose regions or gradient regions the relative errors may be larger.

For the purpose of patient setup and target localization, optical surface scanning, kilovoltage x-ray radiography and cone beam computed tomography (CBCT) as well as magnetic resonance imaging (MRI) are used. Radiotherapy treatment is typically carried out using medical linear accelerators that produce 6, 10 or 15 MV nominal energy x-ray beams or with radioactive brachytherapy sources, such as iodine-125 for low dose rates or iridium-192 for high dose rates. Although modern linacs are equipped with 40–120 kVp and 2.5 MV x-ray beamlines, these beamlines are used solely for imaging. Image-guided treatment necessitates general commissioning and experimental verification of the performance of various imaging and treatment equipment before each treatment fraction. Introduction of NPs into this chain leads to several noteworthy changes of the TPS, imaging, and treatment QA procedures. In the following, we summarize the essential new aspects of QA relevant to NPRT:

(a) imaging of NP distribution for treatment planning;
(b) verification of NP distribution for delivery of treatment;
(c) macroscopic dose calculation for treatment planning;
(d) microscopic dose calculation;
(e) estimation of radiobiological effects at macroscopic and nanoscopic scales.

7.2 Imaging and verification of NP distribution

Determination of NP presence in the tumor and normal tissue is essential for treatment planning purposes as well as for verification of NP distribution during the actual treatment. Distribution of NPs may be quite different depending on how the NP agent is applied: intravenous application with a subsequent tumor cell or tumor microvasculature uptake, application via direct injection into the tumor volume and retention in the intercellular spaces and/or cellular uptake, or via inhalation and concomitant lung deposition and ensuing cellular uptake.

While the presence of NPs in the normal tissue is undesired, it cannot be completely prevented. Ideally, 3D concentration distribution of NPs must be assessed before and during the course of treatment, as it is possible and likely that the NP concentration will not be constant during a treatment fraction or between fractions. The resulting dose distribution has to be computed based on the current NP concentrations in both diseased and normal tissue, and compared to the planning stage dose distribution.

Imaging of NP distribution for treatment planning and for delivery of treatment faces similar challenges and depends on the availability of imaging devices in the treatment simulation and delivery suites. The type of devices and their ability to image NPs may not be identical in simulation versus delivery of treatment. Practical determination of NP agent in the patient body in a clinical setting is not easy because it is limited by the imaging capabilities of clinical x-ray equipment (e.g. CT or CBCT) available on the linacs. The CT-detectable level of NP concentrations depends on kVp energy, size of patient, size of tumor, depth of tumor, tumor versus nearby anatomical structure morphology, concentration of NP agent, and x-ray flux or dose used for imaging. In principle, a small concentration of NP agent seems detectable because of relatively large differences in the attenuation coefficients of high-Z NP versus soft tissue, often reaching multiple orders of magnitude (chapters 1–3). However, a detailed analysis shows that precise measurement of practical NP concentrations with the standard CT might be difficult.

Figure 7.1(a) shows the total attenuation coefficient as a function of energy for water, gold, and a mixture of gold and water for medium to extremely large levels of gold concentrations ($c = 10, 100, 1000$ mg g^{-1}). Noteworthy for $c = 10$ mg g^{-1} is that there seems to be sufficient difference in attenuation for certain energies. However, for more realistic lower concentrations of gold in tissue ($c = 0.1, 0.5, 1$ mg g^{-1}) and for kVp beams (60 kVp–120 kVp) the resulting attenuation coefficient of mixture of gold with water is much smaller, as shown in figure 7.1(b). Figure 7.1(c) shows density of a mixture of gold with water $\rho(c)$ as a function of concentration c(mg g^{-1}) relative to water density (ρ(water) = 1 g cm^{-3}). For small concentrations of gold in water the density of mixture is very close to water (1.011 g cm^{-3}), as seen in figure 7.1(c). This 'dilution' of attenuation enhancement is especially problematic below $c = 1$ mg g^{-1}. While theoretically, one could detect such concentration levels of high-Z NP agent using standard CT, in practice the presence of noise and imaging artifacts have to be considered, which with the standard CT makes it difficult to quantify concentrations on the order of 1 mg g^{-1}.

If NPs are directly injected into the tumor the initial concentrations can be reasonably controlled and much higher concentrations can be delivered than in intravenous administration of NP agent to the whole body. In the case of gold NPs, experimentally investigated concentration range is up to about 30–60 mg g^{-1} tissue. This is sufficiently high to warrant their imaging with CT, for instance. But due to toxicity concerns, the clinical intravenous administration of NP is limited, and their uptake by the tumor may be much smaller ($\ll$1 mg g^{-1}) than can be measured using the standard clinical x-ray techniques.

Dual-energy CT (DECT) and especially multi energy (spectral) MECT with photon counting detectors have been shown to be much more sensitive and specific in the detection of contrast agents (chapter 12). Moreover, they are capable of quantification of contrast agents including new high-Z NP agents. However, so far DECT have not been commonly used for radiotherapy simulation and spectral CT with photon counting detectors is still under development, although promising results have been reported in animal models with various high-Z NP agents (chapter 12).

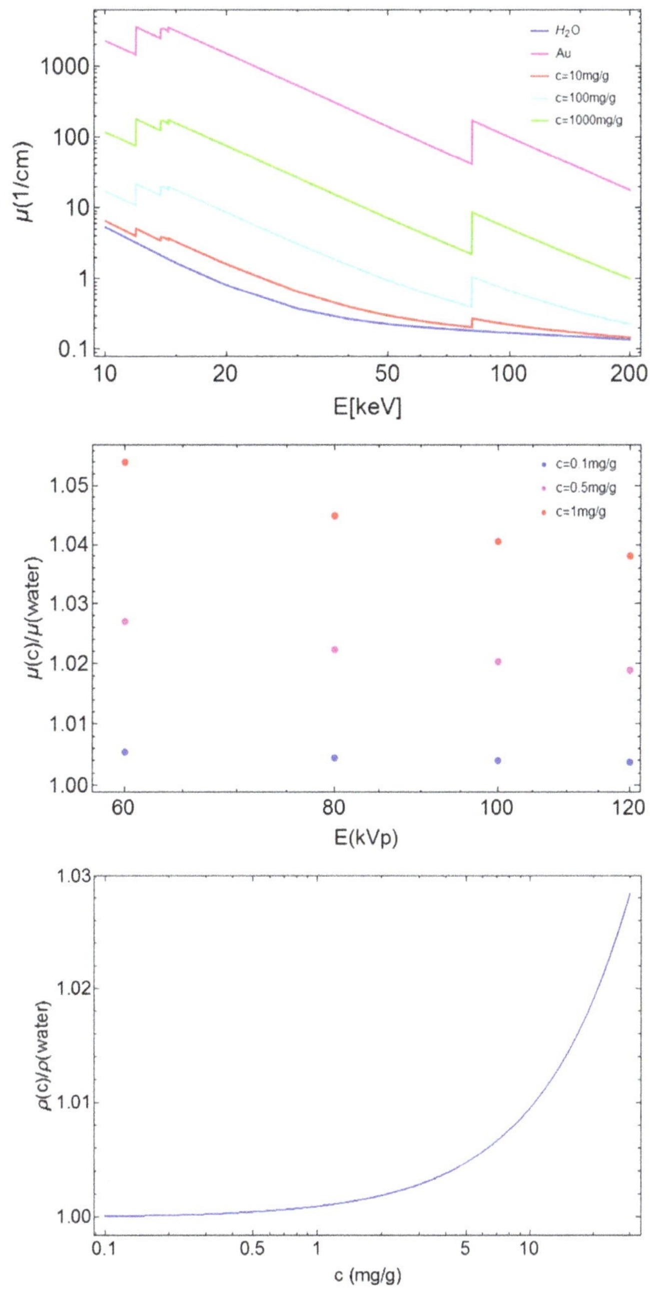

Figure 7.1. (a) Total attenuation coefficient for gold, water, and mixture of gold with water for selected concentrations c = 10, 100, 1000 mg g^{-1}. (b) The total attenuation coefficient $\mu(c)$ of a mixture of gold with water of concentration c = 0.1, 0.5, 1 mg g^{-1} for different kVp energies. The attenuation coefficient of the mixture μ(c) is normalized to the attenuation coefficient for water μ(water). (c) Density of a mixture of gold with water $\rho(c)$ as a function of concentration c (mg g^{-1}) relative to water density (ρ(water) = 1 g cm^{-3}). NIST data tables were used to compute quantities in (a) and (b) (https://physics.nist.gov/PhysRefData/XrayMassCoef/tab3.html and https://physics.nist.gov/PhysRefData/XrayMassCoef/tab4.html).

MRI imaging or x-ray fluorescence CT (XFCT) are potentially much more sensitive than CT (chapter 13). The former modality requires the development of a new hybrid paramagnetic-high-Z NP that can be imaged by MRI and be suitable for significant dose enhancement and yet is non-toxic. Detection of gadolinium-based NPs using MRI simulator or MRI-linac treatment machine is possible (chapter 13), however, quantification of NP concentration may be challenging due to calibration issues in MRI. The latter modality requires the development of x-ray fluorescence imagers and reconstruction techniques that would work with human subjects in clinical environment.

In summary, potential imaging techniques for HZ NPs include: CT, DECT, MECT, MRI and XFCT, in increasing sensitivity order. But quantitative calibration and integration of XFCT or MRI into the clinical workflow may pose problems. At the present stage of clinical technology, DECT and dual energy CBCT appear to be the more likely imaging modalities for clinical implementation of NPRT in simulation and treatment delivery. Spectral CT with photon counting detectors would be recommended once it is developed and available for radiotherapy.

Irrespective of which imaging modality is used, each imaging technique must be calibrated as a function of NP concentration with NP regions of known concentrations in realistic anthropomorphic phantoms. Second, uncertainties in the determination of NP concentration must be identified and their values expressed as a function of NP concentration and other factors, including the size of NP region and its depth, background anatomy or structure of the region with NP, heterogeneous concentration of agent, slice thickness, available x-ray flux at the NP region, and dose from imaging and noise level. There is also a potential but likely weak dependence on the NP size and clustering. Imaging equipment and reconstruction software must be routinely (e.g. weekly or monthly) tested for its ability to determine NP distribution versus the reference data obtained during commissioning stage.

7.3 Macroscopic dose calculation

Assuming that the concentration of NPs inside the tumor has been determined with one of the imaging techniques, the impact of 3D NP distribution and its associated uncertainties on the dose have to be evaluated. There are various scales and various radiobiological effects to consider for dose computation. Note that contemporary clinical imaging is not capable for spatial resolution better than about 1 mm × 1 mm × 1 mm, therefore it cannot provide NP concentration at the cellular level or even microvascular level (5–50 μm). Thus, in this section when we refer to NP distribution and the corresponding dose distribution, we refer to the macroscopic (~>1 mm × 1 mm × 1 mm) distribution in the tissue determined by linac based imaging. Macroscopic dose can be computed in the treatment planning system (TPS). However, depending on the quality of dose modeling in TPS, for small concentrations the macroscopic dose distribution may or may not be accurate. On the other hand, for microscopic or nanoscopic radiation effect computations TPS dose calculation cannot be used even in principle, and a dedicated multi-scale Monte Carlo radiation transport simulation must be used instead [3].

The first-level assessment of dose distribution is naturally at the macroscopic level. However, even in this situation there are several confounding factors to consider when assessing the validity of the dose calculation model and in interpreting the dosimetric results. The NP enhancement agent may be in macroscopic regions and its distribution may be heterogeneous in parts of the tumor or in normal tissue. Therefore, the NP distribution may unevenly impact the macroscopic beam properties: beam flux and spectrum inside and adjacent to the NP-affected regions may be disrupted compared to dose in tissue without high-Z materials.

Specifically, NP regions can harden the x-ray beam, and scattering from NP regions may affect nearby tissues laterally (scatter contribution) and longitudinally (attenuation). Similarly, the macroscopic dose enhancement may also be non-uniform. Because traditional TPS are invariably based on convolution-superposition methods employing rescaled dose deposition kernels in water, they are not designed to compute dose from or inside high-Z materials. Even for bony anatomy, which is an order of magnitude less dense than HZ materials of interest, they are expected to be less accurate. Hence, in a systematic and sound approach, 3D dose calculation should be performed using Monte Carlo simulations to properly account for spectral changes in the beam as it penetrates through the tissues containing NPs. The Monte Carlo computations should be tested against experimental data using phantoms containing high-Z materials and mixtures of high-Z with low-Z materials, as described at the end of this chapter.

In summary, macroscopic dose calculations for clinically achievable low concentrations of NP agent can be carried using TPS dose calculation only after properly testing it against MC dose computations (benchmarking) and diverse experimental setups (validation). For small concentrations of high-Z NP agents administered intravenously, the associated macroscopic radiation effects are likely to be similar to the effects from the standard iodine contrast, and therefore even the TPS dose calculation models may be valid for them after all. However, for directly injected HZ NP agents, the concentrations may be much higher and unvalidated TPS models may be inadequate.

7.4 Radiobiological effect from macroscopic dose enhancement

The impact of macroscopically non-uniform dose enhancement on normal tissue and tumor responses requires consideration of biological effectiveness for the whole organ or tumor. The partial volume effect due to unequal NP enhancement within the tumor or organ could be accounted for by using, for instance, the concept of equivalent uniform dose (EUD) or similar ideas [3, 10]. Parameters of the EUD or similar models must be determined for each tumor and organ type loaded with NP. At present, there are no studies dedicated to such radiation transport and equivalent biological dose effects in NP radiotherapy, except for theoretical studies. For low levels of macroscopic concentrations of NP, one could rely on the model EUD parameters derived in the past for standard radiotherapy without NPs. However, it may not be recommended to extend the macroscopic EUD model parameters to microscopic dose enhancement, as the underlying radiobiology at tissue versus cell levels could be very different and lead to very different cell survival.

7.5 Microscopic dose calculation

At the cellular level, the presence of NPs leads to extremely localized dose enhancement. The real biological impact depends on the distances of NPs to the cellular targets relative to the range of secondary charged particles escaping from the NPs and the diffusion distance of the reactive oxygen species generated by them [2]. Unfortunately, imaging at the cellular level can only be done with cell samples and is not feasible in humans or animals *in vivo*. However, imaging studies confirming NP distributions at the cellular level are essential for the development of biological response models or radiosensitization models due to NPs (chapters 10 and 11).

At the required NP mass density for the effective dose coverage, the number density of NPs may range from 10^{10} to 10^{16} particles per cm^3 of tissue, depending on the size of the NPs. The collision density of these particles by Brownian motion is significant, which can lead to agglomeration and clustering. At the cellular level, clustering of NPs may have an impact on dose enhancement [11]. Because clustering increases the effective size of the NP, it may lead to degradation of enhancement via self-absorption of electrons in the constituent NPs (instead of forming tracks and ionizing the cellular medium, electrons are absorbed in other NP in their bulk). This inefficient use of the high-Z material depends on the cluster size and morphology. Determination of how much radiation is wasted inside the clustered bulk NPs and how much goes to the cellular medium is an essential step for estimating the biological effects and can be obtained only via detailed nano-micro-scale computations [2, 11]. However, the knowledge of the presence of clustering and the size and morphology of the aggregates must be derived from experimental imaging of NP uptake by cells and from NP hydrodynamic transport in bloodstream or diffusion in tissue.

7.6 Radiobiological effect from microscopic dose enhancement

Furthermore, nanoscopic dose enhancement must be computed within a specific cellular target volume and correlated to the cellular survival. The cell survival model must employ stochastic integration over the cellular target volume [10]. Biologically equivalent dose (BED) or EUD concepts can be extended to convert nanoscopic dose enhancement to macroscopic dose in TPS but they must rely on a stochastic modeling of cell survival, accounting for nanoscopic dose variations in a population of cells. Such models can be derived by extending the linear quadratic (LQ) model [3, 9, 10] to account for nanoscopic dose heterogeneity and distribution of NPs or NP clusters among the cells. The effective uniform dose can be derived by employing the same cellular survival for the homogeneous dose and dose with nanoscopic enhancements.

In summary, nano-/micro-scale MC computations are essential for estimation of physical dose enhancement and radiobiological impact using stochastic modeling.

But they have to be used together with experimental parameters derived from cell survival studies with specific cell lines and with clinical outcomes (not available yet). Fluid dynamic transport of NP and NP agglomeration state at the time of the injection and after reaching the tumor tissue may be essential to optimize NP size, distribution and delivery methods (direct or intravenous injection).

7.7 Summary

The major areas for which new QA techniques must be developed are:

(i) imaging of NP distribution for simulation (planning) and delivery of treatment—probably based on DECT or MECT,
(ii) calibration of images to obtain NP concentrations (macroscopic for traditional dose calculation as well as nano-/microscopic for radiobiological estimation),
(iii) macroscopic and nano-/microscopic dose computations in media containing high-*Z* material,
(iv) benchmarking and validation of TPS against Monte Carlo models and experiments,
(v) conversion of dose enhancement to biologically equivalent dose (nanoscale models and macro-scale models using different parameters),
(vi) consideration of particle clustering en-route from injection to tumor.

7.8 Experimental/computation setup

In the following, we will focus on quality assurance for x-ray based imaging (CT, CBCT) and Monte Carlo dose computations.

In macroscopic dose calculations it is relatively easy to obtain the ground truth based on experimental data and compare it to Monte Carlo simulation results as part of validation tests. However, nano- or micro-scale measurements are either not available or are very difficult to acquire and to interpret. For instance, determining NP cluster sizes and distributions or clustered radiation deposition from NPs is very challenging.

There are two main categories of simple experimental setup to consider for testing of imaging and dose calculation in the presence of NPs (figure 7.2):

(A) 3D phantoms with macroscopic inserts containing various uniform or gradually changing concentrations of high-*Z* NPs (low-*Z*–high-Z mixtures);
(B) slab phantoms with high-*Z* films of micrometer or nanometer thickness.

In experiments of type A, phantoms are suitable for calibration of images (Hounsfield Unit versus NP concentration or effective *Z* and *A* values) and macroscopic contrast agent dosimetry. Phantoms in type B experiments are mostly of interest for microdosimetry or dose enhancement or non-equilibrium phenomena at interfaces of high-*Z* materials. Experimental phantoms may contain a detector adjacent to or in the middle of the high-*Z* layers, or outside of it. Detectors can be either internal (measuring dose perturbation at the high-*Z*/low-*Z* interfaces) or

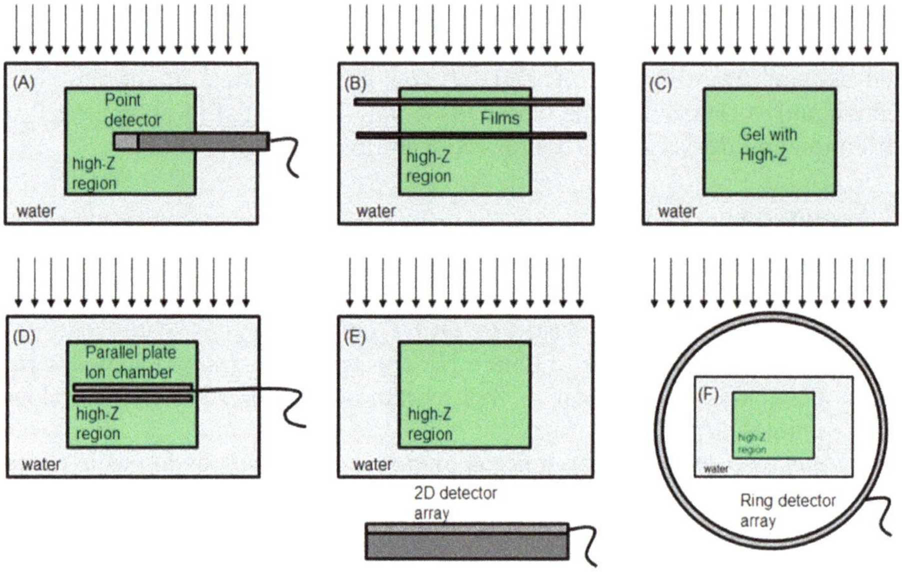

Figure 7.2. Various radiation detection schemes measuring the dose enhancement in macroscopic regions.

external to the phantom (measuring the flux through the phantom). Several possible detectors can be employed in these setups (figure 7.2):

(A) point detectors (ion chamber or diode);
(B) radiosensitive films;
(C) radiosensitive gel;
(D) variable-gap parallel plate ionization chamber with high-*Z* electrode;
(E) 2D detector array (transmission signal);,
(F) photon counting ring detector arrays (x-ray fluorescence, Compton scatter).

7.9 Benchmark and validation tests and data

For the purpose of testing radiation transport computations, several factors impacting dose enhancement have to be accounted for: composite phantom size, depth of the region with NP, energy of incident x-rays, beam collimation, distance from NP or high-*Z* region to target, NP size or region size and the type of simulation. The simplest class of simulation includes 1D radiation transport problems in slab geometry while the most complex are clustering of NPs in or around cellular targets with clustered deposition or damage. There are several versions of 1D radiation transport problems:

(A) high-*Z* layer of nanoscopic thickness (surrogate for a single layer of GNPs) in a homogeneous water phantom; suitable for testing radiation transport at nanoscale with high spatial resolution and interface phenomena (figure 7.3(a));
(B) layers composed of homogeneous mixtures of high-*Z* material and water of microscopic thickness inside surrounding water (surrogate for tumor

microvasculature with a defined NP concentration); suitable for testing transport at microscopic distances and long range phenomena (figure 7.3(b));

(C) high-Z material and water mixtures of macroscopic thickness (surrogate for macroscopic regions with NP with defined concentrations); suitable for testing TPS for macroscopic dose distribution (figure 7.3(c));

(D) similar to (C) but with an external detector measuring transmitted x-ray flux or NP emission flux; suitable for studying imaging (CT, XFCT) (figure 7.3(d)).

For macroscopic and for sub-millimeter regions with NPs, in addition to dose enhancement (DE) other metrics of dose perturbation must also be considered, including dose attenuation (DA) in the upstream and downstream regions with respect to NP region and the incident beam direction (figure 7.3(e)). Monte Carlo simulations supporting cell survival must be carried out with attention to specific macroscopic and microscopic architecture of the experiment (figure 7.4) that accounts for non-equilibrium interfacial effects at different material interfaces.

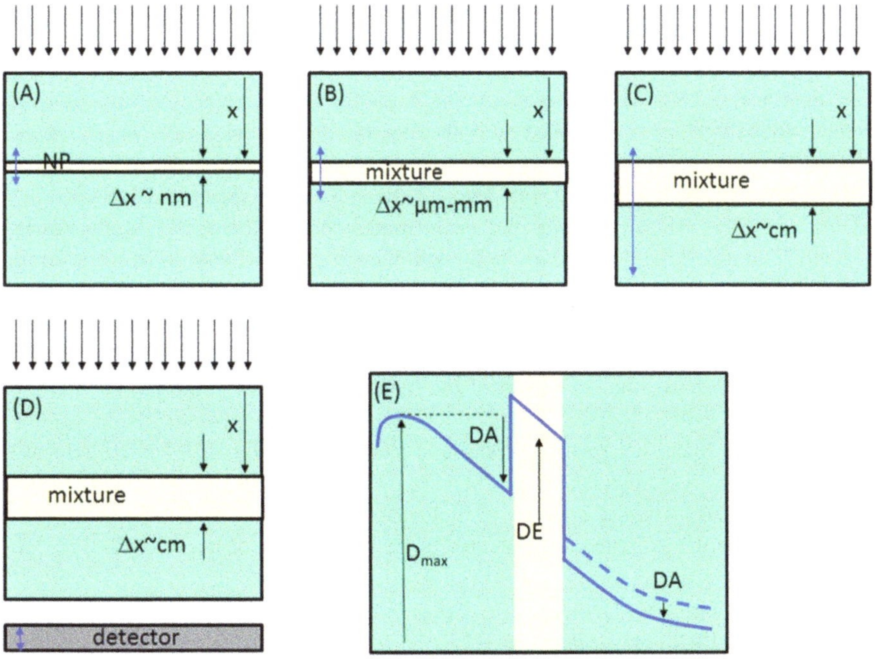

Figure 7.3. Benchmark radiation transport computations: (a) nanoscopic layer simulating a single contiguous layer of NPs individually or in planar clusters, (b) microscopic layer of NP mixed with water in a defined concentration, (c) macroscopic layer of NP mixture, (d) same as (c) but with a detector measuring transmitted flux, (e) schematic dose variation in the phantom with characteristic parameters: maximum dose (Dmax), dose enhancement (DE), dose attenuation (DA) in the upstream and downstream regions with respect to the NP region. The NP region is shaded with yellow and water with blue–green colors. Blue arrows mark the regions of interest.

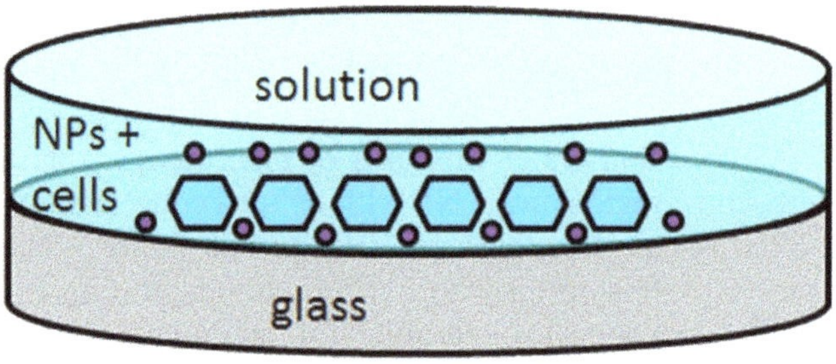

Figure 7.4. Possible experimental setup for radiobiology studies.

In the corresponding chapters 2, 3, we present benchmark data against which dose calculation methods could be tested. The data was generated using the deterministic radiation transport code (CEPXS/ONEDANT) in slab geometry.

References

[1] Peukert D, Kempson I, Douglass M and Bezak E 2018 Metallic nanoparticle radiosensitisation of ion radiotherapy: a review *Phys. Med.* **47** 121–8

[2] Ngwa W, Kumar R, Sridhar S, Korideck H, Zygmanski P, Cormack R A, Berbeco R and Makrigiorgos G M 2014 Targeted radiotherapy with gold nanoparticles: current status and future perspectives *Nanomedicine* **9** 1063–82

[3] Zygmanski P and Sajo E 2016 Nanoscale radiation transport and clinical beam modeling for gold nanoparticle dose enhanced radiotherapy (GNPT) using x-rays *Br. J. Radiol.* **89** 20150200

[4] Ma C M C, Chetty I J, Deng J, Faddegon B, Jiang S B, Li J, Seuntjens J, Siebers J V and Traneus E 2019 Beam modeling and beam model commissioning for Monte Carlo dose calculation-based radiation therapy treatment planning: Report of AAPM Task Group 157 *Med. Phys.* **47** e1–8

[5] Sechopoulos I, Rogers D W O, Bazalova-Carter M, Bolch W E, Heath E C, McNitt-Gray M F, Sempau J and Williamson J F 2017 RECORDS: improved Reporting of montE CarlO RaDiation transport Studies: Report of the AAPM Research Committee Task Group 268 *Med. Phys.* **45** e1–5

[6] Miften M *et al* 2018 Low, tolerance limits and methodologies for IMRT measurement-based verification QA: Recommendations of AAPM Task Group No. 218 *Med. Phys.* **45** e53–83

[7] Li X A *et al* 2012 The use and QA of biologically related models for treatment planning: Short report of the TG-166 of the therapy physics committee of the AAPM *Med. Phys.* **39** 1386–409

[8] Low D A, Moran J M, Dempsey J F, Dong L and Oldham M 2011 Dosimetry tools and techniques for IMRT *Med. Phys.* **38** 1313–38

[9] Ezzell G A *et al* 2009 IMRT commissioning: Multiple institution planning and dosimetry comparisons, a report from AAPM Task Group 119 *Med. Phys.* **36** 5359–73

[10] Zygmanski P, Hoegele W, Tsiamas P, Cifter F, Ngwa W, Berbeco R, Makrigiorgos M and Sajo E 2013 A stochastic model of cell survival for high-*Z* nanoparticle radiotherapy *Med. Phys.* **40** 024102

[11] Gadoue S M, Zygmanski P and Sajo E 2018 The dichotomous nature of dose enhancement by gold nanoparticle aggregates in radiotherapy *Nanomedicine* **13** 809–23

Chapter 8

Optimal nanoparticle concentrations, toxicity and safety and gold nanoparticle design for radiation therapy applications

Rajiv Kumar and Wilfred Ngwa

8.1 Introduction

The advances in nanotechnology field not only enabled new generation of nanoparticles (NPs) to carry multiple diagnostic/therapeutic payloads but also facilitated targeted delivery into specific sites and across complex biological barriers [1, 2]. The concomitant development in the field of nanotechnology and radiation therapy has led to the development of numerous NPs-based platforms for application in the radiation therapy. A number of these NPs-based formulations are used either as radiosensitizers or for carrying radiosensitizing drugs to the target sites. Radiosensitization can be defined as increasing the sensitivity of tumor cells to radiation by means of agents, either drugs or NPs [3, 4]. The physicochemical properties of NPs play a tremendous role in eliciting radiosensitization effect and these properties determine the mechanism by which NPs will radiosensitize the tumor tissue. The use of high atomic number NPs (high Z-materials) as radiosensitizers is well documented. In addition, NPs can act as delivery vehicles for some of the known radiosensitizing drugs or agents (e.g. Docetaxel) [5–8].

To achieve an efficient radiosensitization, either using high Z-NPs or NPs carrying radiosensitizers, require targeting of these NPs to the tumor site. NPs targeting can be achieved either in the passive form, exploiting the well-known EPR effect in tumors or can be actively targeted using the specific over expressed biomarkers [9–12]. A good targeting approach will result in higher accumulation of these NPs in the diseased site sparing the normal tissues and thereby reducing the toxicity to normal tissues. For fabricating such a targeted NPs system with radiosensitizing properties, it becomes imperative to understand the complexity of the disease model, site of tumor, mode of radiosensitization and to correlate these aspects to the physicochemical properties of the NPs, their specificity towards the

doi:10.1088/978-0-7503-2396-3ch8

diseased site over the normal tissue and the long-term fate of these NPs in the body. Combining all these factors together leads to an effort to engineer or design an appropriate NPs system which can address all these concerns as mentioned above.

The engineering of NPs to achieve multifunctionality has led to the complex NPs-based formulations. These complex formulations must be assessed not only in terms of their functional properties, such as therapeutic or imaging efficacy, but also in terms of safety and compatibility in biological systems [13]. The three basic components which play a tremendous role in determining the therapeutic index, biological fate, pharmacokinetics and immune compatibility include size, shape and surface properties of these complex formulations [13, 14]. Apart from this, a careful NP design should consider the disease type, microenvironment of the diseases site, mode of interaction with non-target organs and the fate of these NPs in the *in vivo* environment [5, 15]. Targeted delivery into selective cells is expected to provide significant advancement in disease therapy. One focus for targeted transport is the development of NPs as vectors for efficient and safe delivery. In this regard, this chapter is focused on the importance of NPs design and how these new generations of engineered NPs can dramatically improve radiosensitization while minimizing toxicity.

8.2 Biomedical applications of gold nanoparticles

Colloidal gold nanoparticles (GNPs) have recently received great attention from the nanoscience community due to their unique properties like ease of synthesis, size tunability, surface modifications, biocompatibility and optical properties by virtue of size and high atomic number. For example, their optical scattering magnitude is larger than that of typical quantum dots. The engineering of biocompatible GNPs has grown very rapidly in the last two years because the designed nanoformulation is beneficial for many biological applications such as gene delivery [16], bio-imaging [17–19], photothermal therapy [20, 21], and biosensors [22] and radiation therapy [5, 23]. In addition, the surface of GNPs can be functionalized with various biomolecules for disease specific targeting and sensing. Utilizing the tunable optical properties and functionalities of GNPs for biomedical applications opened new ways to detect and treat cancer. More recently, it has been demonstrated that polyelectrolyte-coated gold nanorods can serve as an siRNA delivery vehicle for the treatment of drug addiction [24].

8.3 Gold nanoparticles are effective, biocompatible tumor-targeting nanocarriers

In addition to the radiotherapy amplification described above, gold nanoplatforms are functionalizable to target tumors [25] and can carry therapeutics [26, 27] for combined chemo-radiation therapy (CRT). GNPs are among the most biocompatible of metallic elemental NPs [28]. Several advantages associated with GNPs make them ideal candidates for use in radiation therapy including: (a) high biocompatibility and inertness [29], (b) ability to absorb more radiation than any other high Z-material between 20 to 100 keV, three times more effective compared to iodine [23],

(c) the ease of fabrication and size tunability (the dose enhancement factor (DEF) depends on the size of the nanoparticles) [30–32], (d) the surface of the GNPs can be easily passivated with different ligands, which not only determine the systemic circulation time, but can also be utilized for conjugating different imaging and targeting agents [31, 33], (e) highly efficient targeting to the tumor sites can be achieved using GNPs with biomolecules conjugated to the NPs, efficient targeting is a key element in the effectiveness of enhancing the radiation dose using GNPs [34] and (f) the added advantage of conjugating an imaging modality to the NP surface can lead to a system which can measure the effectiveness of treatment in real time concomitantly using non-invasive imaging techniques [28, 35, 36].

8.4 Gold nanoparticles in radiation therapy

GNPs amplify the effects of radiation therapy (RT). The interaction of x-rays with gold atoms leads to the emission of low energy electrons, causing a local enhancement in the radiation dose. These 'secondary' electrons can, in turn, provoke a cascade of chemical and biological events including amplified DNA damage, generation of reactive oxygen species (ROS), and disregulation of cell cycle processes, resulting in amplification of cell kill compared with radiation alone. Several studies have clearly demonstrated GNP dose amplification (~2–3×) in combination with radiation [23, 36–39]. Hainfeld *et al* showed improvement in local control with GNP and 250 kVp photons in a mouse model [8]. Our group has demonstrated significant increases in DNA damage in a clinical 6 MV beam [40]. Joh *et al* demonstrated 'vascular dose painting' with GNP and 175 kVp photons in a preclinical glioblastoma multiforme model [41].

This chapter is focused on the GNPs-based enhancement in radiation therapy, NPs design considerations, toxicity and safety aspects. As theoretical considerations have long suggested that heavy metals can augment the efficacy of orthovoltage x-ray therapy. Due to the short ranges of 10–100 keV electrons, it is likely that the dose due to secondary electrons from GNPs may be concentrated in the vicinity of GNPs themselves, leading to an even more dramatic increase in the dose to nearby tumor cells. Until now it has been assumed that radiotherapy (RT) dose boosting from high atomic number (Z) NPs (e.g. platinum and GNPs) would not be significant, partly due to consideration of low concentrations of NPs accumulating in a tumor when administered intravenously.

8.5 Challenges of GNP radiotherapy

Despite the therapeutic potential of this strategy, several challenges have been identified that pose barriers to clinical translation of GNP amplified radiotherapy. (a) The optimum configuration of the gold nanoplatform has yet to be shown in terms of maximizing biological effect. (b) Lack of knowledge of the biological pathways specific to GNP radiosensitization is limiting current attempts to optimize the efficacy. (c) Systemic delivery of untargeted NP formulations limits the amount that reaches the intended target. (d) A crucial step towards clinical translation is the systematic investigation of toxicity after administration. Therefore, understanding the nature of normal tissue interactions will enable further formulation design to mitigate deleterious interactions.

8.6 Design considerations for optimal radiosensitization using GNPs

It has now been well established that engineered nanostructures that are capable of long circulation in the body and delivering therapeutics to targeted sites, requires an understanding of the physicochemical interactions of a synthetic NP with biological systems. A careful NP design should consider the disease type, microenvironment of the diseases site, mode of interaction with non-target organs and the fate of these NPs in an *in vivo* environment. Three 'S's of NPs parameters: size, shape and surface charge are the fundamental parameters which decide the success of any NP-based platform in living systems [14]. Thus, we believe, it is imperative to assess these three properties before engineering a NP for a particular biological application.

8.7 Size and concentration/dose of GNPs

Size of GNPs plays a critical role in determining the efficacy of treatment with radiation [31, 32], simply because of two major factors: (a) smaller size NPs have the higher cross-sectional area and can theoretically have higher dose enhancement effect compared to smaller size NPs. In the case of large size NPs, the ionizing events with the radiation occurs in the bulk of the NPs, reducing the dose of secondary electrons in the surrounding medium around NPs [42, 43] and (b) the size of NPs determines the pharmacokinetics of GNPs in the systemic circulation, clearance and rate of accumulation at tumor site [15, 44]. Therefore, it is imperative to assess both these factors for designing a potent GNP-based platform for application in radiation therapy (figure 8.1). There are several reports published earlier where GNPs of different size and concentrations were used in various *in vitro* and *in vivo* applications [45]. Burns *et al* evaluated size and concentration of GNPs and showed a six-fold dose enhancement with the large size (92 nm) at higher concentration using 50 keV photons [45–47]. Our group reported previously 130% dose enhancement using 50 nm GNPs using low dose rate gamma radiation therapy with ^{125}I brachytherapy seeds [48]. We have also evaluated our new generation of GNP-based platform with keV and MV energies [49, 50]. There are several other groups reporting the use of different size GNPs with radiation [31, 51, 52].

Hainfield *et al* studied combination effect of radiation and GNPs for the first time in mice with subcutaneous EMT-6 mammary carcinoma injected intravenously with 1.9 nm GNPs and treated with radiation. The results showed that mice treated with the combination of GNPs and radiation showed 86% survival rate compared to only 20% survival rate for mice treated with radiation alone [53, 54]. A similar study exploited the use of larger size 13 nm GNPs in combination with clinically relevant MV radiation energies in melanoma mice model and showed a better treatment response for combination therapy [55]. The debate over the use of small size NPs (1.9 nm GNPs used by Hainfield *et al*) versus larger size GNPs (12–50 nm Cho *et al*) requires evaluation of many parameters involved when combining GNPs with radiation. Zheng *et al* have shown that the enhancement effect using GNPs is

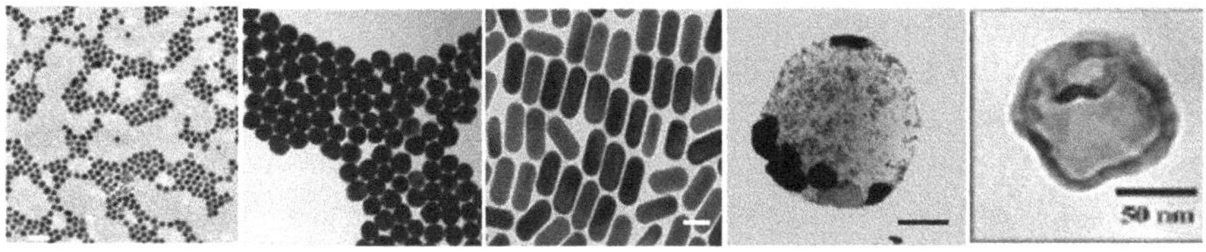

Figure 8.1. Representative TEM images of different GNP formulations synthesized and characterized for various applications. These formulations included spherical particles (2–100 nm), gold nanorods, gold seeded polymeric NPs and hollow gold NPs.

directly proportional to the number of GNPs in the vicinity of DNA [46]. Similarly other factors include the incident x-ray energies as well as DNA:GNP molar ratios and most importantly the disease model [32, 52].

The two *in vivo* studies cited above, involved GNPs of two different sizes (1.9 nm and 12 nm), which apparently look very similar to some of the clinicians and scientific community which are new to the NPs-based radiation dose enhancement field. However, there are very marked distinctions in the physicochemical properties of these NPs, especially in how these two different sizes of NPs behave in systemic circulation. This has been established that small size NPs (<6 nm) will be cleared via renal excretion post intravenous administration, whereas larger NPs (>6 nm) are known to be accumulated in the RES (reticuloendothelial system) leading to less tumor accumulation and undesirable side effects [56]. The fate of larger size NPs with appropriate surface coatings relies either on the degradation of NPs to smaller components which can be excreted via renal route or gradual RES uptake which follows a slow hepatobiliary excretion [57, 58]. Therefore, the smaller size 1.9 nm GNPs, once administered in systemic circulation, undergo clearance from the blood via renal excretion which is very rapid, in the order of minutes. For such small size NPs, the basic requirement is to have very high concentration in the blood to compensate the rapid clearance of the NPs from blood. However, 12 nm GNPs tend to follow a hepatobiliary excretion route which is a slow process and thus bigger size NPs have a better chance in staying a circulation for longer time compared to smaller ones. But it is very critical to state here that there are several other factors that play an important role in clearance of NPs from systemic circulation, such as surface coatings on the NPs, opsonization process, macrophage clearance etc. these are discussed more in depth in the next section.

8.8 Surface charge and multi-functionalities of GNPs

Surface characteristics like functionality and charge of the NPs along with the particle size and composition determine the particle distribution profile and stability in systemic circulation. It is well established that the particle size along with surface composition plays a significant role in various physiological parameters like hepatic filtration, tissue extravasation, tissue diffusion and kidney excretion, and thus determine the biodistribution of the NPs [59]. Thus, it is imperative to study the surface properties and these GNP-based formulations and should be characterized in terms of charge, stability, and adsorption of foreign matter on the NPs' surfaces.

The surface functionalization of GNPs with the amphiphilic polymers like polyethylene glycol (PEG) imparts a very highly hydrophilic surface to the NPs [60, 61]. The PEG coating, also known as 'PEGylation' works in two ways in determining the pharmacokinetics of PEG coated GNPs: (a) *Long circulation time in blood:* the amphiphilic PEG on the surface of GNPs minimizes the interaction with serum proteins/opsonins which are in abundance in the circulating blood. These opsonins if bound to an NP's surface trigger the recruitment of macrophages to clear the NPs from the circulation. Thus, lack of opsonization process (because of the surface decoration of the NPs with PEG) leads to longer systemic circulation time [62, 63]. (b) *Modulate biodistribution and clearance:* as the coatings on the surface of NPs directly impact pharmacokinetics, this results in a longer retention time of NPs in the blood stream and final accumulations in the target sites. Larger size NPs with appropriate surface functionalization with amphiphilic polymers like polyethylene glycol (PEG) are above the renal filtration threshold and possess long blood half-lives [13]. Also, the erosion of surface ligands like PEG slowly results in degradation and clearance of NPs. The surface properties will also determine if the NPs will elicit any immunogenic responses once injected in systemic circulation.

The net charge on the NPs governs both the uptake of NPs into the cells as well as their interaction with the serum proteins. A positive charge on the surface of NPs is known to interact with the negative cell membrane charge and improve the uptake of NPs into the cells [15]. Beddoes *et al* studied the effect of charge on the mechanism of uptake into the cells [64]. Although the positive charge enables the NPs to enter the cells more efficiently, but a net positive charge also results in higher serum protein binding. Thus, to design a potent NPs formulation, it is critical to balance the charge on the NPs surface by appropriate amphiphilic coatings.

Another important aspect of surface coatings on the NPs surface is the feasibility of targeted delivery. The surface of NPs provides a high degree of tunability in terms of surface area to number of free functional ligands which can be modified to provide binding sites for biotargeting agents like antibodies, peptides or small molecule targeting agents [65]. An efficient targeted NP-based delivery platform directly correlates to its high therapeutic efficacy and minimal toxicity.

NPs can home in at the disease sites in two ways: passive accumulation by means of EPR (enhanced permeability and retentivity) effect [66]. Coating of Tween-80 promotes adsorption of proteins, ApoB and E, and thus uptake of NPs by brain capillary endothelial cells via receptor-mediated endocytosis [67, 68]. GNPs have been shown to accumulate in neurons even in the absence of any specific functionalization [24, 69]. Previously, we have studied the effective knockdown of TNF expression using GNPs complexed with TNF-targeting siRNA (or TNFR1- or TNFR2-targeting siRNA) injected stereotactically into rat hippocampus [70]. Active targeting to diseased site can be achieved by conjugating specific biomolecules on the surface of NPs. These biomolecules have specificity towards the specific biomarkers over expressed in cancer cells. There are several reports published previously highlighting the use of antibodies, proteins, peptides, or small molecules.

Multifunctionality added another dimension to the NPs applications in various biological settings. When the surface of NPs is appropriately designed, the availability of functional groups on the NPs surface can be utilized to conjugate different modalities like fluorophores for optical imaging, different chelates like DTPA for MR- or radio-imaging or even conjugating various drugs on the surface of NPs. The first study on exploiting multifunctional GNPs with radiation was based on 2.4 nm dithiolated-diethylene triamine pentaacetic acid–GNPs (DTDTPA–GNPs) in which authors reported that these GNPs were able to penetrate the blood brain barrier via imaging and were able to prolong the survival in 9L gliosarcoma rat model [63]. In another study, small size GNPs were encapsulated in the core polymeric, PEG–PCL, NPs and authors showed concomitant CT imaging and radiosensitization in HT1080 mouse model [71]. In another study, gold nanorods were complexed with SiRNA and these nanoplexes showed as high as 50% tumor regression compared to controls in HNSCC tumor mice models, even at much lower radiation doses than those commonly required in clinical RT [72].

8.9 Toxicity and safety associated with GNP-based radiotherapy

For any given NP-based formulation used in biomedical applications, the composition of the NPs plays a vital role in governing the success of the platform in clinical settings. The NP formulation should be inert, biocompatible and biodegradable, and not only have a sufficient half-life in circulation but also be able to clear out without causing any adverse toxicity. The composition of NPs, especially containing heavy metals, which are known to cause acute or chronic toxicities, must be assessed carefully for any adverse reproductive risks, immunotoxicity, and carcinogenicity to minimize unintended side effects [73]. Biodistribution and clearance profiles are of paramount importance for such side effects [74]. Although GNPs are highly inert and biocompatible, the size and dose of the NPs must be evaluated to assess the toxicity associated with these NPs as the smaller size of NPs are known to be chemically active and higher accumulations in non-target organs can induce severe toxicities when combined with radiation [75]. Several groups studied the toxicity profiles of various GNPs-based formulations, but the majority of the studies were carried out in *in vitro* models concluding that the toxicity potential of GNPs is highly dependent on the size and vary in different cell types [76, 77]. Thus, for designing a GNPs-based platform for radiosensitization, exhaustive toxicology must be performed in the specific animal models.

8.10 AuRad platform

Previously, our group focused on the development of third generation NPs, which were engineered based on the difficult lessons learned from the previous two generations considering all the limitations associated with them for different biological applications. The last section of the chapter is focused on some of the salient features of this potential GNPs-based platform (AuRad platform) and its applications in radiotherapy [5, 78]. Using a rational design consideration for fabricating an NPs-based platform for radiosensitization, we have developed AuRad formulation for application in radiation dose enhancement with the concomitant possibility of optical imaging in small animals for NPs tracking and simultaneous disease progression monitoring.

The salient features of this versatile platform include (a) an optimum size of GNPs; (b) PEGylation of core GNPs (pGNPs) with heterobifunctional polyethylene glycol (PEG); (c) a variety of functional groups on the PEG tip; (d) covalently conjugated fluorophore on the PEG tip linked to pGNPs, (e) high specific targeting using cRGD (for neovascular targeting in pancreatic cancer) and (f) efficient radiation dose enhancement. As synthesized ultrasmall 2–3 nm GNPs were PEGylated with a mixture of heterobifunctional PEG for surface functionality. The hydrodynamic diameter of the GNPs was maintained around 11–12 nm to extend circulation by bypassing rapid renal excretion while avoiding excessive RES accumulation. The functional groups on the surface of the pGNPs were used for conjugating an optical probe (Alexafluor 647) for fluorescence optical imaging. The conjugation of optical probe is a proof of concept for successful surface conjugation to various imaging modalities like magnetic resonance (MR), positron emission tomography (PET) or CT imaging. Figure 8.2 shows the physicochemical characterization data of the AuRad platform [78]. One of the key aspects of small size GNPs is their optimal hydrodynamic diameter, which is optimized to extend circulation, bypassing rapid renal excretion while avoiding excessive reticuloendothelial system (RES) accumulation. These GNPs designed for maximal tumor uptake and optical

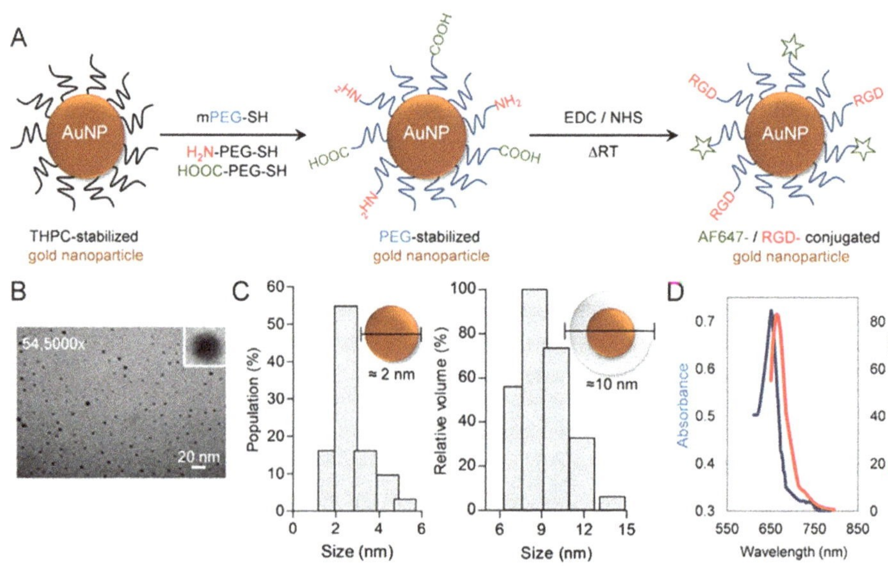

Figure 8.2. Physicochemical characterization of AuRad platform. (a) Schematic representation of synthesis of the third generation of GNPs-based platform 'AuRad' in which ultrasmall GNPs were PEGylated and conjugated with optical probe Alexafluor 647 (AF647) and a targeting peptide *Arg-Gly-Asp* (RGD). (b) TEM image of AuRad platform. (c) The particle size (core and hydrodynamic size) as measured by TEM and DLS, respectively, (core size ≈ 2–3 nm, hydrodynamic size ≈ 8–10 nm). (d) absorption and fluorescence spectra of AuRad platform (λ_{max} of 650/668 nm). Adapted with permission from [78]. Copyright (2015) American Chemical Society.

imaging have great potential in amplifying radiation therapy and to set the foundation to proceed to testing in clinical settings in the near future.

8.11 AuRad Platform targeting tumor vasculature

Previously, we have developed GNPs-based platform 'AuRad' to target the $\alpha_v\beta_3$ integrin receptors. These receptors are known to be over expressed on the endothelial cells of the tumor. It is very well established that the process of angiogenesis results in the formation of neovasculature around the newly formed tumor tissue to supply the essential nutrients for the cancer cells [79]. The endothelial cells associated with neovasculature are anchored to the extracellular matrix via integrins like $\alpha_v\beta_3$ and play an integral role in proliferation, invasion and metastasis of tumor [80]. Thus, a potential strategy to increase the efficiency of tumor diagnosis and efficacy of a therapeutic treatment is to target these over expressed $\alpha_v\beta_3$ integrins. Arg-Gly-Asp (RGD) is a well known peptide that specifically binds to $\alpha_v\beta_3$ integrins and thus can be used to target the endothelial cells of the tumor very efficiently [81].

The functional group on the tip of the PEG coating the surface of GNPs was conjugated to peptide RGD target these over expressing integrins. The targeted AuRad platform was tested in orthotopic and transgenic tumor models of pancreatic and lung cancer, respectively [82]. The targeting efficiency was confirmed by means of live animal imaging using IVIS live animal *in vivo* fluorescence imaging. The results indicated a robust uptake in the tumor post i.v. injection of the NPs. The electron dense nature of GNPs imparts an additional advantage in visualizing the accumulation of GNPs in different tissues using TEM. Thus, we have also performed TEM studies on excised tumors (orthotopic pancreatic tumors and transgenic lung tumors) to visualize the accumulation of GNPs in specific parts of tumors. TEM studies confirmed the accumulation of GNPs specifically in the endothelial cells thereby confirming neovascular targeting of AuRad platform in a pancreatic cancer mouse model (as shown in figure 8.3(a)). Using TEM studies on lung tumor sections, we were able to confirm the localization of GNPs in tumor when GNPs were administered by inhalation/instillation route. Figure 8.3(b) shows that GNPs were not only present in the alveolar spaces but also penetrated the tumor tissue.

8.12 AuRad platform tumor vasculature disruption

Apart from using the AuRad platform for radiosensitization studies in different disease models, our group have exploited the previously established concept of disrupting the tumor vasculature using these third generation GNPs as vascular disrupting agents (VDAs) instead of chemical VDAs [50, 78, 83]. However, chemical VDAs are shown to be effective either alone or in combination with radiation but also marred with severe off-target toxicities [84]. Thus, our targeted AuRad platform can not only target the tumor endothelial cells specifically, but can also elicit localized damage in the presence of radiation and minimize off-target toxicities. We have shown that a 'dual-targeting strategy' using the targeted AuRad platform and

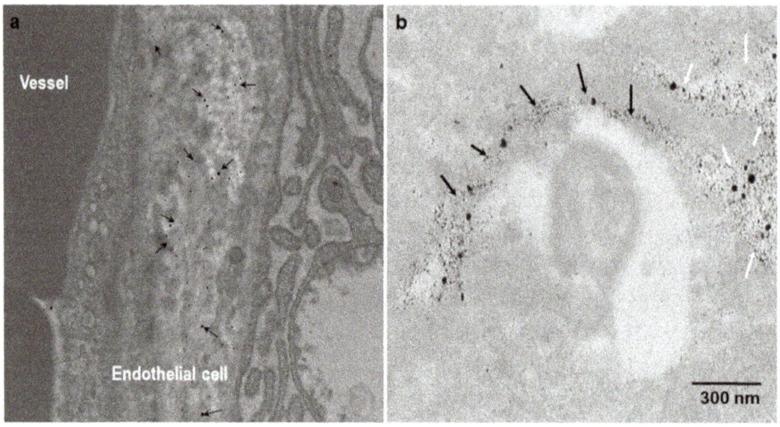

Figure 8.3. TEM image of fixed tumor sections showing accumulation of GNPs in specifically in (a) endothelial cells of the orthotopic Panc 1 pancreatic tumor and (b) the air spaces (white arrows) and migrated to the tumor tissue (black arrows) in lung tumor model.

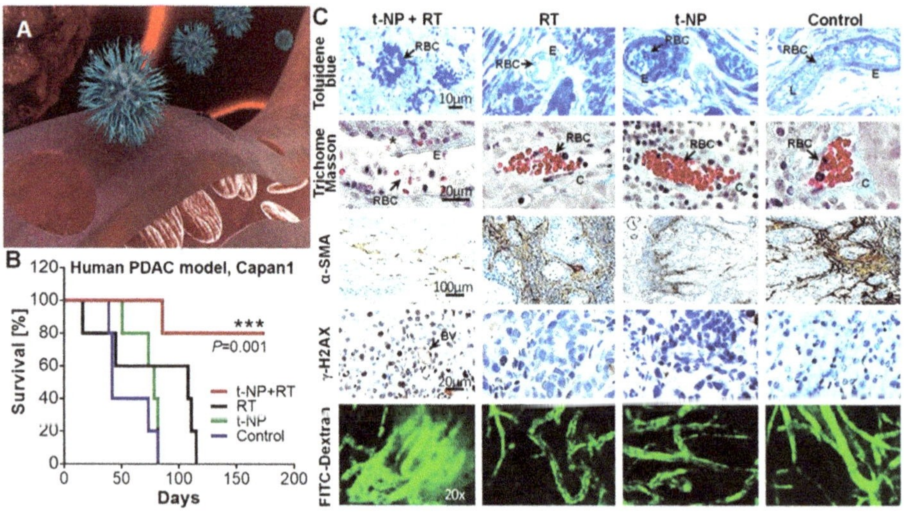

Figure 8.4. (a) Schematic illustration of a tumor angiogenic blood vessel which, after active (vascular) targeting by GNPs to the $\alpha_v\beta_3$ integrin receptors and subsequent irradiation, suffers tumor endothelial disruption. (b) Kaplan–Meier plot depicting survival studies using clinical beam irradiations (6 MV, 10 Gy) demonstrate an improved therapeutic benefit with the t-NP+RT treatment. Log-rank (Mantel-Cox) tests were used for statistical analysis. (c) Histological evidence confirmed the vascular damage at 24 h post-treatment using different qualitative techniques: RBC: red blood cells; E: endothelium; L: lumen; C: collagen; BV: blood vessel. Reproduced from [85]. Copyright the authors 2019. CC BY 4.0.

image guided irradiation resulted in highly localized damage to tumor endothelial cells in mice-bearing (Panc-1) pancreatic tumor xenografts ($\approx$1.2 mg g^{-1} of Au i.v.) [83].

Figure 8.4 presents results published previously by our group, the Kaplan–Meier plot showed 80% survival rate for the combined AuRad and radiation group with an extended survival of ⩾75 days compared to radiation only treatment group. Figure 8.4(c) shows immunostaining studies in which toluidine blue and trichome Masson staining confirmed the rupture of tumor neovessels during combined radiation and NP treatment. Selective rupture (denoted by asterisks in the figure), resulting in non-functional and apoptotic RBCs (arrows) and vascular instability was also observed, in contrast functionally-viable and collagen-sheathed active vessels were present in other control samples. DNA damage studies using γH2aX confirmed radiation-specific damage in the tumor cells and vessels (brown color indicates DNA damage during combined AuRad and radiation treatment). Smooth muscle actins (α-SMA; brown) that support the tumor endothelium was shown to be collapsed during radiation and NP-induced tumor vascular modulation. Functional (or perfusion) damage at 24 h post-radiation, assessed by the FITC-dextran infusion (70 kDa) studies show extensive leakage (or permeation of FITC) in selective, treated vessels in the AuRad plus RT groups. Under all other treatment conditions, the vessels were distinctly labeled, and no signs of passive leakage into the interstitial tumor spaces was evident. These results clearly indicate the immense potential of AuRad platform when combined with radiation therapy. It is worth noting here that these NPs were rationally designed to enable targeting to tumor endothelial cells, inducing localized vascular disruption and minimizing non-target toxicities.

8.13 Summary

More than two decades of research in the field of nanotechnology led to the development of numerous NPs-based formulations for various biomedical applications. GNPs are a vastly studied NPs system and one of the niche areas for GNPs is in radiotherapy applications as a potent radiosensitizing agent. Despite many efforts, the advancement of GNPs from the preclinical findings from the bench to bedside is very slow and challenging. To have an impact on clinical care, it becomes necessary to design these GNPs formulations based on prior learning experiences to have superior physicochemical properties and evaluate in advanced biological systems. These efforts require collaborations between interdisciplinary teams with expertise in nanotechnology, materials sciences, radiation physics, biology, chemistry, radiation oncology etc. Special considerations are required at the onset of designing the NPs platform based on the physicochemical properties required for specific disease models. A rationally engineered GNPs system with optimal design parameters such as size, surface coatings, charge and targeting have tremendous potential in revolutionizing the field of radiation therapy.

References

[1] Pardridge W M 2008 Re-engineering biopharmaceuticals for delivery to brain with molecular Trojan horses *Bioconjug. Chem.* **19** 1327–38

[2] Farokhzad O C and Langer R 2006 Nanomedicine: developing smarter therapeutic and diagnostic modalities *Adv. Drug Deliv. Rev.* **58** 1456–9

[3] Wilson G D, Bentzen S M and Harari P M 2006 Biologic basis for combining drugs with radiation *Semin. Radiat. Oncol.* **16** 2–9

[4] Lawrence T S, Blackstock A W and McGinn C 2003 The mechanism of action of radiosensitization of conventional chemotherapeutic agents *Semin. Radiat. Oncol.* **13** 13–21
[5] Kumar R, Korideck H, Ngwa W, Berbeco R I, Makrigiorgos G M and Sridhar S 2013 Third generation gold nanoplatform optimized for radiation therapy *Transl. Cancer Res.* **2**
[6] Shewach D S and Lawrence T S 1996 Gemcitabine and radiosensitization in human tumor cells *Invest. New Drugs* **14** 257–63
[7] Werner M E, Copp J, Karve S, Cummings N D, Sukumar R, Napier M, Chen R C, Cox A D and Wang A Z 2011 Folate-targeted polymeric nanoparticle formulation of docetaxel is an effective molecularly targeted radiosensitizer with efficacy dependent on the timing of radiotherapy *ACS Nano* **5** 8990–8
[8] Hainfeld J F, Slatkin D N and Smilowitz H M 2004 The use of gold nanoparticles to enhance radiotherapy in mice *Phys. Med. Biol.* **49** N309–15
[9] Debbage P 2009 Targeted drugs and nanomedicine: present and future *Curr. Pharm. Design* **15** 153–72
[10] Mitra S, Gaur U, Ghosh P C and Maitra A N 2001 Tumour targeted delivery of encapsulated dextran-doxorubicin conjugate using chitosan nanoparticles as carrier *J. Control. Release* **74** 317–23
[11] Maeda H 2001 The enhanced permeability and retention (EPR) effect in tumor vasculature: The key role of tumor-selective macromolecular drug targeting *Adv. Enzyme Regul.* **41** 189–207
[12] Wang M and Thanou M 2010 Targeting nanoparticles to cancer *Pharmacol. Res.* **62** 90–9
[13] Kumar R, Roy I, Ohulchanskky T Y, Vathy L A, Bergey E J, Sajjad M and Prasad P N 2010 *In vivo* biodistribution and clearance studies using multimodal organically modified silica nanoparticles *ACS Nano* **4** 699–708
[14] Perrault S D and Chan W C 2010 *In vivo* assembly of nanoparticle components to improve targeted cancer imaging *Proc. Natl Acad. Sci. USA* **107** 11194–9
[15] Albanese A, Tang P S and Chan W C W 2012 The effect of nanoparticle size, shape, and surface chemistry on biological systems *Annu. Rev. Biomed. Eng.* **14** 1–16
[16] Salem A K, Searson P C and Leong K W 2003 Multifunctional nanorods for gene delivery *Nat. Mater.* **2** 668–71
[17] Eghtedari M, Oraevsky A, Copland J A, Kotov N A, Conjusteau A and Motamedi M 2007 High sensitivity of *in vivo* detection of gold nanorods using a laser optoacoustic imaging system *Nano Lett.* **7** 1914–8
[18] Huang X, El-Sayed I H, Qian W and El-Sayed M A 2006 Cancer cell imaging and photothermal therapy in the near-infrared region by using gold nanorods *J. Am. Chem. Soc.* **128** 2115–20
[19] Kopwitthaya A, Yong K T, Hu R, Roy I, Ding H, Vathy L A, Bergey E J and Prasad P N 2010 Biocompatible PEGylated gold nanorods as colored contrast agents for targeted *in vivo* cancer applications *Nanotechnology* **21** 315101
[20] Norman R S, Stone J W, Gole A, Murphy C J and Sabo-Attwood T L 2008 Targeted photothermal lysis of the pathogenic bacteria, Pseudomonas aeruginosa, with gold nanorods *Nano Lett.* **8** 302–6
[21] Ratto F, Matteini P, Rossi F, Menabuoni L, Tiwari N, Kulkarni S K and Pini R 2009 Photothermal effects in connective tissues mediated by laser-activated gold nanorods *Nanomedicine* **5** 143–51
[22] Sudeep P K, Joseph S T and Thomas K G 2005 Selective detection of cysteine and glutathione using gold nanorods *J. Am. Chem. Soc.* **127** 6516–7

[23] Hainfeld J F, Dilmanian F A, Slatkin D N and Smilowitz H M 2008 Radiotherapy enhancement with gold nanoparticles *J. Pharm. Pharmacol.* **60** 977–85
[24] Bonoiu A C, Mahajan S D, Ding H, Roy I, Yong K T, Kumar R, Hu R, Bergey E J, Schwartz S A and Prasad P N 2009 Nanotechnology approach for drug addiction therapy: gene silencing using delivery of gold nanorod-siRNA nanoplex in dopaminergic neurons *Proc. Natl Acad. Sci. USA* **106** 5546–50
[25] Dreaden E C, Austin L A, Mackey M A and El-Sayed M A 2012 Size matters: gold nanoparticles in targeted cancer drug delivery *Ther. Deliv.* **3** 457–78
[26] Cheng J, Gu Y J, Cheng S H and Wong W T 2013 Surface functionalized gold nanoparticles for drug delivery *J. Biomed. Nanotechnol.* **9** 1362–9
[27] Han G, Ghosh P and Rotello V M 2007 Functionalized gold nanoparticles for drug delivery *Nanomedicine* **2** 113–23
[28] Shukla R, Bansal V, Chaudhary M, Basu A, Bhonde R R and Sastry M 2005 Biocompatibility of gold nanoparticles and their endocytotic fate inside the cellular compartment: a microscopic overview *Langmuir* **21** 10644–54
[29] Lasagna-Reeves C, Gonzalez-Romero D, Barria M A, Olmedo I, Clos A, Sadagopa Ramanujam V M, Urayama A, Vergara L, Kogan M J and Soto C 2010 Bioaccumulation and toxicity of gold nanoparticles after repeated administration in mice *Biochem. Biophys. Res. Commun.* **393** 649–55
[30] Chithrani B D and Chan W C W 2007 Elucidating the mechanism of cellular uptake and removal of protein-coated gold nanoparticles of different sizes and shapes *Nano Lett.* **7** 1542–50
[31] Chithrani B D, Ghazani A A and Chan W C W 2006 Determining the size and shape dependence of gold nanoparticle uptake into mammalian cells *Nano Lett.* **6** 662–8
[32] Chithrani D B, Jelveh S, Jalali F, van Prooijen M, Allen C, Bristow R G, Hill R P and Jaffray D A 2010 Gold nanoparticles as radiation sensitizers in cancer therapy *Radiat. Res.* **173** 719–28
[33] Hauck T S, Ghazani A A and Chan W C W 2008 Assessing the effect of surface chemistry on gold nanorod uptake, toxicity, and gene expression in mammalian cells *Small* **4** 153–9
[34] Choi C H J, Alabi C A, Webster P and Davis M E 2010 Mechanism of active targeting in solid tumors with transferrin-containing gold nanoparticles *Proc. Natl Acad. Sci. USA* **107** 1235–40
[35] Mukherjee P, Bhattacharya R, Wang P, Wang L, Basu S, Nagy J A, Atala A, Mukhopadhyay D and Soker S 2005 Antiangiogenic properties of gold nanoparticles *Clin. Cancer Res.* **11** 3530–4
[36] Kumar R, Korideck H, Ngwa W, Berbeco R I, Makrigiorgos G M and Sridhar S 2013 Third generation gold nanoparticle platform optimized for radiation therapy *Transl. Cancer Res.* **2** 228–39
[37] Butterworth K T, McMahon S J, Currell F J and Prise K M 2012 Physical basis and biological mechanisms of gold nanoparticle radiosensitization *Nanoscale* **4** 4830–8
[38] Jain S, Hirst D G and O'Sullivan J M 2012 Gold nanoparticles as novel agents for cancer therapy *Br. J. Radiol.* **85** 101–13
[39] Rahman W N, Bishara N, Ackerly T, He C F, Jackson P, Wong C, Davidson R and Geso M 2009 Enhancement of radiation effects by gold nanoparticles for superficial radiation therapy *Nanomedicine* **5** 136–42

[40] Berbeco R I, Korideck H, Ngwa W, Kumar R, Patel J, Sridhar S, Johnson S, Price B, Kimmelman A and Makrigiorgos G M 2012 DNA damage enhancement from gold nanoparticles for clinical MV photon beams *Radiat. Res.* **178** 604–8

[41] Joh D Y *et al* 2013 Selective targeting of brain tumors with gold nanoparticle-induced radiosensitization *PLoS One* **8** e62425

[42] McMahon S J *et al* 2011 Nanodosimetric effects of gold nanoparticles in megavoltage radiation therapy *Radiother. Oncol.* **100** 412–6

[43] Lin Y, McMahon S J, Paganetti H and Schuemann J 2015 Biological modeling of gold nanoparticle enhanced radiotherapy for proton therapy *Phys. Med. Biol.* **60** 4149–68

[44] Choi H S, Liu W, Misra P, Tanaka E, Zimmer J P, Ipe B I, Bawendi M G and Frangioni J V 2007 Renal clearance of quantum dots *Nat. Biotechnol.* **25** 1165–70

[45] Regulla D F, Hieber L B and Seidenbusch M 1998 Physical and biological interface dose effects in tissue due to x-ray-induced release of secondary radiation from metallic gold surfaces *Radiat. Res.* **150** 92–100

[46] Zheng Y, Hunting D J, Ayotte P and Sanche L 2008 Radiosensitization of DNA by gold nanoparticles irradiated with high-energy electrons *Radiat. Res.* **169** 19–27

[47] Herold D M, Das I J, Stobbe C C, Iyer R V and Chapman J D 2000 Gold microspheres: a selective technique for producing biologically effective dose enhancement *Int. J. Radiat. Biol.* **76** 1357–64

[48] Ngwa W, Korideck H, Kassis A I, Kumar R, Sridhar S, Makrigiorgos G M and Cormack R A 2013 *In vitro* radiosensitization by gold nanoparticles during continuous low-dose-rate gamma irradiation with I-125 brachytherapy seeds *Nanomedicine* **9** 25–7

[49] Ngwa W, Makrigiorgos G M and Berbeco R I 2012 Gold nanoparticle enhancement of stereotactic radiosurgery for neovascular age-related macular degeneration *Phys. Med. Biol.* **57** 6371–80

[50] Berbeco R I, Ngwa W and Makrigiorgos G M 2011 Localized dose enhancement to tumor blood vessel endothelial cells via megavoltage x-rays and targeted gold nanoparticles: new potential for external beam radiotherapy *Int. J. Radiat. Oncol.* **81** 270–6

[51] Butterworth K T, Coulter J A, Jain S, Forker J, McMahon S J, Schettino G, Prise K M, Currell F J and Hirst D G 2010 Evaluation of cytotoxicity and radiation enhancement using 1.9 nm gold particles: potential application for cancer therapy *Nanotechnology* **21** 295101

[52] Jain S *et al* 2011 Cell-specific radiosensitization by gold nanoparticles at megavoltage radiation energies *Int. J. Radiat. Oncol.* **79** 531–9

[53] Hainfeld J F, Dilmanian F A, Zhong Z, Slatkin D N, Kalef-Ezra J A and Smilowitz H M 2010 Gold nanoparticles enhance the radiation therapy of a murine squamous cell carcinoma *Phys. Med. Biol.* **55** 3045–59

[54] Hainfeld J F, Slatkin D N, Focella T M and Smilowitz H M 2006 Gold nanoparticles: a new x-ray contrast agent *Br. J. Radiol.* **79** 248–53

[55] Chang M Y, Shiau A L, Chen Y H, Chang C J, Chen H H and Wu C L 2008 Increased apoptotic potential and dose-enhancing effect of gold nanoparticles in combination with single-dose clinical electron beams on tumor-bearing mice *Cancer Sci.* **99** 1479–84

[56] Choi H S, Liu W, Misra P, Tanaka E, Zimmer J P, Itty Ipe B, Bawendi M G and Frangioni J V 2007 Renal clearance of quantum dots *Nat. Biotechnol.* **25** 1165–70

[57] Ballou B, Lagerholm B C, Ernst L A, Bruchez M P and Waggoner A S 2004 Noninvasive imaging of quantum dots in mice *Bioconjug. Chem.* **15** 79–86

[58] Fitzpatrick J A, Andreko S K, Ernst L A, Waggoner A S, Ballou B and Bruchez M P 2009 Long-term persistence and spectral blue shifting of quantum dots *in vivo* *Nano Lett.* **9** 2736–41
[59] Moghimi S M, Hunter A C and Andresen T L 2012 Factors controlling nanoparticle pharmacokinetics: an integrated analysis and perspective *Annu. Rev. Pharmacol. Toxicol.* **52** 481–503
[60] Rifkin R M, Gregory S A, Mohrbacher A and Hussein M A 2006 Pegylated liposomal doxorubicin, vincristine, and dexamethasone provide significant reduction in toxicity compared with doxorubicin, vincristine, and dexamethasone in patients with newly diagnosed multiple myeloma: a Phase III multicenter randomized trial *Cancer* **106** 848–58
[61] Otsuka H, Nagasaki Y and Kataoka K 2003 PEGylated nanoparticles for biological and pharmaceutical applications *Adv. Drug Deliv. Rev.* **55** 403–19
[62] Alexis F, Pridgen E, Molnar L K and Farokhzad O C 2008 Factors affecting the clearance and biodistribution of polymeric nanoparticles *Mol. Pharm.* **5** 505–15
[63] Alric C, Serduc R, Mandon C, Taleb J, Le Duc G, Le Meur-Herland A, Billotey C, Perriat P, Roux S and Tillement O 2008 Gold nanoparticles designed for combining dual modality imaging and radiotherapy *Gold Bull.* **41** 90–7
[64] Beddoes C M, Case C P and Briscoe W H 2015 Understanding nanoparticle cellular entry: A physicochemical perspective *Adv. Colloid Interface Sci.* **218** 48–68
[65] Salvati A, Pitek A S, Monopoli M P, Prapainop K, Bombelli F B, Hristov D R, Kelly P M, Aberg C, Mahon E and Dawson K A 2013 Transferrin-functionalized nanoparticles lose their targeting capabilities when a biomolecule corona adsorbs on the surface *Nat. Nanotechnol.* **8** 137–43
[66] Maeda H, Wu J, Sawa T, Matsumura Y and Hori K 2000 Tumor vascular permeability and the EPR effect in macromolecular therapeutics: a review *J. Control. Release* **65** 271–84
[67] Kreuter J, Shamenkov D, Petrov V, Ramge P, Cychutek K, Koch-Brandt C and Alyautdin R 2002 Apolipoprotein-mediated transport of nanoparticle-bound drugs across the blood-brain barrier *J. Drug Target.* **10** 317–25
[68] Michaelis K, Hoffmann M M, Dreis S, Herbert E, Alyautdin R N, Michaelis M, Kreuter J and Langer K 2006 Covalent linkage of Apolipoprotein E to albumin nanoparticles strongly enhances drug transport into the brain *J. Pharmacol. Exp. Ther.* **317** 1246–53
[69] Sousa F *et al* 2010 Functionalized gold nanoparticles: a detailed *in vivo* multimodal microscopic brain distribution study *Nanoscale* **2** 2826–34
[70] Gerard E, Spengler R N, Bonoiu A C, Mahajan S D, Davidson B A, Ding H, Kumar R, Prasad P N, Knight P R and Ignatowski T A 2015 Chronic constriction injury-induced nociception is relieved by nanomedicine-mediated decrease of rat hippocampal tumor necrosis factor *Pain* **156** 1320–33
[71] Al Zaki A, Joh D, Cheng Z L, De Barros A L B, Kao G, Dorsey J and Tsourkas A 2014 Gold-loaded polymeric micelles for computed tomography-guided radiation therapy treatment and radiosensitization *ACS Nano* **8** 104–12
[72] Masood R, Roy I, Zu S, Hochstim C, Yong K T, Law W C, Ding H, Sinha U K and Prasad P N 2012 Gold nanorod-sphingosine kinase siRNA nanocomplexes: a novel therapeutic tool for potent radiosensitization of head and neck cancer *Integr. Biol.* **4** 132–41
[73] Oberdorster G 2001 Pulmonary effects of inhaled ultrafine particles *Int. Arch. Occup. Environ. Health* **74** 1–8
[74] Choi H S and Frangioni J V 2010 Nanoparticles for biomedical imaging: fundamentals of clinical translation *Mol. Imaging* **9** 291–310

[75] Alkilany A M and Murphy C J 2010 Toxicity and cellular uptake of gold nanoparticles: what we have learned so far? *J. Nanopart. Res.* **12** 2313–33
[76] Tsoli M, Kuhn H, Brandau W, Esche H and Schmid G 2005 Cellular uptake and toxicity of Au55 clusters *Small* **1** 841–4
[77] Pan Y, Neuss S, Leifert A, Fischler M, Wen F, Simon U, Schmid G, Brandau W and Jahnen-Dechent W 2007 Size-dependent cytotoxicity of gold nanoparticles *Small* **3** 1941–9
[78] Kunjachan S *et al* 2015 Nanoparticle mediated tumor vascular disruption: a novel strategy in radiation therapy *Nano Lett.* **15** 7488–96
[79] Gil P R and Parak W J 2008 Composite nanoparticles take aim at cancer *ACS Nano* **2** 2200–5
[80] Rajangam K, Behanna H A, Hui M J, Han X, Hulvat J F, Lomasney J W and Stupp S I 2006 Heparin binding nanostructures to promote growth of blood vessels *Nano Lett.* **6** 2086–90
[81] Cheng Z, Wu Y, Xiong Z, Gambhir S S and Chen X 2005 Near-infrared fluorescent RGD peptides for optical imaging of integrin alphavbeta3 expression in living mice *Bioconjug. Chem.* **16** 1433–41
[82] Hao Y, Altundal Y, Moreau M, Sajo E, Kumar R and Ngwa W 2015 Potential for enhancing external beam radiotherapy for lung cancer using high-Z nanoparticles administered via inhalation *Phys. Med. Biol.* **60** 7035–43
[83] Kunjachan S *et al* 2018 Targeted drug delivery by radiation-induced tumor vascular modulation *bioRxiv* https://www.biorxiv.org/content/10.1101/268714v1.full
[84] Hinnen P and Eskens F A 2007 Vascular disrupting agents in clinical development *Br. J. Cancer* **96** 1159–65
[85] Kunjachan S *et al* 2019 Selective priming of tumor blood vessels by radiation therapy enahnces nanodrug delivery *Sci. Rep.* **9** 15844

IOP Publishing

Nanoparticle Enhanced Radiation Therapy
Principles, methods and applications
Erno Sajo and Piotr Zygmanski

Chapter 9

Translational nanomaterials for cancer radiation therapy

Shady Kotb and Sijumon Kunjachan

9.1 Introduction

With over 10 million new cases every year worldwide, cancer remains one of the most difficult to treat diseases, exhibiting significant morbidity and mortality [1]. Radiotherapy (RT) is an oft-administered non-surgical treatment method for cancer with more than 50% of patients receiving it either alone or in combination with chemotherapy. However, RT is limited in its ability to deliver optimal therapeutic doses to tumor tissue without inducing peripheral tissue damage [2, 3]. Numerous solutions have been proposed to overcome this issue: (i) implementation of advanced RT techniques such as intensity modulated radiation therapy (IMRT) [4], stereotactic radiotherapy [5], and volumetric-modulated arc radiotherapy (VMAT) [4–6]; (ii) by using heavy metal nanoparticles (also known as radiosensitizers) to target the cancerous tissues and improve the radiation cross-section compared to soft tissue. Overall, technological advances in advanced RT treatments methods and innovative nanoparticle-based solutions have dramatically improved the field of radiation therapy along with radiobiological imaging [7, 8].

9.1.1 Silica-based nanoparticles

Silica nanoparticles do not possess any innate imaging or therapeutic properties unlike gadolinium or gold-based nanoparticles. However, they are prominent due to their biocompatibility, ease of synthesis at low cost and further functionalization [18]. One of the most promising functionalized silica NPs was proposed by Wiesner research group at Cornel university, where they developed platforms known as Cornell dots [19]. The Cornell dots (C'dots) are comprised of ultrasmall polyethylene glycol coated fluorescent core–shell silica nanoparticles with either drug or radioactive markers covalently attached to the surface [20]. C'dots are currently under clinical trials at different phases. A trial has been conducted for patients with metastatic melanoma where the particles were labeled with ^{124}I for positron emission tomography imaging and modified with cRGDY peptides for targeting. The safety, pharmacokinetics, clearance properties and radiation dosimetry were assessed after intravenous administration in patients. Findings were consistent with well-tolerated inorganic particles with no toxicities or adverse events [19].

9.1.2 Superparamagnetic iron oxide nanoparticles (SPIONs)

SPIONs are commercially approved metal oxide nanoparticles. They hold huge potential in a vast variety of biomedical applications including magnetic resonance imaging, targeted delivery of drugs or genes, tissue engineering, targeted hyperthermia of tumor, T2 contrast agent producing negative contrast and chelation therapy [21–24]. SPIONs are divided into three main categories based on their hydrodynamic size: oral SPIONs of 300 nm, standard SPIONs of 150 nm and ultrasmall SPIONs of >50 nm. SPIONs of size 10–100 nm are considered optimal for intravenous administration. Nanoparticles of ~200 nm are sequestered by the spleen and liver [25]. Despite the dramatic versatility and therapeutic benefits, SPIONs show significant toxicities such as inflammation, cell apoptosis, impaired mitochondrial function and generation of reactive oxygen species [26]. Thus, there is an immediate need to address the safety and biocompatibility issues that pertain to the *in vivo* use of SPIONs in various clinically relevant *in vivo* applications.

9.1.3 Quantum dots (QDs)

QDs are semiconductor nanoparticles made from the group II, VI elements (e.g. CdSe and CdTe). QDs possess a crystalline structure that ranges from 2–10 nm in diameter [27]. The inorganic nanoparticle core provides a rigid platform for the development of QDs probes. Manipulation of the core chemical composition, size and structure control the photophysical properties of the probe [28]. However, bare nanoparticles cannot interact with biological systems and do not possess any biological functionality. Careful design using suitable chemical materials that can encapsulate the QD core and shield it from inadvertent degradation can yield biocompatible and beneficial probes for medical applications.

QDs exhibit many supreme characteristics compared to conventional fluorophores, including size-tunability and spectrally narrow light emission along with efficient light absorption throughout the wide spectrum. In fact, these characteristics facilitate their use in multiple imaging modalities and therapy. QDs are used in *in vitro* applications such as molecular pathology, real-time monitoring of molecular processes, and labeling of intracellular targets in live cells [29–31]. At the *in vivo* scale, QDs are used for noninvasive fluorescence, CT, PET and SPECT imaging [32–34].

9.2 High-*Z* metals and radiosensitization

In contrast to low atomic number elements found predominately in living systems, the presence of high-*Z*-species interacting with highly ionizing radiation implies a new physicochemical mode of action. Due to the photoelectric effect, high atomic metals can undergo ionization with high efficiency, leading to unstable atomic rearrangement that is stabilized by the emission of low energy photons and electrons (Auger emission). Multiple Auger emissions can occur from a single ionization event and can cause an Auger cascade. Electrons produced by the Auger emission possess a few kilovolts of energy as a result, leading to their deposition in close vicinity and damaging several tissues or initiating complex biological effects [7, 15]. Most common radiosensitizing elements that have been studied includes bismuth ($Z = 83$), gold ($Z = 79$), platinum ($Z = 78$), hafnium ($Z = 72$), gadolinium ($Z = 64$) and silver ($Z = 47$).

9.2.1 Platinum nanoparticles

Given the atomic number of platinum (Pt), which is almost close to that of gold, they exhibit several properties that are similar. Porcel *et al* proposed a new strategy based on the combination of platinum nanoparticles with radiation by C^{6+} fast ions used in hadron therapy [40]. It was observed that Pt strongly enhanced lethal damage in DNA with an efficacy factor close to 2 for its DNA double strand breaks. The enhanced sensitization of Pt nanoparticles was due to the energy deposition in the close vicinity of the metal. Along with Pt nanoparticles, molecular forms of platinum such as cis-diamminedichloro-platinum (II) (CDDP) are reportedly used in glioma treatment [41, 42]. CDDP molecules react with the nucleophilic sites of DNA and forms DNA adducts, thus acting as a chemotherapeutic agent because of its DNA binding property. Numerous *in vivo* studies involving platinum compounds and medical x-rays have been performed in tumor-bearing mice or rats. However, these experiments demonstrated a small increase in life span due to their relatively low uptake in the tumor [43–45]. A study by Biston and colleagues used CDDP with monochromatic synchrotron x-rays (78.8 kV) to optimize a chemo-radiotherapy protocol in Fisher rats bearing glioma tumors [46]. Findings from this study suggested that chemo-radiotherapy is far more efficient than radiotherapy or chemotherapy alone by a factor of 1.4.

9.2.2 Gold nanoparticles

Gold nanoparticles (AuNPs) have chemical and physical properties that make them attractive to be used as radiation dose amplifiers and to improve therapeutic index of radiation therapy. This includes low toxicity, high surface area, biocompatibility and ease of fabrication into ranges of various size and shape [47]. An additional important property of AuNPs is the ease with which they can be functionalized through established thiol chemistry on the nanoparticle surface [48] Drugs may be linked to AuNPs using a number of strategies including covalent or non-covalent linking, encapsulation into nano matrixes, and electrostatic adsorption [49]. These approaches have the potential to improve the biodistribution and pharmacokinetics. Early evidence of using AuNPs as radiosensitizers was demonstrated by Hainfeld and colleagues in mice bearing subcutaneous EMT-6 mammary carcinomas. They used 1.9 nm thiol-coated Aurovist nanoparticles in combination with 250 kV x-rays [50]. Following systemic delivery of nanoparticles at a dose of 2.7 g Au kg^{-1}, Hainfeld and colleagues observed complete tumor regression. This was also coupled with an increase in survival from 20% for x-ray irradiated to 86% for animals irradiated in combination with AuNPs. The same group further published interesting tumor growth delay in an aggressive human glioblastoma cancer model. Non-functionalized AuNPs of 11 nm size were administrated intravenously 15 h prior to radiation treatment. The AuNPs efficiently crossed the blood brain barrier to accumulate in the tumor at tumor : brain ratio of 19:1. The combined treated of AuNP and radiation resulted in 50% long-term survival [51].

Stephan Roux and colleagues have developed different types of Au-NP platforms for combined imaging and radiotherapy [52–54]. They developed formulations with diethylene triamine pentaacetic acid (DTPA) grafted AuNPs (2.4 nm) that passively accumulated in the tumor tissue and rapidly cleared without significant reticuloendothelial retention. When tested in osteosarcoma-bearing animals treated with microbeam radiation therapy, they improved the median survival from 42.5 days to 61 days [52]. The apparent regression and disappearance of tumor was evident in six of the seven animals tested, demonstrating major improvement in overall survival. For preclinical prostate cancer model (PC3), animals treated with AuNP conjugated with diethylene triamine pentaacetic acid (DTDTPA) survived by 31% when compared to the animals that received only radiation from 220 kV source [53].

Although these findings clearly show the efficacy of AuNPs as radiosensitizers, there are concerns about AuNP toxicity for therapeutic purposes [55–57]. Moreover, it is difficult to draw direct comparison between studies performed due to the sheer number of variables presented (size, surface coating, charge, and concentration). Nevertheless, there is no clinical trial currently in progress for AuNPs due to its low tumor uptake, lack of targeting specificity, and the induction of cytotoxicity and oxidative stress due to the elevated amount of ROS [58].

9.2.3 Hafnium oxide nanoparticles

Hafnium oxide nanoparticles were the first clinically-administered nanoparticles in the humans. They were engineered as 50 nm-sized spheres, bearing a negative surface charge in aqueous solution at pH 6–8, also known as NBTXR3 [59]. The intratumoral distribution of NBTXR3 was demonstrated, with the dispersion of nanoparticles in 3D and its persistence in the tumor structure [60]. Radioenhancement of NBTXR3 nanoparticles was tested in HCT 116, NCT-H460-LUC2, PANC-1, Hs913T and 42-MG-BA *in vitro* with x-ray 200 kV [59]. Further, antitumor activities demonstrated a marked advantage in terms of survival, tumor-specific growth delay and local control in both mesenchyme and epithelial human tumor xenograft models using high-energy source (6 MV) compared to radiation alone [60]. NBTXR3 has entered clinical trials phase I for hepatocellular carcinoma (HCC) and soft tissue sarcoma, Phase I/II trials in liver cancers (HCC and liver metastases) and head and neck cancer [59].

The combination of radiobiological imaging and RT treatment is a classic example of *theranostics*—a new term in the field of cancer therapy. Theranostics is a combination of *therapeutics* and *diagnosis*. It can be defined as an integrated system that provides therapy and aids in the diagnosis and monitoring of therapy through imaging [9]. In a broader sense, theranostic systems and strategies facilitate to correlate and identify responders and non-responders by imaging and provide personalized integrated treatment.

9.3 Theranostics nanoparticles

Improving the outcome of cancer treatment by combining chemical/biochemical agents with radiotherapy has been of interest to oncologists for many decades [10, 11]. The clinical studies of radiation in combination with drug (chemotherapy and/or radiosensitizers) have been generically divided into the following categories: (a) spatial cooperation, in which each treatment modality accounts for a different anatomic site, e.g. adjuvant therapy after the treatment of the primary tumor; (b) toxicity in-dependence, in which each agent can be given in full dose because the toxicities do not overlap or enhance one another; (c) protection of normal tissue; (d) enhancement of tumor response, in which drug-radiation interaction may be additive or supraadditive [12, 13].

With rapid developments in nanoscale, future of therapeutic nanoparticles started flourishing [14, 15]. Nanoparticles have several advantages in comparison to their respective molecular agents: (a) they exhibit specific physicochemical properties due to their nanometer size [15]; (b) they are tuned for better biodistribution and accumulation in the body and tumor; (c) ability to be targeted to the tumor using *active* or *passive* tumor targeting methods [16]; (c) their potential to act as multimodal agents and facilitate imaging, diagnosis and therapy, either as a standalone therapy or in combinations [17].

9.3.1 Gadolinium nanoparticles

Gadolinium ($Z = 64$) is one of the most widely used contrast agents for MRI imaging. It's most common oxidation state is +3 as with most lanthanides, and it is favored with the presence of seven unpaired electrons that generate dipoles interaction with water to exhibit long electron relaxation time [61]. Gadolinium-based contrast agents impact proton relaxation time in the following manner: protons in the human body (water) produce energy when subjected to radio-frequency waves, which is amplified to transform into an MRI signal. More than a large volume of ~10 million MRI studies use gadolinium per year [62].

Gadolinium (Gd) possess two main roles in cancer therapy: (a) it acts as MRI contrast agent to enhance the T1 weighted image contrast; (b) Gd is a radiosensitizer that enhances radiotherapy (RT). When subjected to radiation, Gd ($Z = 64$) undergo photoelectric effect and K-shell vacancies are created and subsequently filled with higher orbital electrons. The electron reorganization of atoms yield a cascade of either photoelectrons or auger electrons that have low energy depending on the shell (K,L,M) of ejection [63]. Released energy is deposited close to the site of production leading to complex biological damage. It is worth noting that the interaction mechanism of Gd with the ionizing radiation is highly dependent on the photon energy. Gd-based agents also act as promising candidates for MR-guided radiotherapy. The most extensively reported and developed gadolinium compound for either MRI contrast agent or radiosensitization includes motexafin gadolinium, magnevist and DOTAREM.

Paramagnetic metal chelates, as previously mentioned, increase the relaxation rate of surrounding water protons. However, commercially available contrast agents have several shortcomings: (i) they rapidly extravasate from blood vessels to the interstitial space, making them inadequate for imaging cardiovascular system; (ii) they have a short circulation time, precluding accumulation in tumors; (iii) they show poor contrast at high magnetic field; and (iv) they are only effective at high concentration, causing problems with Gd^{3+} leakage or accumulation causing nephrogenic systemic fibrosis [64]. Two major approaches have been proposed to overcome the considerable drawbacks: increasing the number of gadolinium units, for instance by incorporating the chelates in polymers [66], dendrimers [67], nanogels [68], or nanoparticles [69] and optimizing the chemical structures of the chelates, essentially by increasing the rotational correlation time [62, 65, 70].

Different formulations of gadolinium nanoparticles have been researched and reported over the years for both imaging and radiation-enhancement purposes. Studies have used polymer complexes of Gd^{3+} chemically conjugated to a polysiloxane ring complexed with DOTA. This platform, known as AGuIX has been widely tested in mice, rats and non-human mammalian models for both imaging and radiosensitization. This exemplary theranostic platform is currently tested in humans for clinical trials.

9.3.2 Bismuth complexes and nanoparticles

Bismuth (Bi) is a heavy metal ($Z = 83$) having similar properties to lead (Pb) and tin (Sn). However, what differentiates Bi from Pb or Sn is its low toxicity in a specific chelating form [35]. Thus, both metal bismuth and its complexes are commonly considered as biologically safe. The first bismuth-containing medicine was reported in 1786 for the treatment of dyspepsia [36]. More bismuth complexes were further explored in the treatment of various gastrointestinal disorders and microbial infections. Moreover, the use of radioactive ^{212}Bi and ^{213}Bi compounds as targeted radiotherapeutic agents for cancer therapy has indicated anticancer activities of Bi complexes [37]. The biological activities of bismuth complexes rely on both the ligand and the coordination geometry of the complexes. Recently, Bi nanoparticles have drawn great attention for their application in biological sciences, including their use in bioimaging and x-ray radiosensitization [38, 39]. Bi nanoparticles displayed higher radiation dose enhancement than gold and platinum nanoparticles for a given size, concentration and target location. Bi nanoparticles in the tumor (350 mg g^{-1}) and when irradiated by a 50 kV source, demonstrated 1.25- and 1.29-times higher radiation dose enhancement than gold or platinum nanoparticles. Auger electrons from bismuth nanoparticles provided 2–2.4 times more radiation enhancement than gold or platinum [39].

9.4 Mechanism of action

At a mechanistic level, there are at least four major pathways that cause radiosensitization: (a) localized absorption of x-rays by the nanoparticles, leading to an increase in physical dose enhancement, (b) direct damage of DNA or other cellular structures due to the generation of photoelectrons or auger electrons, (c) generation of reactive oxygen species and its indirect damage on the cells, some of which may have effects that go beyond a few μm, and (d) different intracellular signaling pathways that are dependent on reactive oxygen species, transforming growth factor-β and interleukin-8. All these may lead to or initiate programmed cell death.

Despite the theoretical predictions, there are several possibilities for additional chemical and biological process in nanoparticle-mediated radiosensitization. One of the main mechanisms of radiation-induced cell death is free radical mediated DNA damage predominantly by hydroxyl formed due to water radiolysis. Hydroxyl radicals readily react with biological molecules including cellular DNA to initiate radiation induced apoptosis. Functional radicals can typically include the super oxides (O_2^-), hydrogen peroxide (H_2O_2) and hydroxyl (OH^-) molecules, which indirectly cause cell damage, by oxidation of lipids, proteins, DNA, and cytoplasm. This further results in mitochondrial dysfunction and apoptotic and necrotic cell death [55, 71, 72]. Of note, H_2O_2 has a long range of action (up to a few μm), high stability, and can act as a source of many ROS generations, further undergoing different chemical reactions. A thorough and full understanding of all factors is extremely important prior to designing a drug or nanoparticle system that can increase the cell damage and maximize the therapeutic benefit.

9.5 Bystander effect

For a long time, it was generally believed that radiation outcomes such as cell death, DNA damage, chromosomal aberrations and mutagenesis result from direct ionization of cell structures, particularly the DNA. Indirect damage through the generation of ROS and hydrolysis of water that are attributed to irreparable DNA damage was also considered a major mechanism of action [1, 8, 9]. However, emerging evidence that shows non-targeted effects such as ionizing radiation-induced bystander effects (RIBE) presents a paradigm shift in our understanding of radiation mechanisms. It is highly likely that multiple pathways are involved in cell signaling and the response is in accordance with the stimulated signaling pathways [73–75]. It appears that RIBE may be transmitted either by direct cell-to-cell contact or through soluble factors [76]. However, the bystander effect shows non-linear dose response and is more pronounced at low doses of radiation. The bystander effect has been observed in a variety of treatment endpoints, including induction of DNA damage, instability of chromosomes, mutations and cell death or apoptosis. At least two main factors play a major role in RIBE: the quality of the radiation and the formation of ROS after radiation exposure. RIBE can partially explain the radiosensitization property of different high-Z metals as ROS—in particular hydrogen peroxide—have been implicated in various mediated bystander responses using a variety of endpoints [73].

References

[1] Peer D *et al* 2007 Nanocarriers as an emerging platform for cancer therapy *Nat. Nanotechnol.* **2** 751–60

[2] Li G, Wang J, Hu W and Zhang Z 2015 Radiation-induced liver injury in three-dimensional conformal radiation therapy (3D-CRT) for postoperative or locoregional recurrent gastric cancer: risk factors and dose limitations *PLoS One* **10** e0136288

[3] Prezado Y *et al* 2015 Tolerance to dose escalation in minibeam radiation therapy applied to normal rat brain: long-term clinical, radiological and histopathological analysis *Radiat. Res.* **184** 314–21

[4] Yang J C, Terezakis S A, Dunkel I J, Gilheeney S W and Wolden S L 2016 Intensity-modulated radiation therapy with dose painting: a brain-sparing technique for intracranial germ cell tumors *Pediatr. Blood Cancer* **63**

[5] Devoid H-M *et al* 2016 Recent advances in radiosurgical management of brain metastases *Front. Biosci. Sch. Ed.* **8** 203–14

[6] Lee J, Park J M, Wu H-G, Kim J H and Ye S-J 2015 The effect of body contouring on the dose distribution delivered with volumetric-modulated arc therapy technique *J. Appl. Clin. Med. Phys. Am. Coll. Med. Phys.* **16** 5810

[7] McMahon S J *et al* 2011 Biological consequences of nanoscale energy deposition near irradiated heavy atom nanoparticles *Sci. Rep.* **1** 18

[8] Sharma H, Mishra P K, Talegaonkar S and Vaidya B 2015 Metal nanoparticles: a theranostic nanotool against cancer *Drug Discov. Today* **20** 1143–51

[9] Jeelani S *et al* 2014 Theranostics: a treasured tailor for tomorrow *J. Pharm. Bioallied Sci.* **6** S6–8

[10] Zhang J *et al* 2014 Phase II study of low-dose paclitaxel with timed thoracic radiotherapy followed by adjuvant gemcitabine and carboplatin in unresectable stage III non-small cell lung cancer *Lung Cancer* **83** 67–72

[11] Eisbruch A *et al* 1999 Bromodeoxyuridine alternating with radiation for advanced uterine cervix cancer: a phase I and drug incorporation study *J. Clin. Oncol.* **17** 31–40

[12] Steel G G 1988 The search for therapeutic gain in the combination of radiotherapy and chemotherapy *Radiother. Oncol. J. Eur. Soc. Ther. Radiol. Oncol.* **11** 31–53

[13] Steel G G and Peckham M J 1979 Exploitable mechanisms in combined radiotherapyche-motherapy: the concept of additivity *Int. J. Radiat. Oncol. Biol. Phys.* **5** 85–91

[14] Kumar P, Gulbake A and Jain S K 2012 Liposomes a vesicular nanocarrier: potential advancements in cancer chemotherapy *Crit. Rev. Ther. Drug Carrier Syst.* **29** 355–419

[15] Coulter J A, Hyland W B, Nicol J and Currell F J 2013 Radiosensitising nanoparticles as novel cancer therapeutics—pipe dream or realistic prospect? *Clin. Oncol.* **25** 593–603

[16] Maeda H, Wu J, Sawa T, Matsumura Y and Hori K 2000 Tumor vascular permeability and the EPR effect in macromolecular therapeutics: a review *J. Control. Release* **65** 271–84

[17] Ricciardi L *et al* 2014 Multifunctional material based on ionic transition metal complexes and gold-silica nanoparticles: synthesis and photophysical characterization for application in imaging and therapy *J. Photochem. Photobiol. B* **140** 396–404

[18] Bradbury M S, Pauliah M, Zanzonico P, Wiesner U and Patel S 2016 Intraoperative mapping of sentinel lymph node metastases using a clinically translated ultrasmall silica nanoparticle: SLN mapping using ultrasmall fluorescent silica particles *Wiley Interdiscip. Rev. Nanomed. Nanobiotechnol.* **8** 535–53

[19] Phillips E *et al* 2014 Clinical translation of an ultrasmall inorganic optical-PET imaging nanoparticle probe *Sci. Transl. Med.* **6** 260ra149

[20] Yoo B *et al* 2015 Ultrasmall dual-modality silica nanoparticle drug conjugates: Design, synthesis, and characterization *Bioorg. Med. Chem.* **23** 7119–30

[21] Rosen J E, Chan L, Shieh D-B and Gu F X 2012 Iron oxide nanoparticles for targeted cancer imaging and diagnostics *Nanomed. Nanotechnol. Biol. Med.* **8** 275–90

[22] Ito A, Shinkai M, Honda H and Kobayashi T 2005 Medical application of functionalized magnetic nanoparticles *J. Biosci. Bioeng.* **100** 1–11

[23] Liu G *et al* 2006 Nanoparticle iron chelators: a new therapeutic approach in Alzheimer disease and other neurologic disorders associated with trace metal imbalance *Neurosci. Lett.* **406** 189–93

[24] Gupta A K and Gupta M 2005 Synthesis and surface engineering of iron oxide nanoparticles for biomedical applications *Biomaterials* **26** 3995–4021

[25] Huber D L 2005 Synthesis, properties, and applications of iron nanoparticles *Small Weinh. Bergstr. Ger.* **1** 482–501

[26] Singh N, Jenkins G J S, Asadi R and Doak S H 2010 Potential toxicity of superparamagnetic iron oxide nanoparticles (SPION) *Nano Rev.* **1**

[27] Soo Choi H *et al* 2007 Renal clearance of quantum dots *Nat. Biotechnol.* **25** 1165–70

[28] Zrazhevskiy P, Sena M and Gao X 2010 Designing multifunctional quantum dots for bioimaging, detection, and drug delivery *Chem. Soc. Rev.* **39** 4326–54

[29] Bruchez M, Moronne M, Gin P, Weiss S and Alivisatos A P 1998 Semiconductor nanocrystals as fluorescent biological labels *Science* **281** 2013–6

[30] Chan W C and Nie S 1998 Quantum dot bioconjugates for ultrasensitive nonisotopic detection *Science* **281** 2016–8

[31] Byers R J *et al* 2007 Semiautomated multiplexed quantum dot-based *in situ* hybridization and spectral deconvolution *J. Mol. Diagn.* **9** 20–9

[32] Yong K-T *et al* 2009 Imaging pancreatic cancer using bioconjugated InP quantum dots *ACS Nano* **3** 502–10

[33] Graves E E, Weissleder R and Ntziachristos V 2004 Fluorescence molecular imaging of small animal tumor models *Curr. Mol. Med.* **4** 419–30

[34] Panthani M G *et al* 2013 *In vivo* whole animal fluorescence imaging of a microparticle-based oral vaccine containing (CuInSe*x*S2-*x*)/ZnS core/shell quantum dots *Nano Lett.* **13** 4294–8

[35] Luo Y *et al* 2012 *In vitro* cytotoxicity of surface modified bismuth nanoparticles *J. Mater. Sci., Mater. Med.* **23** 2563–73

[36] Yang N and Sun H 2010 *Biological Chemistry of Arsenic, Antimony and Bismuth* ed H Sun (New York: Wiley) pp 53–81

[37] Wang Y *et al* 2015 Bio-coordination of bismuth in *Helicobacter pylori* revealed by immobilized metal affinity chromatography *Chem. Commun.* **51** 16479–82

[38] Su X-Y, Liu P-D, Wu H and Gu N 2014 Enhancement of radiosensitization by metalbased nanoparticles in cancer radiation therapy *Cancer Biol. Med.* **11** 86–91

[39] Hossain M and Su M 2012 Nanoparticle location and material dependent dose enhancement in x-ray radiation therapy *J. Phys. Chem. C Nanomater. Interfaces* **116** 23047–52

[40] Porcel E *et al* 2010 Platinum nanoparticles: a promising material for future cancer therapy *Nanotechnology* **21** 85103

[41] Kelland L 2007 The resurgence of platinum-based cancer chemotherapy *Nat. Rev. Cancer* **7** 573–84

[42] Screnci D and McKeage M J 1999 Platinum neurotoxicity: clinical profiles, experimental models and neuroprotective approaches *J. Inorg. Biochem.* **77** 105–10
[43] Yang W *et al* 2011 Convection enhanced delivery of carboplatin in combination with radiotherapy for the treatment of brain tumors *J. Neurooncol.* **101** 379–90
[44] Twentyman P R, Kallman R F and Brown J M 1979 The effect of time between Xirradiation and chemotherapy on the growth of three solid mouse tumors. III. Cis-diamminedichloroplatinum *Int. J. Radiat. Oncol. Biol. Phys.* **5** 1365–7
[45] Vinchon-Petit S *et al* 2010 External irradiation models for intracranial 9L glioma studies *J. Exp. Clin. Cancer Res.* **29** 142
[46] Biston M-C *et al* 2004 Cure of Fisher rats bearing radioresistant F98 glioma treated with cis-platinum and irradiated with monochromatic synchrotron x-rays *Cancer Res.* **64** 2317–23
[47] Her S, Jaffray D A and Allen C 2015 Gold nanoparticles for applications in cancer radiotherapy: Mechanisms and recent advancements *Adv. Drug Deliv. Rev.* **109** 84–101.
[48] Jadzinsky P D, Calero G, Ackerson C J, Bushnell D A and Kornberg R D 2007 Structure of a thiol monolayer-protected gold nanoparticle at 1.1 A resolution *Science* **318** 430–3
[49] Vigderman L and Zubarev E R 2013 Therapeutic platforms based on gold nanoparticles and their covalent conjugates with drug molecules *Adv. Drug Deliv. Rev.* **65** 663–76
[50] Hainfeld J F, Slatkin D N and Smilowitz H M 2004 The use of gold nanoparticles to enhance radiotherapy in mice *Phys. Med. Biol.* **49** N309–15
[51] Hainfeld J F, Smilowitz H M, O'Connor M J, Dilmanian F A and Slatkin D N 2013 Gold nanoparticle imaging and radiotherapy of brain tumors in mice *Nanomedicine* **8** 1601–9
[52] Laurent G *et al* 2016 Minor changes in the macrocyclic ligands but major consequences on the efficiency of gold nanoparticles designed for radiosensitization *Nanoscale* **8** 12054–65
[53] Butterworth K T *et al* 2016 Preclinical evaluation of gold-DTDTPA nanoparticles as theranostic agents in prostate cancer radiotherapy *Nanomedicine* **11** 2035–47
[54] Miladi I *et al* 2014 The *in vivo* radiosensitizing effect of gold nanoparticles based MRI contrast agents *Small Weinh. Bergstr. Ger.* **10** 1116–24
[55] Geng F *et al* 2011 Thio-glucose bound gold nanoparticles enhance radio-cytotoxic targeting of ovarian cancer *Nanotechnology* **22** 285101
[56] Liu C-J *et al* 2010 Enhancement of cell radiation sensitivity by pegylated gold nanoparticles *Phys. Med. Biol.* **55** 931
[57] Chithrani D B *et al* 2010 Gold nanoparticles as radiation sensitizers in cancer therapy *Radiat. Res.* **173** 719–28
[58] Taggart L E, McMahon S J, Currell F J, Prise K M and Butterworth K T 2014 The role of mitochondrial function in gold nanoparticle mediated radiosensitisation *Cancer Nanotechnol.* **5** 5
[59] Marill J *et al* 2014 Hafnium oxide nanoparticles: toward an *in vitro* predictive biological effect? *Radiat. Oncol. Lond. Engl.* **9** 150
[60] Maggiorella L *et al* 2012 Nanoscale radiotherapy with hafnium oxide nanoparticles *Future Oncol. Lond. Engl.* **8** 1167–81
[61] Caravan P, Ellison J J, McMurry T J and Lauffer R B 1999 Gadolinium(III) chelates as MRI contrast agents: structure, dynamics, and applications *Chem. Rev.* **99** 2293–352
[62] Caravan P 2006 Strategies for increasing the sensitivity of gadolinium based MRI contrast agents *Chem. Soc. Rev.* **35** 512–23
[63] Taupin F *et al* 2015 Gadolinium nanoparticles and contrast agent as radiation sensitizers *Phys. Med. Biol.* **60** 4449–64

[64] Perazella M A 2009 Current status of gadolinium toxicity in patients with kidney disease *Clin. J. Am. Soc. Nephrol.* **4** 461–9
[65] Terreno E, Castelli D D, Viale A and Aime S 2010 Challenges for molecular magnetic resonance imaging *Chem. Rev.* **110** 3019–42
[66] Li Y *et al* 2012 Macromolecular ligands for gadolinium MRI contrast agents *Macromolecules* **45** 4196–204
[67] Lim J *et al* 2012 Gadolinium MRI contrast agents based on triazine dendrimers: relaxivity and *in vivo* pharmacokinetics *Bioconjug. Chem.* **23** 2291–9
[68] Lux J *et al* 2013 Metal chelating crosslinkers form nanogels with high chelation stability *J. Mater. Chem. B* **1** 6359–64
[69] Lux F, Roux S, Perriat P and Tillement O 2011 Biomedical applications of nanomaterials containing gadolinium *Curr. Inorg. Chem.* **1** 117–29
[70] Botta M and Tei L 2012 Relaxivity enhancement in macromolecular and nanosized GdIII-based MRI contrast agents *Eur. J. Inorg. Chem.* **2012** 1945–60
[71] Butterworth K T, McMahon S J, Taggart L E and Prise K M 2013 Radiosensitization by gold nanoparticles: effective at megavoltage energies and potential role of oxidative stress *Transl. Cancer Res.* **2** 269–79
[72] Misawa M and Takahashi J 2011 Generation of reactive oxygen species induced by gold nanoparticles under x-ray and UV Irradiations *Nanomed. Nanotechnol. Biol. Med.* **7** 604–14
[73] Ebert M A, Suchowerska N, Jackson M A and McKenzie D R 2010 A mathematical framework for separating the direct and bystander components of cellular radiation response *Acta Oncol. Stockh. Swed.* **49** 1334–43
[74] Hei T K *et al* 2008 Mechanism of radiation-induced bystander effects: a unifying model *J. Pharm. Pharmacol.* **60** 943–50
[75] Facoetti A *et al* 2009 Experimental and theoretical analysis of cytokine release for the study of radiation-induced bystander effect *Int. J. Radiat. Biol.* **85** 690–9
[76] Yang H, Asaad N and Held K D 2005 Medium-mediated intercellular communication is involved in bystander responses of x-ray-irradiated normal human fibroblasts *Oncogene* **24** 2096–103

Chapter 10

Gold nanoparticle enhanced radiosensitivity of cells: considerations and contradictions from model systems and basic investigations of cell damaging for radiation therapy

Martin Falk, Michael Wolinsky, Marlon R Veldwijk, Georg Hildenbrand and Michael Hausmann

Most cancer patients are currently treated with radiotherapy (Atun *et al* 2015) and/or chemotherapy, which besides surgery have been very effective and successful therapy approaches for many types of cancer. The primary precondition for successful radiotherapy (and/or chemotherapy) (Wenz *et al* 2001) is a higher sensitivity of cancer cells than normal cells to DNA damage by radiation and their lower DNA repair capacity. This is fulfilled in many cases. For instance, due to improper cell cycle checkpoints or deficient repair pathways (Löffler *et al* 2007), cancer cells become genetically unstable and accumulate genomic alterations making tumors more and more vulnerable to DNA damaging agents compared to non-cancer cells. Damage tolerance is of relevance here as well, and most likely quite in favor for the tumor cells. Cancer cells often become radio-resistant since genomic instability accelerates their evolution and overgrowth of aggressive cell clones. Highly radio-resistant tumors are difficult to be eradicated without also seriously damaging the normal tissue and organs in tumor surroundings (Tomita *et al* 2018, Lam *et al* 2018, Gu *et al* 2018). In these cases, a crucial question for improved cancer treatment therefore is, how to enhance the radiation treatment effects in the (radio-resistant) tumor cells while preserving the normal, non-tumorous surrounding tissues as much as possible. This issue also becomes of fundamental importance for tumors located in very close proximity to organs with central vital functions. In the worst situation, the radio-resistance and problematic location appear in combination, as for instance in the case of the most aggressive and highly radio-resistant tumor (Zhou *et al* 2007) starting in the brain known as glioblastoma

doi:10.1088/978-0-7503-2396-3ch10

multiforme (Davis 2016). Investigations of such tumors require the development of special model systems (Struve *et al* 2015).

SkBr3 cells (Engel and Young 1978) as used in the data presented here in detail were involved as a model for breast cancer with Her2/neu up-regulation, on which the radiation effects are studied in combination with antibody and/or chemo-treatment (Lacroix and Leclercq 2004).

Many promising strategies are under development to improve radiotherapy. Spatial dose fractionation, time dose fractionation, micro/mini-beam irradiation, heavy-ion irradiation (Durante *et al* 2017, González and Prezado 2018, Jánváry *et al* 2018, Zhang *et al* 2018, Sammer *et al* 2017, Prezado *et al* 2009, Jezkova *et al* 2018, Girst *et al* 2016), and application of normal cell radio-protectants (Hofer *et al* 2017a, 2017b) and/or tumor cell radio-sensitizers (Hofer *et al* 2016) are already being used and combined in practice. One of the radio-sensitizing approaches often discussed is to selectively potentiate radiation toxicity only in tumor cells by incorporation of metal nanoparticles either into the tumor tissue or even into the tumor cells (Štefančiková *et al* 2016, Ngwa *et al* 2014, 2017, Hildenbrand *et al* 2018, Kuncic and Lacombe 2018, Lux *et al* 2018, Li *et al* 2017, Sancey *et al* 2014, Pagáčová *et al* 2019). Due to high electron content and photoelectric absorption cross-section, metal (high-Z material; Z = atomic number of the element) nanoparticles emit showers of secondary electrons upon irradiation (Nikjoo *et al* 2008, Hossain and Su 2012). Launched electrons then generate clouds of highly dense ionization processes, enhancing radiation-induced cell damage followed by cell death (Zygmanski *et al* 2013a).

Even under physiological conditions the DNA in the cell nucleus is sensitive to many environmental stressing conditions (Falk *et al* 2014a, 2014b, Rittich *et al* 2004, Freneau *et al* 2018) and can be considerably damaged even with relatively low doses of ionizing radiation (Falk *et al* 2010, Hausmann *et al* 2017). As serious damaging effects of ionizing radiation on (cancer) cells are mostly mediated through fragmentation of nuclear chromatin by inserting single strand (SSB) and double strand (DSB) DNA breaks (Schipler and Iliakis 2013), nanoparticle radio-sensitizing effects have been ascribed to an increase of DSBs generated with the same radiation dose in the presence of nanoparticles (Hildenbrand *et al* 2018). Clustered and thus complex DSBs can hardly be repaired without any remaining damage consequences (Jezkova *et al* 2018, Bobkova *et al* 2018, Mladenov *et al* 2016, Mladenov *et al* 2013) and are known as the main factor responsible for the enhanced radiobiological efficiency (RBE) of densely ionizing high LET radiation. According to this hypothesis, at a given dose of a given radiation type, nanoparticles boost cell killing by locally amplifying the dose within the cell volume (Porcel *et al* 2010), which is followed by additional DNA damage processes. Indeed, an increase of SSBs and DSBs has been reported relative to untreated samples (i.e. without nanoparticle incorporation) in nuclear DNA of cells irradiated in the presence of various metal nanoparticles (Porcel *et al* 2010).

In general, nanoparticles are preferentially internalized by and enriched in tumor tissue due to the phenomenon known as enhanced permeability and retention (EPR). This enhancement effect reasons that, in radiotherapy, nanoparticles may be selectively targeted to tumor cells (Maeda 2010, 2011, Fang *et al* 2011, Prabhakar *et al* 2013, Bertrand *et al* 2014, Chithrani 2010a, Chithrani *et al* 2010b). Furthermore, several types of nanoparticles can simultaneously be used as imaging contrast agents in theranostics (Hainfeld *et al* 2013). Nanoparticles can be also functionalized to better select and infiltrate tumor cells (only) or to target cellular organelles specifically (Hildenbrand *et al* 2018, Bertrand 2014). Such surface modifications include attachment of antibodies, drugs, labelling with purposefully designed oligonucleotide sequences etc. Another advantage especially for microscopic driven research may be that nanoparticles can also be used as imaging tags, thereby avoiding photo-bleaching (He *et al* 2008, Moser *et al* 2016) experienced with classic fluorochromes (see also chapter 11 'Super-Resolution Microscopy of Nanogold-Labelling' in this book).

The aforementioned properties of nanoparticles and the nanoparticle-mediated radio-sensitization were experimentally confirmed both in cells obtained from different organs and tissues (Burger *et al* 2014, Hildenbrand *et al* 2018, Pagáčová *et al* 2019), and animal models (Hainfeld *et al* 2013). Increased cell death compared to non-incubated controls was also observed in several studies when nanoparticles were added to cell cultures prior to irradiation (Štefančiková *et al* 2016, Porcel *et al* 2010, Lacombe *et al* 2017). In parallel, experiments with isolated DNA showed higher radiation-induced fragmentation of the DNA molecule in the presence of various nanoparticles (Porcel *et al* 2010). However, efforts to repeat these findings for cell systems only provided contradictory results, as is further discussed for gold nanoparticles. Among many high-*Z* materials, gold nanoparticles have attracted scientific attention due to their unique characteristics, including good biocompatibility, advantageous physical and chemical properties (e.g. chemical stability, simple synthesis, and ability to locally amplify radiation dose, to serve as contrast agents, and to blink after laser excitation (figure 10.1), etc). It should also be noted that gold nanoparticles of less than 12 nm in diameter can penetrate the blood–brain barrier (Oberdorster *et al* 2004, Sarin *et al* 2008, Sonavane *et al* 2008) and those smaller than about 50 nm can be easily internalized by cells (Conner and Schmid 2003, Chithrani *et al* 2006), although larger ones are in general not excluded from incorporation. More important, there seems to be an optimum for retention around 50 nm. Much smaller will be taken up readily, yet can also leave the cell more efficiently. As such, gold nanoparticles promise potentially wide applicability in research and medicine. Many different studies demonstrated that gold nanoparticles open new opportunities for improvement in treatment of cancer and various non-malignant diseases, i.e. for radiotherapy or drug delivery, diagnostics, chemical sensing, biological imaging, etc (Alkilany and Murphy 2010). However, research on the relationship between physical and chemical properties of gold nanoparticles and their biological effects is still in its infancy. This is mostly due to the fact that, in the nano-range of about 1–100 nm, the physico-chemical properties (electronic, magnetic, optical, mechanical, etc) and biological interactions of nanoparticles extremely depend on their size, shape, and surface modification, which complicates systematic research.

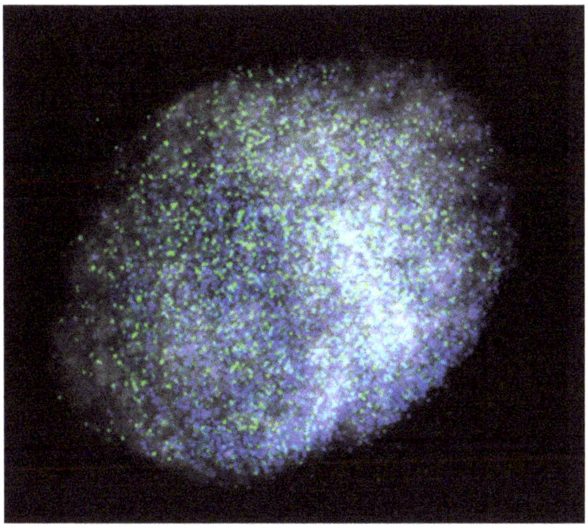

Figure 10.1. Example of an SkBr3 cell after treatment with gold nanoparticles. The image shows an overlay of a widefield image of the cell and a localization microscopy image of 10 nm gold nanoparticles (blue–green points). By means of high laser illumination power, surface plasmons are induced leading the gold nanoparticles to blink. The on–off of particle fluorescence allows the precise nano-scaled localization of each particle. For details about the imaging mechanisms of localization microscopy see chapter 11.

It is in fact not so easy to understand the nanoparticle-mediated radio-sensitization and radio-response of cells and a lot of open questions are under debate (Pagáčová *et al* 2019). It seems that using different cell models, different types and sizes of particles, or different radiation qualities and doses is contributing to this inconsistent, sometimes confusing image. Another shortcoming with respect to DNA damaging followed from *in situ*/*in vivo* experiments: nanoparticles of all sizes up to about 50 nm are able to cross the cell membrane and penetrate the cellular cytosol; however, even those of very small dimensions, e.g. of 2–3 nm in diameter, do not pervade the cell nucleus (Štefančiková *et al* 2014, 2016, Hildenbrand *et al* 2018, Moser *et al* 2016) unless they are specifically modified and treated according to a certain transfection protocol for this purpose. Nevertheless even there, the nanoparticles were primarily perinuclear (Burger *et al* 2014). Nanoparticles of different materials and sizes enter cells by pinocytosis (reviewed in Yameen *et al* 2014) and remain retained inside the cytoplasm. There they can accumulate not only in particle aggregates but also in endoplasmic vesicles (endosomes) and lysosomes (Štefančiková *et al* 2014, 2016, Fernando *et al* 2010). In some cases, nanoparticles may also be found to co-localize preferentially with/in the endoplasmic reticulum (Hildenbrand *et al* 2018, Cartiera *et al* 2009) and/or Golgi apparatus (reviewed in Yameen *et al* 2014) or nearby the cell membrane (own unpublished results). Mitochondria, however, the only organelles in human cells that contain their own DNA except for the nucleus, are not primary targets for nanoparticles or nanoparticle aggregates.

These sometime contradicting findings occurring under certain experimental conditions only put into play a plethora of cellular and biophysical processes that could potentially participate in nanoparticle-mediated tumor cell radio-sensitization. It is therefore not excluded that different types and sizes of nanoparticles do not follow a common mode of action, both in terms of the type of cell damage and its potentially underlying mechanism (reviewed in Fröhlich 2013). Contradictories on the radio-sensitization mediated by (various) gold nanoparticles and the mechanism of this phenomenon, as they follow from the comparison of irradiated cell viability (Clonogenic Assay) and their DNA integrity (Super-Resolution Microscopic Analysis of γH2AX Foci), are discussed in detail below.

10.1 Cell viability upon cell irradiation in the presence of nanoparticles—colony formation assay (CFA)

Irrespective of the underlying mechanism, some types of nanoparticles added to culture medium significantly reduce clonogenic survival of cells either by themselves (cytotoxicity) or upon irradiation (radio-sensitization). After cell irradiation with doses known to be high for a given cell type, irradiated cells can die immediately by necrosis or apoptosis due to irreparable DNA damage and extensive harm to all cellular structures (membranes, organelles). However, the majority of irradiated cells usually survive the initial period after irradiation and enter senescence or die later because of their inability to accomplish mitosis. These cells can continue to live for some period of time but cannot multiply—they are clonogenically inactivated, i.e. 'mitotically dead'. Conclusions based simply on cell viability measurements other than CFA after irradiation can be therefore misleading. The assay that can discriminate between surviving cells capable of producing progeny and mitotically dead cells and quantify their fractions was already proposed by Puck and Marcus in 1956 (Puck and Markus 1956) and is currently accepted as the gold standard method in (radio)biology. Referred to as clonogenic assay or colony formation assay (CFA), this method is often used as primary approach to follow survival of irradiated cells (or anyhow treated cells) and also to confirm results of other tests of cell viability, like flow cytometric quantification of annexin V/propidium iodide positivity (apoptosis induction), methyl-thiazol-tetrazolium [MTT-] test, or trypan blue exclusion test. Before discussing the results of clonogenic assay relevant for nano-particle radio-sensitization, a brief introduction of the method will be provided.

The data of clonogenic assays are usually represented as the so called survival curves, showing the fraction of cells that are able to generate a colony (perform at least 5–6 divisions) dependent on radiation dose. An example of such curves is provided in figure 10.2. Typically, the survival curves follow the linear-quadratic dependence, described by the equation

$$\mathrm{SF} = \exp\left(-\alpha D - \beta D^2\right),$$

where SF is the survival fraction of cells and α and β are the linear and quadratic parameters, respectively. D is the radiation dose.

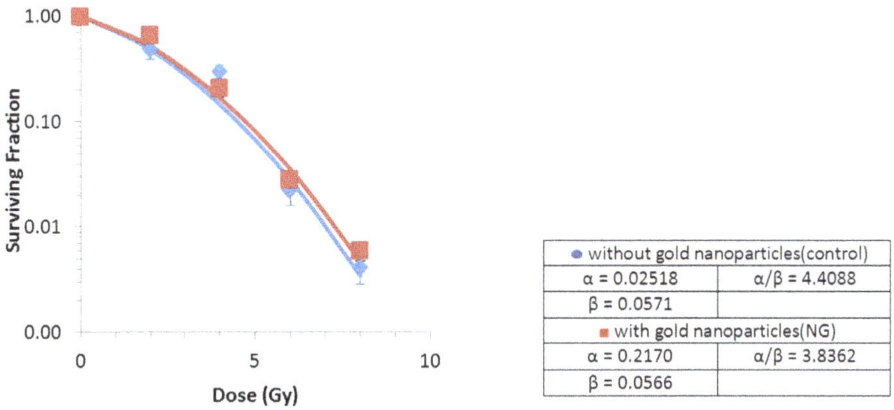

Figure 10.2. Clonogenic survival of SkBr3 cells after irradiation with indicated doses of 6 MV x-rays in the presence (■) and absence (◆) of 10 nm gold nanoparticles, respectively. A semi-logarithmic plot of cell survival is shown. Red corresponds to SkBr3 cells, treated with gold nanoparticles and irradiated. Blue corresponds to SkBr3 cells, irradiated, but not treated with gold nanoparticles. Error bars are the standard deviation of surviving fractions across three replicates. No differences in the survival fractions were found with and without gold nanoparticle incorporation. The table shows the α and β values are coefficients of the fit curve SF = exp $(-\alpha D - \beta D^2)$.

Many individual studies reported different effects of various gold nanoparticles on clonogenic survival of cells, leading to contradictory conclusions on their cytotoxicity (Pan *et al* 2007, Alkilany and Murphy 2010, Coulter *et al* 2012, Soenen *et al* 2012, Youkhana *et al* 2017, Benton *et al* 2018, Martínez-Torres *et al* 2018, Yang *et al* 2018, Patil *et al* 2019); and the same holds true for nanoparticle-mediated radio-sensitization by gold (and other types of) nanoparticles (Herold *et al* 2000, Jain *et al* 2011, Coulter *et al* 2012, Chen *et al* 2015, Taggart *et al* 2016, Paro *et al* 2017, Kim *et al* 2017, Yang *et al* 2018). Hence, we are still far from understanding the structure function relationship between the physical and chemical properties of nanoparticles and consequently their interactions with cells and organisms.

Challenges with interpretation of results on nanoparticle-mediated cell radio-sensitization can be illustratively demonstrated on our experimental dataset for SkBr3 cells, as presented below. Clonogenic assay (figure 10.2) indicated the contradictions between investigations of radiation-sensitizing effects due to gold nanoparticle incorporation. We found no significant difference between the survival curves for cells irradiated with or without pure gold nanoparticle (10 nm) incorporation. This well agrees with the findings on HeLa cells after application of unmodified 10 nm gold nanoparticles recently published by Burger *et al* (2014) but is the opposite of some other cell survival studies (Wolfe *et al* 2015, Paro *et al* 2017, Kim *et al* 2017) in which also different sizes were used. Interestingly, our experiments also in some way contrast the results of Hildenbrand *et al* (2018) for the same cell line, where the counting of γH2AX foci (accepted as the most sensitive surrogate DSB marker, see below next section) revealed a small additional increase in DSB numbers in cells that were incubated with gold nanoparticles prior to irradiation with different x-rays doses. This contradiction motivated us to analyze γH2AX foci on single cell level, too. If tumor cells are either tolerant toward DNA damage or effective enough in DNA (strand break) repair, clonogenic survival would not be altered even if gold nanoparticles enhanced DNA damage by ionizing radiation.

10.2 DNA damage upon cell irradiation in the presence of nanoparticles—super-resolution microscopic analysis of γH2AX foci

The phosphorylation of the histone variant H2AX (Turinetto and Giachino 2015) is a key factor highlighting double stranded DNA breaks after cell exposure to ionizing radiation. In minutes after irradiation, H2AX becomes phosphorylated on serine 139 (then called γH2AX) Rogakou *et al* 1998) in a vicinity of about 1 Mb around a DNA double strand break. With this tagging also other repair proteins are accumulated at the damaged side. Importantly, labelling of γH2AX by fluorescent antibodies allows visualization of DSBs as microscopically visible repair foci. Since this γH2AX focus formation is a sensitive and early indicator of DSBs both *in vitro* and *in vivo* (Kuo and Yang 2008), it has been proven useful as a measure for this most serious type of DNA damage (Löbrich and Jeggo 2010), also in cases of low doses where other established methods such as for instance pulse-field gel electrophoresis (PFGE) or comet assay lose their accuracy (Banath *et al* 2004 and Löbrich and Jeggo 2017). Since the relationship between DSBs and γH2AX foci is close to 1:1, the counting of γH2AX foci has been established as a potent method in biological dosimetry (Löbrich *et al* 2010).

At a dose of about 1 Gy about 1%–2% of H2AX histone protein molecules become phosphorylated leading to the formation of hundreds to thousands of γH2AX molecules at repair foci. It has been shown that different cell types have different background levels of γH2AX (Dikomey *et al* 1998), which results in different γH2AX focus responses. The relative dose-dependency of focus numbers after DNA damage induction does not seem to be influenced by different radiation sensitivity of cells, whereas the intensity of the single foci (= number of antibody-labelled γH2AX molecules) differs in different cell lines (MacPhail *et al* 2003). Recently, it has been shown that the counting of single fluorescently labelled γH2AX molecules by super-resolution light microscopy can bring about deeper insights into DNA damage induction and focus formation (Natale *et al* 2017, Hausmann *et al* 2018). The number of γH2AX labelling tags increases with dose and decreases during repair in a compatible way to γH2AX foci. However, the analysis of distances between the labelling points indicates focus sub-structures (clusters) that seem to be characteristic for individual breaks and their chromatin surroundings (Hofmann *et al* 2018).

In the example presented here, γH2AX was specifically labelled in cell nuclei using fluorescent antibodies and the fluorescence was detected by single molecule localization microscopy (see chapter 11), which is a technique of super-resolution fluorescence light microscopy (Cremer and Masters 2013) that circumvents the

Abbe–Rayleigh boundary conditions of diffraction and offers effective optical resolution down to the order of 10 nm. The fundamental concept of the technique is optical isolation of molecular objects (for instance individual fluorophores of antibodies). Switching the fluorophores between two different spectral states, e.g. on and off (Thompson *et al* 2002), allows a temporal isolation and thus a spatial separation of single (molecule) signals. From a reversible dark state, fluorescent molecules can randomly return to the emission state and emit their photons when they are irradiated by laser light (Lemmer *et al* 2008, Lemmer *et al* 2009, Kaufmann *et al* 2009). Each of the emitting fluorophores is represented by an Airy disc in the microscopic image. The barycentre of such an Airy disc approximates the location of the emitting single molecule. This allows the precise determination of spatial object positions and the calculation of spatial distances between single molecules with a precision and thus optical resolution in the 10 nm regime (Deschout *et al* 2014). All coordinates of fluorescent molecules can be merged into a matrix and visualized in a 'pointillist', super-resolution image (figure 10.3) (Hausmann *et al* 2017).

Thirty minutes after irradiation with 2 Gy and 4 Gy x-rays, the SkBr3 cells were fixed, labelled with specific fluorescent antibodies against γH2AX, and the labelling points were counted in relation to the non-irradiated control. The data were compared also for cells with and without gold nanoparticle incorporation. For each type of the six different treatments, 35–40 cell nuclei of stained cells were visualized and their composite images analyzed (see Materials and Methods, section 10.5). The position of the fluorescent label was precisely determined and the coordinates were transferred into a density image where the intensity of each point refers to the numbers of its next neighbors (figure 10.3).

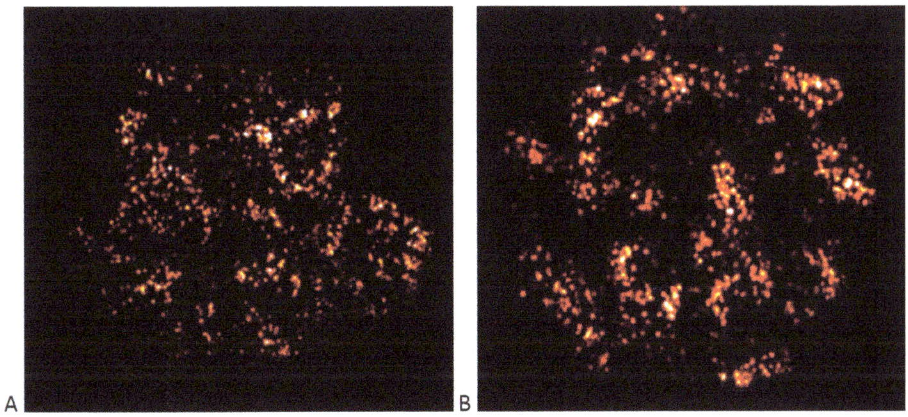

Figure 10.3. Example of an SkBr3 cell nucleus after (a) irradiation with a dose of 4 Gy of 6 MV x-rays and (b) treatment with 10 nm gold nanoparticles and irradiation with a dose of 4 Gy of 6 MV x-rays. The figure shows a localization microscopy image of γH2AX fluorescent labeling points obtained after visualization with the specific antibody. The intensity of signals encodes the relative number of next neighbors. For details about the imaging mechanisms of localization microscopy see chapter 11.

The results show that the numbers of γH2AX signals in irradiated cell nuclei grow with radiation dose (figure 10.4). It is also evident that the incorporation of gold nanoparticles by themselves increases the numbers of γH2AX signals, i.e. even without irradiation. This may be due to a toxicity effect of the particles or a cell stress provoked by particle load in the cytoplasm. Hence, it is not surprising that this effect seems to synergistically work with radiation stress so that in all cases the number of γH2AX molecules was higher for cells with gold nanoparticles than for those without. If one would subtract this 0 Gy nanogold effect from the data of the nanogold treated and irradiated cells, no difference would occur any longer between the irradiated specimens with and without gold nanoparticle incorporation. This means that the results based on the amount of single labelling tags of γH2AX molecules did not reveal any significant difference between irradiated specimens treated and not treated with gold nanoparticles.

In the next step, we analyzed whether presence of gold nanoparticles influences clustering of γH2AX signals. γH2AX clusters were analyzed as described in Krufczik *et al* (2017), (Hausmann *et al* 2018). Clusters were interactively determined and defined by the presence of at least 45 signal points within a circular region of 200 nm radius around any point (figure 10.5). The counting of γH2AX clusters in each cell (figure 10.6) revealed that their number grows with radiation dose. An additional (although not significant) increase of γH2AX cluster numbers was

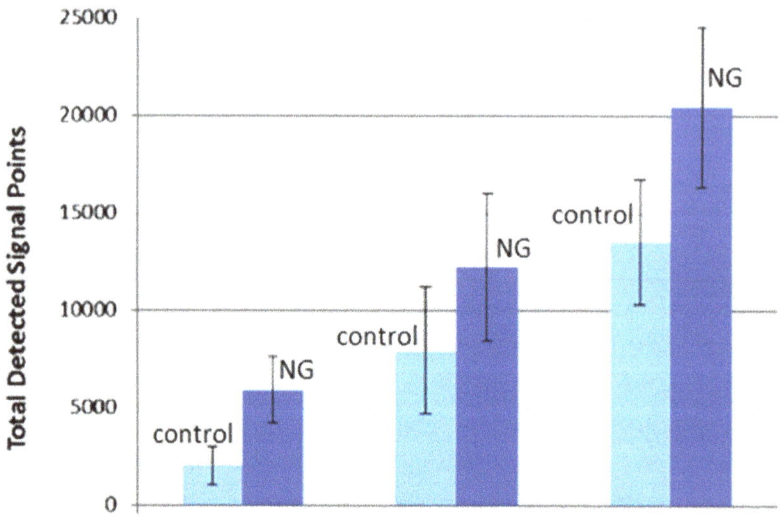

Figure 10.4. Numbers of γH2AX signal points detected in cells for indicated treatments, i.e. exposures to different doses of 6 MV x-rays (dose rate 6.67 Gy min^{-1}) combined or not combined with 10 nm gold nanoparticle incubation. The columns represent the mean γH2AX signal detected in cell nuclei 30 min after irradiation. Light blue columns are the mean signal points in cells not treated with gold nanoparticles ('control'). The dark blue columns are the mean signal points from cells incubated with gold nanoparticles ('NG'). Error bars show the standard deviation of signal numbers.

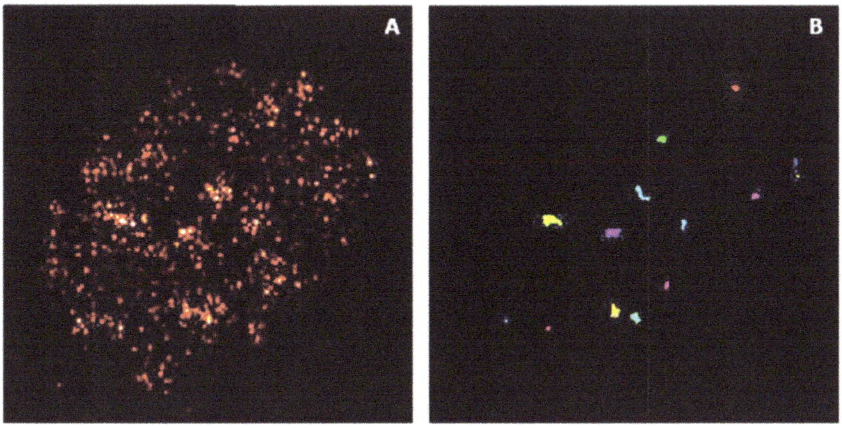

Figure 10.5. Determination of clusters: (a) signal density image of γH2AX labelling tags in a SkBr3 cell nucleus irradiated with 2 Gy of x-rays but not treated with gold nanoparticles. (b) Clusters highlighted by contiguous areas of different colors. The cluster parameters of minimum 45 points in a radius of 200 nm around a labeling tag were interactively determined.

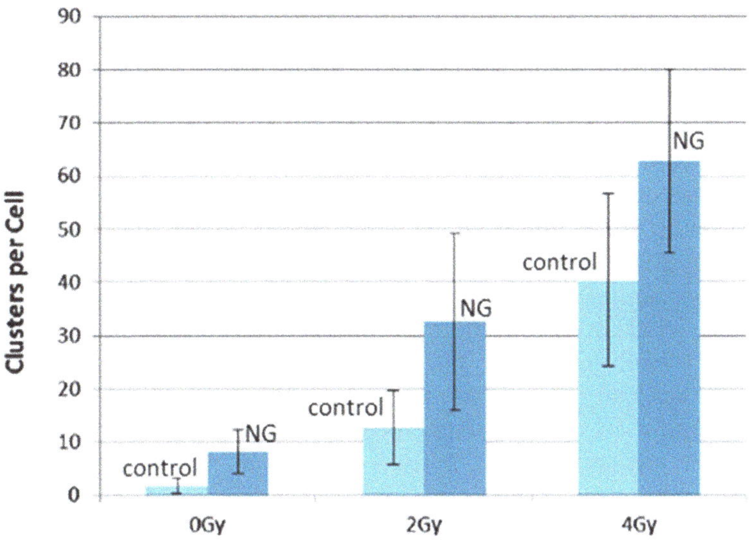

Figure 10.6. Numbers of γH2AX clusters in SkBr3 cell nuclei observed for indicated treatments. The columns represent the mean numbers of γH2AX signal clusters per cell nucleus obtained from 35 to 40 cell nuclei analyzed for each treatment. The light blue columns show the mean number of clusters in cell nuclei not treated with gold nanoparticles ('control'). The dark blue columns show the mean number of clusters in cell nuclei treated with gold nanoparticles ('NG'). Error bars show the standard deviation of cluster numbers per cell.

observed in irradiated cells treated with gold nanoparticles as compared to irradiated but untreated controls. This observation points to more serious damage introduced to the (nuclear) DNA by the combined action of radiation and nanoparticles.

To summarize, the mechanisms of radiation interaction with nanoparticles, specifically gold nanoparticles, and the radiation response of differently radio-sensitive cells remain elusive. Standard procedures such as clonogenic assay provide the crucial information on survival of nanoparticle-treated cells upon irradiation but do not consider initial DNA damage unless it forces them to die. Hence, with the 'survival' approaches, the results on DNA damage induction may be more influenced by damage tolerance or improved repair capacity of various cancer cells than the presence or absence of nanoparticles. The counting of γH2AX foci may help to directly access radiation-induced nanoparticle enhanced damage of chromatin since it can be performed just after damage induction on the single cell level. These approaches could be supported by the application of novel super-resolution light microscopy techniques which offer a more detailed view on the damaging process and DNA lesion complexity. New super-resolution microscopy techniques thus significantly broaden our experimental opportunities and bring about new chances to better understand the mechanisms of radiation effect enhancement by nanoparticles in tumor cells and to allow methodological translation of this knowledge into cancer radiation therapy.

Beyond the aforementioned nanoparticle damaging effects, another open question has for instance to be accessed: how could nanoparticles be modified to directly access the cell nucleus or even target tumor-related genome sites? So far, only an unspecific transfer into the cell nucleus has been reported. It seemed to result in an additional decrease of cell survival after irradiation as compared to cells irradiated with nanoparticles in the cytosol only (Aliru *et al* 2017). This may be due to short-range Auger electrons inducing additional damaging effects. But for 6 MV x-rays, it does not seem to be very relevant as short-ranged Auger electrons in gold are irrelevant at those energies. On the other hand, if nanoparticles would not easily pass the nuclear membrane, other organelles relevant for cell survival could be preferentially targeted and damaged (Hildenbrand *et al* 2018) as discussed in the following paragraph. The final and rather 'philosophical' question therefore is, if we really want to target nanoparticles to the nucleus. Would the increase in tumor cell dying given by the ability of nanoparticles to penetrate the cell nucleus be sufficient to compensate the increased risk of genome damage in normal cells, also to some extent infiltrated by nanoparticles?

10.3 Nanoparticle-mediated radio-sensitization of tumor cells independent of nuclear DNA damage

Radio-sensitizing effects of nanoparticles that are not dependent on amplified DNA damage in cells irradiated in the presence of nanoparticles remain mostly unexplored as holds true also for cytoplasmic effects of irradiation only. The first extra-nuclear target one can think of in relation to nanoparticle mediated radio-sensitization are mitochondria, since they are the only cytoplasmic organelles in human cells that contain DNA and produce energy for cell processes. Thus, the same physical mechanism as that already proposed to damage the cell nucleus (nuclear DNA)—based on electron showers emission and local dose amplification by scattering—can also harm mitochondria. However, most studies did not observe co-localization of randomly non-targetedly incorporated nanoparticles with this organelle, leaving the mitochondria-based hypothesis rather theoretical; hence, damage to mitochondria would be probably overweighed by effects on the nucleus or other cellular targets. Moreover, incorporation into mitochondria would require that the gold nanoparticles pass two additional membranes. Nevertheless, mitochondria damage was considered as an important aspect of nanoparticle-mediated tumor cell radiosensitization for instance by Taggart *et al* (2014) or Ghita *et al* (2017).

Endoplasmic reticulum is another important cytoplasmic organelle potentially affected by nanoparticles. Similar to mitochondria though, studies localizing nanoparticles to this space are rather exceptional; nevertheless, induction of endoplasmic reticulum stress by nanoparticles has been described in several studies (Chen *et al* 2014, Noël *et al* 2016, Gunduz *et al* 2017).

In addition, targeting of modified targeting nanogold probes tagged with multiple DNA oligonucleotides or PNA chains that are aiming against RNAs of genes that are up-regulated in tumor cells and accumulated in the endoplasmic reticulum could represent a new therapeutic approach. In these cases, RNA tagging would lead to a preferred accumulation of gold nanoparticles in the endoplasmatic reticulum and damage the protein synthesizing machinery. The SmartFlare probes (Seferos *et al* 2007, Prigodich *et al* 2012), based on this design, were originally proposed for RNA targeting and visualization (the gold core serves just as a carrier for the dye). However, SmartFlare binding to a gene product in the endoplasmic reticulum would also concentrate nanoparticles in this organelle and around the cell nucleus. Thus, in tumor cell types where certain genes are considerably up-regulated, targeting of nanoparticles to over-transcribed RNAs of these genes could ensure nanoparticle accumulation in the tumor cells only. Upon irradiation, this will selectively reduce the radio-resistance of cancer cells as compared to normal counterparts without extra-ordinary gene up-regulation.

In contrast to mitochondria and endoplasmatic reticulum, frequent studies localized nanoparticles to lysosomes that represent the place of their final destination in the cells. Co-localization studies showed that lysosomes accumulate substantial amounts of nanoparticles as compared to other cellular compartments. Nanoparticles appear also in the free cytoplasm, with some of them forming a sort of rim around the cell nucleus, and in endosomes (before being released into lysosomes). Several groups showed that nanoparticles internalized in lysosomes can increase cell dying upon irradiation independently of the nuclear DNA damage enhancement (Boya and Kroemer 2008, Serrano-Puebla and Boya 2018). This finding, confirmed also by clonogenic assay that still represents the gold standard method in radiobiology for this purpose, was quite surprising as scientists originally only considered lysosomes as cellular thresh bins clearing the cells from extracellular agents and redundant or damaged cellular components (autophagy). However, as discovered later, lysosomes also participate in important regulatory cell pathways, most importantly cell death initiation (Boya and Kroemer 2008, Serrano-Puebla and Boya 2018).

Hence, in principle two ways, though still hypothetical, could explain activation of cell death by nanoparticles irradiated inside lysosomes. Lysosomes contain many different hydrolytic enzymes, including proteases, nucleases, phosphatases, phospholipases, glycosidases and sulfatases (Boya and Kroemer 2008, Serrano-Puebla and Boya 2018). Massive disintegration of many lysosomes—for instance by harmful free radicals generated by irradiated nanoparticles, can therefore release large amounts these enzymes into the cytoplasm and its direct damage. Although aggressive lysosomal enzymes usually work at low pH that is actively being maintained only in lysosomes, if the leakage is extensive enough, the cytoplasm cannot further buffer its pH, becomes acidified, and digested together with all the organelles contained. This leads to fast death of the cell by necrosis.

Less extensive disruption of lysosomes by irradiated nanoparticles may then contribute to dying of irradiated cells indirectly. Under these circumstances, only limited amounts of proteases enter the cytoplasm. Among them, cathepsin B, cathepsin D and cathepsin L remain active at neutral pH and activate proapoptotic effectors, such as caspases, and mitochondria. This pathway can thus translate local effects of short-lived secondary electrons and reactive oxygen species produced by irradiated nanoparticles into global cell signaling and finally cell death by apoptosis (Boya and Kroemer 2008). In fact, some nanoparticles produce ROS even without irradiation, which may also result in lysosome damage, in turn manifested as cytotoxicity. Production of free radicals by nanoparticles (Soenen *et al* 2012, Martínez-Torres *et al* 2018) and lysosome-mediated nanoparticle enhanced cell death by both the direct and the indirect mechanisms upon irradiation have already been proposed in the literature (Štefančíiková *et al* 2016); however, their experimental confirmation remains a matter of future research. Just to emphasize the importance of lysosomes—the former trash bins—for the cell life, a hypothesis was proposed (Settembre *et al* 2012) based on data that lysosomes sense the physiological and nutritional condition of the cells and signal this information to the nucleus, where it is used to coordinate gene expression programs. Altogether, compelling evidence indicates that lysosomes have a much broader role than previously thought—they play a key role in maintaining cell homeostasis by regulating cellular clearance, energy production (Settembre *et al* 2012, Lim and Zoncu 2016), and cell death signaling associated with apoptosis and/or autophagy (Boya and Kroemer 2008, Settembre *et al* 2013, Lim and Zoncu 2016). Lysosomes thus serve as regulating knots interconnecting several important pathways of the cell signaling network and their damage can have far-reaching consequences even upon relatively mild stimuli.

10.4 Conclusions

To conclude, within the present situation of nanoparticle research many contradictions remain on the mechanism of nanoparticle-mediated tumor cell radiosensitization as well as on the relationship between their physical and chemical properties and biological effects, including cytotoxicity. This is not very surprising concerning the variability of nanoparticles (material, size, shape, composition, surface modifications and functionalization) and biological systems (cell types, cell origin etc) as well as different radiation qualities and types or evaluation procedures used in experiments.

In the experiments presented here, a standard cell model was used for gold nanoparticle induced radio-sensitization. However, cell death was not increasing. This may be due to several effects simultaneously disturbing cell functions; thereby not increasing DNA damaging as would be indicated by the outcome of cell survival. Such processes are discussed above without finding any preference. The results of cell survival, however, did not reflect results of γH2AX cluster analyses. This may be conclusive with the hypothesis that application of the particles may increase DNA damaging and influence the repair process by a delayed synthesis of repair proteins. Survival curves are measured over a long period in which a short delay in repair would not matter. Recent preliminary results (data not shown) did not support this hypothesis. So these findings of uninfluenced cell survival and increase of γH2AX clusters are also compatible with an accompanied, increased repair activity, typical for radio-resistant cell types (Bobkova *et al* 2018).

On the other hand, depending on the cell type used, nanoparticles seem to be isolated and distributed over the cytosol, or clustered either nearby the endoplastmatic reticulum or the cell membrane (Hildenbrand *et al* 2018; unpublished own results). This might have an influence on radiation scattering and thus on cell survival of individual cells. The number of nanoparticles and their distances to specific cellular targets (e.g. DNA in cell nuclei) as well as the ability to correctly repair DNA damage is not the same for all cells. This may lead to stochastic effects in $SF = \exp(-\alpha D - \beta D^2)$. From the mathematical perspective, in the presence of nanoparticles this simple prediction of SF cannot be used further and a more complex stochastic framework (Zygmanski *et al* 2013b) must be applied. Variations in SF are due to the situation in which some cellular targets may be damaged or even over-damaged, and others under-damaged. Experimental cell survival studies are based on bulge measurements for a population of cells. But these populations are a mixed bag. Stochastic effects apply differently to a uniform sample and differently to heterogeneous populations (Gadoue *et al* 2018). Thus, SMLM or other super-resolution, single cell techniques acquiring detailed information about sub-cellular modifications may be techniques that could bring new light into the shadow of lacking understanding of nanoparticle induced cell damaging mechanisms.

Nevertheless, it becomes evident that functional structuralization of cells and their biological behavior play an important role in the process initiated by nanoparticles in cells prior to and after irradiation. Super-resolution optical microscopy methods, as also demonstrated in the present contribution, thus represent new experimental approaches that promise new important discoveries in the field which could support so far well-established techniques in biological dosimetry as clonogenic assay or others. Since clonogenic growth is the most important result for the clinical outcome, a better understanding of DNA damage might support methods to modify cell treatment towards further reduction of tumor cell survival.

10.5 Materials and methods

10.5.1 Cell culture, gold nanoparticle incorporation, and specimen irradiation

SkBr3 human breast adenocarcinoma cells, obtained from ATCC (American Type Culture Collection, Manassas, VA, USA), were cultivated in flat-bottom T75 flasks in McCoy's Medium supplemented with 10% FBS without any antibiotics. Cells were incubated in a chamber at 37 °C and 95% air/5% CO_2. Every three to four days the cells were harvested and reseeded 1:10 in flasks: The cells were washed with PBS and incubated in 2 ml of a solution of 3× Trypsin/EDTA at 37 °C for 5 min Once all cells were detached from the bottom of the flask, fresh media was added and the cell suspension was homogenized by pipette. Upon reaching approximately 70%–90% visible confluence of cells, they again were harvested, counted, and diluted to obtain 10^4 cells ml^{-1} in each well of a six-well culture plate, and incubated overnight, allowing cells to adhere to the bottom of each well.

Then the medium was removed from each well, and cells were washed with PBS. Each well received 2.5 ml of fresh McCoy's Medium containing no FBS. Each well for gold nanoparticle incorporation received 8 μl colloidal gold nanoparticle (10 nm diameter, $5 \cdot \times 10^{12}$ particles ml^{-1}) suspension ('NG') in 2.5 ml of FBS-free media. Untreated control wells only received FBS-free media. Cells were then incubated in these well-plates for 18 h at 37 °C.

In addition, SkBr3 cells were also grown on clean coverslips in well-plates according to the same protocol. After 18 h incubation, cells adhered to coverslips were washed with PBS, and fresh McCoy's medium containing 10% FBS was added.

Each well-plate was irradiated at room temperature by 6 MV x-rays (dose: 2 Gy, 4 Gy) delivered from a clinical linear accelerator (LINAC, Synergy, Elekta AB, Stockholm, Sweden; dose rate 6.67 Gy min^{-1}). During irradiation, the well-plates were positioned in such a way that the surface of the media in each well was about 100 cm distant from the radiation source. Each well-plate was put on top of eight 1 cm thick RW3 phantom plates with one 1 cm thick PMMA plate placed on top to homogenize backscatter effects (figure 10.7).

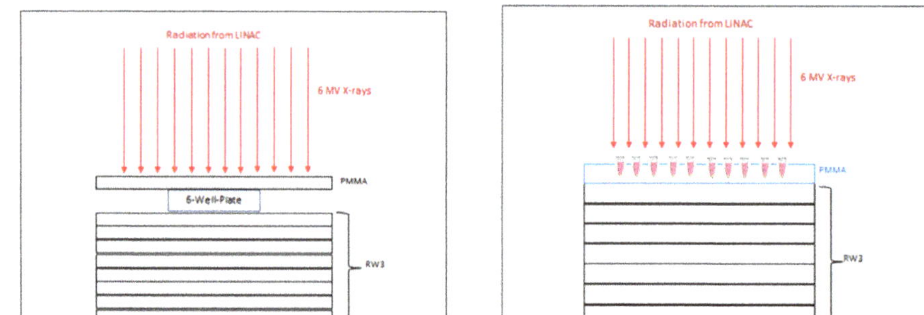

Figure 10.7. Schematic representation of the setup for cell irradiation in the clinical linear accelerator. (a) Set-up for the localization microscopy experiments. (b) Set-up for clonogenic assays.

Following irradiation, cells were incubated at 37 °C for 30 min, after which the media was removed from all wells in all plates and replaced with PBS for 5 min at room temperature. Then the cells were fixed in 3.7% formaldehyde (prepared from paraformaldehyde) for 30 min at room temperature. After fixation, cells were washed three times with PBS and stored in PBS containing 0.05% sodium azide for further processing.

10.5.2 Clonogenic assay (colony forming assay)

The following clonogenic assay (also known as colony forming assay; CFA) procedure was adapted from a protocol described in Burger *et al* (2014). SkBr3 cells were grown in well plates as described above. After 18 h incubation, medium was removed from each well and cells were washed with PBS. Cells were then incubated in 1 ml 3× Trypsin/EDTA per well at 37 °C for 5 min Once all cells were detached from the bottom of the wells, 2 ml of fresh McCoy's Medium with 10% FBS were added to each well and the cell suspension was homogenized by pipette. From each well the cell suspension was transferred to two separate 15 ml tubes, one for untreated cells ('control') and the other for cells treated with gold nanoparticles (NG). The number of cells in each tube was counted with a hemo-cytometer viewed under the microscope.

The content of each 15 ml tube was diluted with a specific volume of fresh McCoy's medium with 10% FBS calculated to achieve the desired cell number in 400 μl, the volume consequently transferred into a single micro-centrifuge tube for each radiation dose. This process created 10 micro-centrifuge tubes, each containing 400 μl of liquid, where five tubes contained cells treated with gold nanoparticles and five tubes untreated cells, one for each radiation dose.

All 10 micro-centrifuge tubes were sealed and centrifuged at 290 g for 5 min The cells were irradiated in the closed micro-centrifuge tubes by 6 MV x-rays delivered from a linear accelerator (LINAC, Synergy, Elekta AB, Stockholm, Sweden; dose rate 6.67 Gy min^{-1}) at room temperature. During irradiation, the tubes were positioned in such a way that the surface of the media in each well was about 100 cm distant from the radiation source. The tubes were put on top of eight 1 cm thick RW3 phantom plates (figure 10.7).

After irradiation, cell pellets were thoroughly re-suspended by pipette to ensure homogeneity and individual dispersal of cells within each tube. 100 μl was then transferred from each tube into one of three corresponding T25 flasks. Assuming homogenous resuspension, each flask received one quarter of the cells seeded into each micro-centrifuge tube. 5 ml of fresh McCoy's medium with 10% FBS was then added to each flask.

Cells were incubated at 37 °C and 95% air/5% CO_2 for 14 days to allow sufficient colony growth. After the two weeks of incubation, the medium was removed from the flasks; the cells were washed with PBS and fixed with 3.7% formaldehyde (prepared from paraformaldehyde), followed by 70% ethanol fixation for 10 min each. For visualization of colonies, adherent cells were then stained with Coomassie dye for 40 s, rinsed with cold water, and subsequently dyed with Giemsa solution for

40 min Stained colonies, of at least 50 cells, were visualized under the microscope and counted. The surviving fraction of cells in each flask was determined by dividing the number of colonies per cells seed by the plating efficiency of the cells. Plating efficiency (PE) of the SkBr3 cell line used in these experiments had already been determined by growing the cells (without treatment or radiation) in McCoy's Medium with 10% FBS at various densities and counting the colonies that formed after two weeks. Surviving fractions (SF) were plotted for each treatment at each dose (D) and survival curves fitted using the linear-quadratic model ($SF = e^{-(\alpha D+\beta D^2)}$).

10.5.3 γH2AX immunostaining

Immunostaining of γH2AX was performed according to the protocol described recently (Krufczik *et al* 2017). Coverslips containing fixed cells were washed with 1× PBS + Mg/Ca to remove residual sodium azide. The coverslips, each within the well of a six-well plate, were submerged in 2 ml of permeabilization solution (0.2% Triton-X in 1× PBS + Mg/Ca) and the plate was shaken for 3 min at room temperature. Cells were then washed three times with 1× PBS + Mg/Ca for 5 min each before being incubated in blocking solution (2% BSA in 1× PBS + Mg/Ca) for 30 min. Cells were then incubated with 100 μl of primary mouse-anti-phospho-histone H2AX (Ser139) antibody solution (clone JBW301, Merck Chemicals GmbH, Darmstadt, Germany; 1:500 in 2 % BSA in 1× PBS + Mg/Ca) for 18 h at 4 °C in a humidified chamber. After incubation, cells were washed three times with 1× PBS + Mg/Ca for 5 min each, and then incubated with 100 μl of the secondary Alexa Fluor® 647 labelled goat-anti-mouse IgG antibody solution (Merck Chemicals GmbH, Darmstadt, Germany; 1:500 in 2 % BSA (in 1× PBS + Mg/Ca)for 30 min in a 37 °C humidified chamber. Cells were then washed three times with 1× PBS + Mg/Ca for 5 min before being fixed in 2% formaldehyde (freshly prepared from paraformaldehyde) at 37 °C for 10 min. The cells were incubated for 21 h in a 37 °C humidified chamber. The cells were washed three times in 2× SSC at 37 °C for 10 min each. Coverslips were then soaked in 1× PBS + Mg/Ca and the cells allowed to equilibrate for 5 min. The cells were then incubated in 100 μl 4′,6-diamidino-2-phenylindole (DAPI) solution (100–500 ng ml^{-1} in 1× PBS) for 5 min at room temperature in the dark. After DAPI staining, coverslips were again washed with 1× PBS + Mg/Ca before being placed cell side down onto 20 μl of ProlongGold (ThermoFischer, Massachusetts, USA, ProLong® Gold Antifade Mountant, P36930) on a microscope slide. Coverslips were sealed on slides and stored in darkness at 4 °C until being used for localization microscopy.

10.5.4 Single molecule localization microscopy

Single molecule localization microscopy (SMLM) was used to count γH2AX labelling tags and to determine the frequency distributions of γH2AX foci/clusters within SkBr3 cell nuclei. For data acquisition, the setup from the light microscopy facility of the German Cancer Research Centre (DKFZ) was used (in detail described elsewhere (Krufczik *et al* 2017, Hausmann *et al* 2017, 2018, Eryilmaz *et al* 2018). The microscope has an oil-objective (100×/NA 1.46) and four lasers 405 nm/491 nm/561 nm/642 nm with maximal laser powers of 120 mW/200 mW/200 mW/140 mW, respectively. An in-built electron multiplier (EM-gain) enhances signals detected by the EmCCD camera (80 nm/px). In order to minimize drifts, the microscope was installed on a Smart-Table, compensating for vibrations, and provided with a water-cooling system to keep constant temperature.

Cells in this experiment were imaged using the 405 nm and 642 nm lasers to visualize DAPI and γH2AX stains, respectively. At least 35 cells from each treatment were imaged. Individual cell nuclei were selected by uniform shape as visualized by DAPI staining (using the 405 nm laser). Images were cropped to isolate and encompass an entire cell nucleus. 2000 image frames were acquired at each wavelength with an exposure time of 100 ms per image.

Super-resolution signal coordinates were calculated using Matlab-based in-house software as described elsewhere (Hausmann *et al* 2017, Krufczik *et al* 2017, Pilarczyk *et al* 2017, Stuhlmüller *et al* 2015, Kaufmann *et al* 2009). Background levels were multiplied by threshold factors for more rigorous background subtraction. The intensity barycenter determined the x-, y-coordinates of a signal point with a certain localization error. For quantitative super-resolution data analyses, the total number of signal points and all-to-all point distances between signal points were calculated. Resulting single-cell data were summarized for each experimental setup for further statistical analysis. Cluster analysis was performed according to interactively determined parameters. (figure 10.5): Pixel size = 10 nm, radius = 20 pixels, maximum distance for all distances = 200 nm, maximum distance for next neighbors = 200 nm. The minimal neighbor value (N) was determined to $N = 45$. The mean number of clusters per cell was calculated.

Acknowledgement

The authors thank PD Dr Carsten Herskind, Department of Radiation Oncology, Mannheim, for using his laboratory for cell culture work and Dr Felix Bestvater, German Cancer Research Center, Heidelberg, for using the localization microscope setup. The authors also thank Adriana Grbenicek, Miriam Bierbaum, Philipp Metzler and Jin-Ho Lee for their support and discussions. The discussion with Piotr Zygmanski about stochastic effects is acknowledged improving several perspectives of the manuscript. The work was supported by the Heidelberg University Mobility Grant for International Research Cooperation within the excellence initiative II of the Deutsche Forschungsgemeinschaft (DFG) to M H, and by the Mobility project DAAD-19–03 to M H and M F.

References

Aliru M L, Aziz K, Bodd M, Sanders K, Mahadevan L S K, Sahoo N, Tailor R C and Krishnan S 2017 Targeted gold nanoparticles enhance radiation effects in pancreatic tumor models *Int. J. Radiat. Oncol. Biol. Phys.* **99** E574–5

Alkilany A M and Murphy C J 2010 Toxicity and cellular uptake of gold nanoparticles: what we have learned so far? *J. Nanopart. Res.* **12** 2313–33

Atun R *et al* 2015 Expanding global access to radiotherapy *Lancet Oncol.* **16** 1153–86
Banath J P, MacPhail S H and Olive P L 2004 Radiation sensitivity, H2AX phosphorylation, and kinetics of repair of DNA strand breaks in irradiated cervical cancer cell lines *Cancer Res.* **64** 7144–9
Benton J Z, Williams R J, Patel A, Meichner K, Tarigo J, Nagata K, Pethel T D and Gogal R M Jr 2018 Gold nanoparticles enhance radiation sensitization and suppress colony formation in a feline injection site sarcoma cell line, *in vitro Res. Vet. Sci.* **117** 104–10
Bertrand N, Wu J, Xu X, Kamaly N and Farokhzad O C 2014 Cancer nanotechnology: The impact of passive and active targeting in the era of modern cancer biology *Adv. Drug Deliv. Rev.* **66** 2–25
Bobkova E *et al* 2018 Recruitment of 53BP1 proteins for DNA repair and persistence of repair clusters differ for cell types as detected by single molecule localization microscopy *Int. J. Molec. Sci.* **19** 3713
Boya P and Kroemer G 2008 Lysosomal membrane permeabilization in cell death *Oncogene* **27** 6434–51
Burger N, Biswas A, Barzan D, Kirchner A, Hosser H, Hausmann M, Hildenbrand G, Herskind C, Wenz F and Veldwijk M R 2014 A method for the efficient cellular uptake and retention of small modified gold nanoparticles for the radiosensitization of cells *Nanomed. Nanotechnol. Biol. Med.* **10** 1365–73
Cartiera M S, Johnson K M, Rajendran V, Caplan M J and Saltzman W M 2009 The uptake and intracellular fate of PLGA nanoparticles in epithelial cells *Biomaterials* **30** 2790–8
Chen R, Huo L, Shi X, Bai R, Zhang Z, Zhao Y, Chang Y and Chen C 2014 Endoplasmic reticulum stress induced by zinc oxide nanoparticles is an earlier biomarker for nano-toxicological evaluation *ACS Nano.* **8** 2562–74
Chen F, Zhang X H, Hu X D, Zhang W, Lou Z C, Xie L H, Liu P D and Zhang H Q 2015 Enhancement of radiotherapy by ceria nanoparticles modified with neogambogic acid in breast cancer cells *Int. J. Nanomed.* **10** 4957–69
Chithrani B D, Ghazani A A and Chan W C 2006 Determining the size and shape dependence of gold nanoparticle uptake into mammalian cells *Nano Lett.* **6** 662–8
Chithrani D B 2010a Nanoparticles for improved therapeutics and imaging in cancer therapy *Recent Pat. Nanotechnol.* **4** 171–80
Chithrani D B, Jelveh S, Jalali F, van Prooijen M, Allen C, Bristow R G, Hill R P and Jaffray D A 2010b Gold nanoparticles as radiation sensitizers in cancer therapy *Radiat. Res.* **173** 719–28
Conner S D and Schmid S L 2003 Regulated portals of entry into the cell *Nature* **422** 37–44
Coulter J A *et al* 2012 Cell type-dependent uptake, localization, and cytotoxicity of 1.9 nm gold nanoparticles *Int. J. Nanomed.* **7** 2673–85
Cremer C and Masters B R 2013 Resolution enhancement techniques in microscopy *Eur. Phys. J. H* **38** 281–344
Davis M E 2016 Glioblastoma: Overview of disease and treatment *Clin. J. Oncol. Nurs.* **20** S2–8
Deschout H, Cella Zanacchi F, Mlodzianoski M, Diaspro A, Bewersdorf J, Hess S T and Braeckmans K 2014 Precisely and accurately localizing single emitters in fluorescent microscopy *Nat. Methods* **11** 253–66
Dikomey E, Dahm-Daphi J, Brammer I, Martensen R and Kaina B 1998 Correlation between cellular radiosensitivity and non-repaired double-strand breaks studied in nine mammalian cell lines *Int. J. Radiat. Biol.* **73** 269–78

Durante M, Orecchia R and Loeffler J S 2017 Charged-particle therapy in cancer: clinical uses and future perspectives *Nat. Rev. Clin. Oncol.* **14** 483–95

Engel L W and Young N A 1978 Human breast carcinoma cells in continuous culture: a review *Cancer Res.* **38** 4327–39

Eryilmaz M, Schmitt E, Krufczik M, Theda F, Lee J-H, Cremer C, Bestvater F, Schaufler W, Hausmann M and Hildenbrand G 2018 Localization microscopy analyses of MRE11 clusters in 3D-conserved cell nuclei of different cell lines *Cancers* **10** 25

Falk M *et al* 2014a Determining omics spatiotemporal dimensions using exciting new nanoscopy techniques to assess complex cell responses to DNA damage: part A—radiomics *Crit. Rev. Eukaryot. Gene Expr.* **24** 205–23

Falk M *et al* 2014b Determining omics spatiotemporal dimensions using exciting new nanoscopy techniques to assess complex cell responses to DNA damage: part B—structuromics *Crit. Rev. Eukaryot. Gene Expr.* **24** 225–47

Falk M, Lukasova E and Kozubek S 2010 Higher-order chromatin structure in DSB induction, repair and misrepair *Mutat. Res.* **704** 88–100

Fang J, Nakamura H and Maeda H 2011 The EPR effect: unique features of tumor blood vessels for drug delivery, factors involved, and limitations and augmentation of the effect *Adv. Drug Deliv. Rev.* **63** 136–51

Fernando L P, Kandel P K, Yu J, McNeill J, Ackroyd P C and Christensen K A 2010 Mechanism of cellular uptake of highly fluorescent conjugated polymer nanoparticles *Biomacromolecules* **11** 2675–82

Freneau A, Dos Santos M, Voisin P, Tang N, Bueno Vizcarra M, Villagrasa C, Roy L, Vaurijoux A and Gruel G 2018 Relation between DNA double-strand breaks and energy spectra of secondary electrons produced by different x-ray energies *Int. J. Radiat. Biol.* **94** 1075–84

Fröhlich E 2013 Cellular targets and mechanisms in the cytotoxic action of non-biodegradable engineered nanoparticles *Curr. Drug Metab.* **14** 976–88

Gadoue S M, Zygmanski P and Sajo E 2018 The dichotomous nature of dose enhancement by gold nanoparticle aggregates in radiotherapy *Nanomedicine* **13** 809–23

Ghita M, McMahon S J, Taggart L E, Butterworth K T, Schettino G and Prise K M 2017 A mechanistic study of gold nanoparticle radiosensitisation using targeted microbeam irradiation *Sci. Rep.* **7** 44752

Girst S *et al* 2016 Proton minibeam radiation therapy reduces side effects in an *in vivo* mouse ear model *Int. J. Radiat. Oncol.* **95** 234–41

González W and Prezado Y 2018 Spatial fractionation of the dose in heavy ions therapy: an optimization study *Med. Phys.* **45** 2620–7

Gu H, Huang T, Shen Y, Liu Y, Zhou F, Jin Y, Sattar H and Wei Y 2018 Reactive oxygen species-mediated tumor microenvironment transformation: the mechanism of radioresistant gastric cancer *Oxid. Med. Cell. Longev.* **2018** 5801209

Gunduz N, Ceylan H, Guler M O and Tekinay A B 2017 Intracellular accumulation of gold nanoparticles leads to inhibition of macropinocytosis to reduce the endoplasmic reticulum stress *Sci. Rep.* **7** 40493

Hainfeld J F, Smilowitz H M, O'Connor M J, Dilmanian F A and Slatkin D N 2013 Gold nanoparticle imaging and radiotherapy of brain tumors in mice *Nanomedicine* **8** 1601–9

Hausmann M *et al* 2017 Challenges for super-resolution localization microscopy and biomolecular fluorescent nano-probing in cancer research *Int. J. Mol. Sci.* **18** 2066

Hausmann M, Wagner E, Lee J-H, Schrock G, Schaufler W, Krufczik M, Papenfuß F, Port M, Bestvater F and Scherthan H 2018 Super-resolution localization microscopy of radiation-induced histone H2AX-phosphorylation in relation to H3K9-trimethylation in HeLa cells *Nanoscale* **10** 4320–31

He H, Xie C and Ren J 2008 Nonbleaching fluorescence of gold nanoparticles and its applications in cancer cell imaging *Anal. Chem.* **80** 5951–7

Herold D M, Das I J, Stobbe C C, Iyer R V and Chapman J D 2000 Gold microspheres: a selective technique for producing biologically effective dose enhancement *Int. J. Radiat. Biol.* **76** 1357–64

Hildenbrand G *et al* 2018 Dose enhancement effects of gold nanoparticles specifically targeting RNA in breast cancer cells *PLoS One* **13** e0190183

Hofer M *et al* 2016 Two new faces of amifostine: protector from dna damage in normal cells and inhibitor of dna repair in cancer cells *J. Med. Chem.* **59** 3003–17

Hofer M, Hoferová Z, Depeš D and Falk M 2017a Combining pharmacological countermeasures to attenuate the acute radiation syndrome-a concise review *Molecules* **22** 834

Hofer M, Hoferová Z and Falk M 2017b Pharmacological modulation of radiation damage. does it exist a chance for other substances than hematopoietic growth factors and cytokines? *Int. J. Mol. Sci.* **18** 1385

Hofmann A, Krufczik M, Heermann D W and Hausmann M 2018 Using persistent homology as a new approach for super-resolution localization microscopy data analysis and classification of γH2AX foci/clusters *Int. J. Mol. Sci.* **19** 2263

Hossain M and Su M 2012 Nanoparticle location and material dependent dose enhancement in x-ray radiation therapy *J. Phys. Chem. C Nanomater. Interfaces* **116** 23047–52

Jain S *et al* 2011 Cell-specific radiosensitization by gold nanoparticles at megavoltage radiation energies *Int. J. Radiat. Oncol. Biol. Phys.* **79** 531–9

Jánváry L Z, Ferenczi Ö, Takácsi-Nagy Z, Bajcsay A and Polgár C 2018 [Application of CyberKnife stereotactic radiosurgery in the treatment of head and neck cancer] *Magy. Onkol.* **62** 180–5

Jezkova L *et al* 2018 Particles with similar LET values generate DNA breaks of different complexity and reparability: a high-resolution microscopy analysis of γH2AX/53BP1 foci *Nanoscale* **10** 1162–79

Kaufmann R, Lemmer P, Gunkel M, Weiland Y, Müller P, Hausmann M, Baddeley D, Amberger R and Cremer C 2009 SPDM—single molecule superresolution of cellular nanostructures *Proc. SPIE* **7185** 71850J1–19

Kim E H, Kim M S, Song H S, Yoo S H, Sai S, Chung K, Sung J, Jeong Y K, Jo Y and Yoon M 2017 Gold nanoparticles as a potent radiosensitizer in neutron therapy *Oncotarget* **8** 112390–400

Krufczik M, Sievers A, Hausmann A, Lee J-H, Hildenbrand G, Schaufler W and Hausmann M 2017 Combining low temperature fluorescence DNA-hybridization, immunostaining, and super-resolution localization microscopy for nano-structure analysis of ALU elements and their influence on chromatin structure *Int. J. Mol. Sci.* **18** 1005

Kuncic Z and Lacombe S 2018 Nanoparticle radio-enhancement: principles, progress and application to cancer treatment *Phys. Med. Biol.* **63** 02TR01

Kuo L J and Yang L X 2008 γ-H2AX—a novel biomarker for DNA double-strand breaks *In Vivo* **22** 305–10

Lacombe S, Porcel E and Scifoni E 2017 Particle therapy and nanomedicine: state of art and research perspectives *Cancer Nanotechnol.* **8** 9

Lacroix M and Leclercq G 2004 Relevance of breast cancer cell lines as models for breast tumours: an update *Breast Cancer Res. Treat.* **83** 249–89

Lam W W, Oakden W, Murray L, Klein J, Iorio C, Screaton R A, Koletar M M, Chu W, Liu S K and Stanisz G J 2018 Differentiation of normal and radioresistant prostate cancer xenografts using magnetization transfer-prepared MRI *Sci. Rep.* **8** 10447

Lemmer P, Gunkel M, Baddeley D, Kaufmann R, Urich A, Weiland Y, Reymann J, Müller P, Hausmann M and Cremer C 2008 SPDM: Light microscopy with single-molecule resolution at the nanoscale *Appl. Phys. B* **93** 1–12

Lemmer P *et al* 2009 Using conventional fluorescent markers for far-field fluorescence localization nanoscopy allows resolution in the 10 nm range *J. Microsc.* **235** 163–71

Li S, Porcel E, Remita H, Marco S, Réfrégiers M, Dutertre M, Confalonieri F and Lacombe S 2017 Platinum nanoparticles: An exquisite tool to overcome radioresistance *Cancer Nanotechnol.* **8** 4

Lim C Y and Zoncu R 2016 The lysosome as a command-and-control center for cellular metabolism *J. Cell Biol.* **214** 653–64

Löbrich M and Jeggo P A 2017 A process of resection-dependent non-homologous end joining involving the goddess Artemis *Trends Biol. Sci.* **42** 690–701

Löbrich M, Shibata A, Beucher A, Fisher A, Ensminger M, Goodarzi A A, Barton O and Jeggo P A 2010 γ-H2AX foci analysis for monitoring DNA double-strand repair: Strengths, limitations and optimization *Cell Cycle* **9** 662–9

Löffler H, Bochtler T, Fritz B, Tews B, Ho A D, Lukas J, Bartek J and Krämer A 2007 DNA damage-induced accumulation of centrosomal Chk1 contributes to its checkpoint function *Cell Cycle* **6** 2541–8

Lux F *et al* 2018 AGuIX® from bench to bedside-Transfer of an ultrasmall theranostic gadolinium-based nanoparticle to clinical medicine *Br. J. Radiol.* **92** 20180365

MacPhail S H *et al* 2003 Expression of phosphorylated histone H2AX in cultured cell line following exposure to x-rays *Int. J. Radiat. Biol.* **79** 351–8

Maeda H 2010 Tumor-selective delivery of macromolecular drugs via the EPR effect: Background and future prospects *Bioconjug. Chem.* **21** 797–802

Maeda H and Matsumura Y 2011 EPR effect based drug design and clinical outlook for enhanced cancer chemotherapy *Adv. Drug Deliv. Rev.* **63** 129–30

Martínez-Torres A C, Zarate-Triviño D G, Lorenzo-Anota H Y, Ávila-Ávila A, Rodríguez-Abrego C and Rodríguez-Padilla C 2018 Chitosan gold nanoparticles induce cell death in HeLa and MCF-7 cells through reactive oxygen species production *Int. J. Nanomed.* **13** 3235–50

Mladenov E, Magin S, Soni A and Iliakis G 2013 DNA double-strand break repair as determinant of cellular radiosensitivity to killing and target in radiation therapy *Front. Oncol.* **3** 113

Mladenov E, Magin S, Soni A and Iliakis G 2016 DNA double-strand-break repair in higher eukaryotes and its role in genomic instability and cancer: cell cycle and proliferation-dependent regulation *Semin. Cancer Biol.* **37–38** 51–64

Moser F *et al* 2016 Cellular uptake of gold nanoparticles and their behavior as labels for localization microscopy *Biophys. J.* **110** 947–53

Natale F *et al* 2017 Identification of the elementary structural units of the DNA damage response *Nat. Commun.* **8** 15760

Ngwa W *et al* 2017 Smart radiation therapy biomaterials *Int. J. Radiat. Oncol. Biol. Phys.* **97** 624–37

Ngwa W, Kumar R, Sridhar S, Korideck H, Zygmanski P, Cormack R A, Berbeco R and Makrigiorgos G M 2014 Targeted radiotherapy with gold nanoparticles: Current status and future perspectives *Nanomedicine* **9** 1063–82

Nikjoo H, Uehara S, Emfietzoglou D and Brahme A 2008 Heavy charged particles in radiation biology and biophysics *New J. Phys.* **10** 075006

Noël C, Simard J C and Girard D 2016 Gold nanoparticles induce apoptosis, endoplasmic reticulum stress events and cleavage of cytoskeletal proteins in human neutrophils *Toxicol. in Vitro* 12–22

Oberdorster G *et al* 2004 Translocation of inhaled ultrafine particles to the brain *Inhal. Toxicol.* **16** 437–45

Pan Y, Neuss S, Leifert A, Fischler M, Wen F, Simon U, Schmid G, Brandau W and Jahnen-Dechent W 2007 Size-dependent cytotoxicity of gold nanoparticles *Small* **3** 1941–9

Paro A D, Shanmugam I and van de Ven A L 2017 Nanoparticle-mediated x-ray radiation enhancement for cancer therapy *Methods Mol. Biol.* **1530** 391–401

Patil Y M, Rajpathak S N and Deobagkar D D 2019 Characterization and DNA methylation modulatory activity of gold nanoparticles synthesized by pseudoalteromonas strain *J. Biosci.* **44** pii:15

Pagáčová E *et al* 2019 Challenges and contradictions of metal nano-particle applications for radio-sensitivity enhancement in cancer therapy *Int. J. Mol. Sci.* **20** 588

Pilarczyk G, Nesnidal I, Gunkel M, Bach M, Bestvater F and Hausmann M 2017 Localisation microscopy of breast epithelial ErbB-2 receptors and gap junctions: Trafficking after gamma-irradiation, Neuregulin-1b and Herceptin application *Int. J. Mol. Sci.* **18** 362

Porcel E, Liehn S, Remita H, Usami N, Kobayashi K, Furusawa Y, Le Sech C and Lacombe S 2010 Platinum nanoparticles: a promising material for future cancer therapy? *Nanotechnology* **21** 85103

Prabhakar U, Maeda H, Jain R K, Sevick-Muraca E M, Zamboni W, Farokhzad O C, Barry S T, Gabizon A, Grodzinski P and Blakey D C 2013 Challenges and key considerations of the enhanced permeability and retention effect for nanomedicine drug delivery in oncology *Cancer Res.* **73** 2412–7

Prezado Y, Renier M and Bravin A 2009 A new method of creating minibeam patterns for synchrotron radiation therapy: a feasibility study *J. Synchrotron Radiat.* **16** 582–6

Prigodich A E, Randeria P S, Briley W E, Kim N J, Daniel W L, Giljohann D A and Mirkin C A 2012 Multiplexed nanoflares: mRNA detection in live cells *Anal. Chem.* **84** 2062–6

Puck T T and Markus P I 1956 Action of x-rays on mammalian cells *J. Exp. Med.* **103** 653–66

Rittich B, Spanová A, Falk M, Benes M J and Hrubý M 2004 Cleavage of double stranded plasmid DNA by lanthanide complexes *J. Chromatogr. B Anal. Technol. Biomed. Life Sci.* **800** 169–73

Rogakou E P, Pilch D R, Orr A H, Ivanova V S and Bonner W M 1998 DNA double-starnd breaks induce histone H2AX phosphorylation on serine 139 *J. Biol. Chem.* **273** 5858–68

Sammer M, Greubel C, Girst S and Dollinger G 2017 Optimization of beam arrangements in proton minibeam radiotherapy by cell survival simulations *Med. Phys.* **44** 6096–104

Sancey L *et al* 2014 The use of theranostic gadolinium-based nanoprobes to improve radiotherapy efficacy *Br. J. Radiol.* **87** 20140134
Sarin H *et al* 2008 Effective transvascular delivery of nanoparticles across the blood-brain tumor barrier into malignant glioma cells *J. Transl. Med.* **2008** 1–15
Schipler A and Iliakis G 2013 DNA double-strand-break complexity levels and their possible contributions to the probability for error-prone processing and repair pathway choice *Nucl. Acids Res.* **41** 7589–605
Seferos D S, Giljohann D A, Hill H D, Prigodich A E and Mirkin C A 2007 Nano-flares: probes for transfection and mRNA detection in living cells *J. Am. Chem. Soc.* **129** 15477–9
Serrano-Puebla A and Boya P 2018 Lysosomal membrane permeabilization as a cell death mechanism in cancer cells *Biochem. Soc. Trans.* **46** 207–15
Settembre C *et al* 2012 A lysosome-to-nucleus signalling mechanism senses and regulates the lysosome via mTOR and TFEB *EMBO J.* **31** 1095–108
Settembre C, Fraldi A, Medina D L and Ballabio A 2013 Signals for the lysosome: a control center for cellular clearance and energy metabolism *Nat. Rev. Mol. Cell Biol.* **14** 283–96
Soenen S J *et al* 2012 Cytotoxic effects of gold nanoparticles: a multiparametric study *ACS Nano* **6** 5767–83
Sonavane G, Tomoda K and Makino K 2008 Biodistribution of colloidal gold nanoparticles after intravenous administration: effect of particle size *Colloids Surf. B Biointerfaces* **66** 274–80
Štefančíiková L, Lacombe S, Salado D, Porcel E, Pagáčová E, Tillement O, Lux F, Depeš D, Kozubek S and Falk M 2016 Effect of gadolinium-based nanoparticles on nuclear DNA damage and repair in glioblastoma tumor cells *J. Nanobiotechnol.* **14** 63
Stefančíiková L *et al* 2014 Cell localisation of gadolinium-based nanoparticles and related radiosensitising efficacy in glioblastoma cells *Cancer Nanotechnol.* **5** 6
Struve N *et al* 2015 EGFRvIII does not affect radiosensitivity with or without gefitinib treatment in glioblastoma cells *Oncotarget* **20** 33867–77
Stuhlmüller M, Schwarz-Finsterle J, Fey E, Lux J, Bach M, Cremer C, Hinderhofer K, Hausmann M and Hildenbrand G 2015 In situ optical sequencing and nano-structure analysis of a trinucleotide expansion region by localization microscopy after specific COMBO-FISH labelling *Nanoscale* **7** 17938–46
Taggart L E, McMahon S J, Currell F J, Prise K M and Butterworth K T 2014 The role of mitochondrial function in gold nanoparticle mediated radiosensitisation *Cancer Nanotechnol.* **5** 5
Taggart L E, McMahon S J, Butterworth K T, Currell F J, Schettino G and Prise K M 2016 Protein disulphide isomerase as a target for nanoparticle-mediated sensitisation of cancer cells to radiation *Nanotechnology* **27** 215101
Thompson R E, Larson D R and Webb W W 2002 Precise nanometer localization analysis for individual fluorescent probes *Biophys. J.* **82** 2775–83
Tomita K, Kuwahara Y, Takashi Y, Igarashi K, Nagasawa T, Nabika H, Kurimasa A, Fukumoto M, Nishitani Y and Sato T 2018 Clinically relevant radioresistant cells exhibit resistance to H_2O_2 by decreasing internal H_2O_2 and lipid peroxidation *Tumour Biol.* **40** 1010428318799250
Turinetto V and Giachino C 2015 Multiple facets of histon variant H2AX: a DNA double-strand-break marker with several biological functions *Nucl. Acids Res.* **43** 2489–98
Wenz F, Tiefenbacher U, Willeke F and Weber K-J 2001 Auf der Suche nach der *Therapeutischen breite* in der Radioonkologie *Oncol. Res. Treat.* **24** 51–5

Wolfe T, Chatterjee D, Lee J, Grant J D, Bhattarai S, Tailor R, Goodrich G, Nicolucci P and Krishnan S 2015 Targeted gold nanoparticles enhance sensitization of prostate tumors to megavoltage radiation therapy *in vivo Nanotechnol. Biol. Med.* **11** 1277–83

Yang C, Bromma K, Sung W, Schuemann J and Chithrani D 2018 Determining the radiation enhancement effects of gold nanoparticles in cells in a combined treatment with cisplatin and radiation at therapeutic megavoltage energies *Cancers* 10 pii: E150

Yameen B, Choi W I, Vilos C, Swami A, Shi J and Farokhzad O C 2014 Insight into nanoparticle cellular uptake and intracellular targeting *J. Control. Release* **190** 485–99

Youkhana E Q, Feltis B, Blencowe A and Geso M 2017 Titanium dioxide nanoparticles as radiosensitisers: an *in vitro* and phantom-based study *Int. J. Med. Sci.* **14** 602–14

Zhang H *et al* 2018 *In vitro* radiobiological advantages of hypofractionation compared with conventional fractionation: early-passage NSCLC cells are less aggressive after hypofractionation *Radiat. Res.* **190** 584–95

Zhou H, Miki R, Eeva M, Fike F M, Seligson D, Yang L, Yoshimura A, Teitell M A, Jamieson C A M and Cacalano N A 2007 Reciprocal regulation of SOCS1 and SOCS3 enhances resistance to ionizing radiation in glioblastoma multiforme *Clin. Cancer Res.* **13** 2344–53

Zygmanski P, Hoegele W, Tsiamas P, Cifter F, Ngwa W, Berbeco R, Makrigiorgos M and Sajo E 2013a A stochastic model of cell survival for high-Z nanoparticle radiotherapy *Med. Phys.* **40** 024102

Zygmanski P, Liu B, Tsiamas P, Cifter F, Petersheim M, Hesser J and Sajo E 2013b Dependence of Monte Carlo microdosimetric computations on the simulation geometry of gold nanoparticles *Phys. Med. Biol.* **58** 7961–77

Part II

Imaging

Chapter 11

Super-resolution microscopy of nanogold-labelling

Michael Hausmann, Götz Pilarczyk, Emanuel Maus, Jürgen Hesser and Georg Hildenbrand

For super-resolution microscopy (electron microscopy as well as super-resolution optical microscopy), nanoparticles like nanogold particles can be used as labels of organelles or cells, or they can also be attached to specific antibodies instead of fluorochromes. This universal application in so far two different 'worlds of microscopy' shows the potential of such labelling systems for bridging the gap between super-resolution microscopy techniques in biological and bio-medical research. In this article we will show some principle considerations that have to be kept in mind for investigations of the biological nano-world.

11.1 Electron microscopy

Transmission electron microscopy developed in the 1930s and continuously improved in the following decades is one of the best super-resolving techniques in biology and life-sciences leading to deep insights into supra-molecular organization of molecular complexes and organelles in cells and cell nuclei. For imaging, electrons are accelerated by an electric field with a voltage of 80 kV–120 kV. The electrons are elastically or inelastically scattered by the sample so that they do not reach the same detection plane (focal plane) as the non-scattered electrons, thus leading to a contrast between object structures and environment. Since this Rutherford scattering of electrons at atom nuclei is strongly depending on the atomic number of the scattering elements, high atomic numbers improve contrasting and resolution.

Unfortunately, cell specimens do not provide regions with high atomic numbers so that advanced specimen preparation techniques are required: (1) The cell specimen has to be fixed by glutaraldehyde or vitrified by shock cryo-fixation in liquid ethane. (2) For dehydration, supercritical drying via ethanol and acetone

doi:10.1088/978-0-7503-2396-3ch11

series can be applied. (3) Then the specimen is embedded in resin block and thinned into micro-slices of a few hundred nm. (4) Biological samples (cells, tissues, etc) need high atomic number stains to enhance contrast. Compounds of heavy metals such as osmium, lead, uranium or gold may be used to selectively deposit electron dense atoms in or on the sample in desired cellular or protein region.

Heavy metal staining is mostly addressing biological structures in a general and less specific way. Nanogold particles can be further used as highly scattering points (molecular sized tags) in a heavy metal (e.g. osmium) sputtered biological specimen (figure 11.1(a)). So, electron microscopy is well suited to imaging nanogold particles due to their high electron density. However, transmission electron microscopy requires a rather complicated and time-consuming sample preparation which can be circumvented by light microscopy (see below).

In order to label molecular compounds (Ngwa *et al* 2017) specifically as for instance proteins, chromatin sides, receptors, etc, specific antibodies, oligonucleotides, or peptides can be used that highlight single target molecules. Such highly specific tags can be visualized by electron microscopy using nanogold particles bound to a secondary antibody against the primary antibody specifically labelling a given target side. Typically the size of such nanogold particles varies between 2 nm and 25 nm. If different primary and secondary antibodies are applied in one specimen, nanogold tags of different sizes allow the simultaneous labelling and lead to a 'multi-colour' approach in electron microscopy.

For example, in biological radiation research Rübe *et al* have established such a gold-labelling technique for identification and localization of different repair components and proteins in cell nuclei and tissue samples exposed to ionizing radiation like x-rays or heavy ions (Rübe *et al* 2011, Lorat *et al* 2015). Using differently sized nanogold particles, damaged sides were analysed by specific

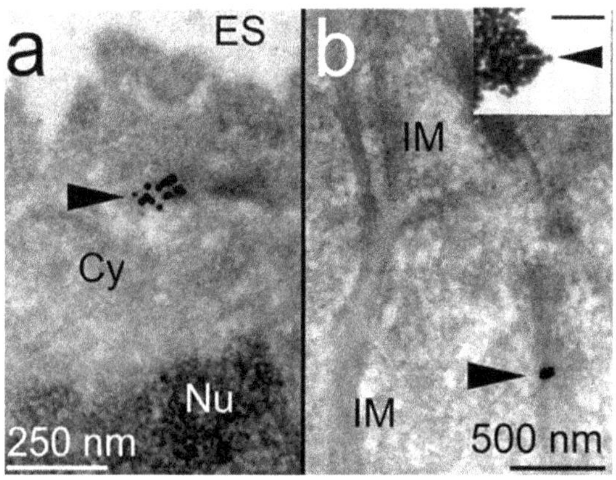

Figure 11.1. Transmission electron microscopy images of cell sections: (a) nanogold particles are visualized in the cytosol (Cy) but not in the cell nucleus (Nu) nor in the extracellular space (ES). (b) Nanogold particles specifically decorated with oligonucleotides against mRNA of the Her2/neu gene show an accumulation in the vicinity of components of the intracellular membrane apparatus (IM). The insert (scale bar 100 nm) shows the resolution of particle clusters in individual nanogold particles of about 10 nm in diameter.

labelling of H2AX phosphorylation sides (γH2AX) simultaneously with the recruitment of proteins like 53BP1, Ku78, Ku80, XRCC1 etc, which are prominent proteins in certain repair pathways.

Another example is shown in figure 11.1(b) where nanogold particles of 13 nm core diameter are decorated with oligonucleotides (figure 11.2) specific for a RNA sequence of a given gene transcript (Seferos *et al* 2007). Here the RNA stretches of the Her2/neu gene transcript were specifically addressed resulting in labelling within the folded membrane of the SkBr3 (breast cancer) cells used (Hildenbrand *et al* 2018).

11.2 Light microscopy and localization microscopy

The physical properties of nanogold particles allow them to be used with a wide range of imaging techniques. This not only allows for quantification of the uptake and distribution in a cell but also for specific visualization when attached to appropriately combined labelling molecules (Ngwa *et al* 2017).

In contrast to macroscopic bodies of gold, colloidal solutions of nanogold particles show characteristic colors from yellow to far red depending on the size of the particles. This had already been observed and described by Michael Faraday in the mid-19th century and explains the common color of old church windows and glass. The physical reason for the chromaticity of the nanogold particles is dipole surface plasmon resonance (figure 11.3(a)). If a nanogold particle is illuminated by visible light, the electromagnetic field of the light wave is inducing coherent collective oscillations of the free electrons relative to the fixed positive atom nuclei. The frequency of the oscillation is depending on the dielectric permittivity of the particle and the surrounding medium as well as on the size and the shape of the particle. The light with the wavelength that is in resonance with the surface plasmon oscillation has an absorption maximum (figure 11.3(b)). With increasing size the resonant absorption wavelength is also increasing. Nanogold particles attached to labelling molecules are also showing a shift in the resonant absorption wavelength. This physical phenomenon reasons to the application of specific nanogold/nanosilver labeled antibodies as fluorescence markers in (scanning) near-field optical microscopy (Bazylewski *et al* 2017).

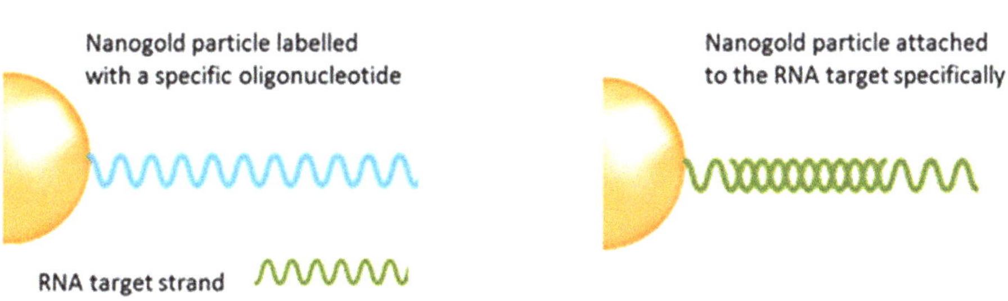

Figure 11.2. Specific oligonucleotide sequences are coupled to the nanogold particle via –SH bridges. These sequences bind to the complementary target sequence.

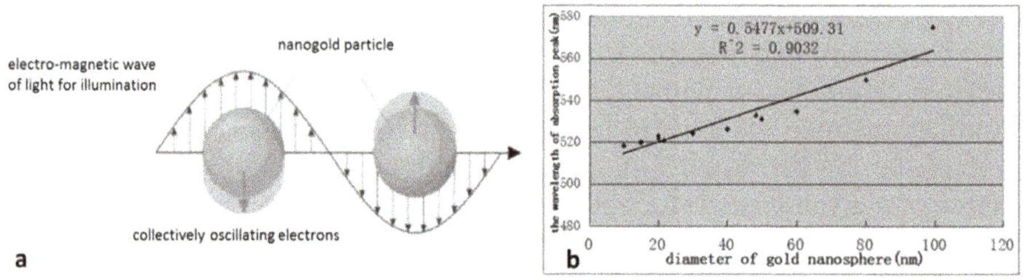

Figure 11.3. (a) Schematic representation of the induction of dipole surface plasmon oscillations in nanogold particles. (b) Measurements of the position of the light absorption maximum versus nanogold particle size.

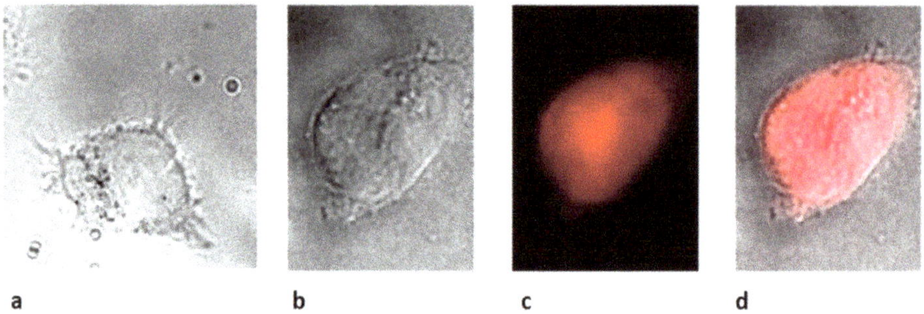

Figure 11.4. Light microscopy images of HeLa cells with nanogold particles incorporated; (a) wide-field image of a HeLa cell with clusters of nanogold particles of a size of 25 nm in diameter (black dots); (b) wide-field image of a HeLa cell with nanogold particles of a size of 10 nm in diameter which are visualized by the red emission in (c); (d) merged image of (b) and (c).

The collective oscillation of the electron cloud in a nanogold particle is inducing an electric dipole field around the particle perpendicularly orientated to the exciting electromagnetic wave. This field can reflect the nano-shape of the particle and influences the direct molecular neighborhood of the particle. This interaction can also cause a modulation of the surface plasmon resonance leading to off–on of the light emitted from the nanogold particle. This stochastic switching of nanogold particles can be triggered by the intensity of the illuminating light resulting into particle blinking, a prerequisite for localization microscopy (see below).

In figure 11.4 examples of HeLa-cells are shown that have incorporated nanogold particles of a size of 10 nm and 25 nm, respectively, in diameter. In the wide-field images the clusters of 25 nm particles are visible as black dots, whereas the 10 nm particles cannot be resolved but show a red color staining all over the cellular cytoplasm.

As mentioned above, the surface plasmon resonance oscillation can be modulated so that the particle light emission starts blinking on a time scale of seconds to minutes. This blinking effect can be used for signal discrimination in super-resolution localization microscopy (SMLM) (Cremer *et al* 2011) nowadays applied for analyses of molecular architectures of receptors in cell membranes (Boyd *et al* 2016, Pilarczyk *et al* 2017), radiation induced damage of chromatin and protein recruitment during DNA repair (Hausmann *et al* 2017, 2018), or chromatin loops in chromosomal aberrations (Stuhlmüller *et al* 2015). In contrast to transmission electron microscopy, SMLM has the advantage that standard preparation techniques established in light microscopy can be used, which allows 3D cell maintenance and omits steps of sputtering and mechanical sectioning making the light microscopy preparation techniques faster and more straightforward.

The embodiment of SMLM used here in combination with nanogold labelling was originally based on the application of fluorescent proteins and standard fluorescent dyes. It can be switched between spectral 'on' and 'off' states (Lemmer *et al* 2008, 2009) to achieve temporal isolation and thus spatial separation of single-molecule/single-particle signals. From a reversible dark state, the fluorescent molecules/light emitting nanogold particles can randomly return to the emission state and emit their photons when irradiated by light at resonance wavelengths. Each of the emitting fluorophores is represented by an Airy disc in the microscopic image. The centre-of-mass (barycentre) of such a disc approximates the location of the emitting molecule/particle. This allows not only the precise determination of object positions but also the calculation of particle uptake (Burger *et al* 2014, Moser *et al* 2016) their spatial distances in the 10 nm regime. Using the matrix of the coordinates of light emitting tags, all acquired positions and distances of fluorescent molecules/nanogold particles can be analyzed without generation of an image (Hausmann *et al* 2017). From this matrix, an artificial 'pointillist', super-resolution image can also be prepared (figure 11.5), in which the effective resolution is only depending on the localization precision of the particle. A detailed description of the instrumental setup is given elsewhere (Hausmann *et al* 2018, Eryilmaz *et al* 2018).

The ability to precisely count the number of nanogold particles and to determine nanogold particle localization with nm-precision provides insights of uptake pathways (Moser *et al* 2016) as well as potentially identifying the nanogold particle location within the sample as a cause of radiation mediated damaging (Hildenbrand

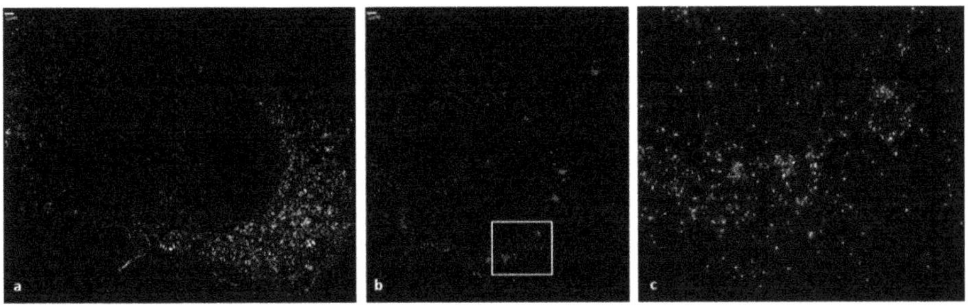

Figure 11.5. Super-resolution localization microscopy images of SkBr3 cells with nanogold particles incorporated; (a) unspecific distribution in the cytoplasm of nanogold particles of a size of 10 nm in diameter (white dots); (b) nanogold particles specifically decorated with oligonucleotides against mRNA of the Her2/neu gene (see also figure 11.2) show an accumulation in the vicinity of the cell nuclei presumptively in the intracellular membrane apparatus. (c) The insert highlighted in (b) shows the resolution of single particles arranged in linear-like organization (see for comparison figure 11.1(b)).

et al 2018) (for further application details see also chapter 10, figures 10.3 and 10.5, of Martin Falk *et al* in this book). Specific labelling and accurate imaging will help to achieve precise dose deposition and may also be a tool for providing better understanding of mechanisms behind radio-sensitization (Pagáčová *et al* 2018). However, when applying SMLM for absolute counting of nanogold particles and measurements of particle arrangements, special care has to be taken to discriminate self-fluorescent background from real particle signals. This is especially true if one tries to exit the particles in the absorption maximum which is mostly in the blue–green spectrum where also protein complexes and organelles may fluoresce.

This caveat for image processing of SMLM will be explained by the following example: in the experiments nanogold particles were counted that were either randomly distributed in the cytoplasm or specifically labelled with oligonucleotides for mRNA of the Her2/neu gene and therefore accumulated in the intracellular membranes. By these absolute measurements, it could be answered by which procedure the number of persisting particles is higher and therefore more damaging during radiation treatments. The preliminary results presented in table 11.1 show that SMLM evaluation of particle numbers after illuminating the samples by a laser with 491 nm excitation wavelength is contradictory. The control does even show higher signal numbers than the samples with nanogold incorporated. This contradiction could be overcome if the specimen was illuminated at 642 nm where self-fluorescence could be neglected. Since the induction of surface plasmon resonance is not only depending on the particle size but also on the cellular environment, absorption measurements verified that in a cellular system the absorption peaks are often disappearing towards a broad absorption band.

Nevertheless the application of nanogold particles as specific molecular tags offers broad potentials in super-resolution microscopy since it has become possible not only to do conventional diffraction limited far-field microscopy simultaneously

Table 11.1. Super-resolution localization microscopy of MCF-7 cells of a breast cancer cell line: signals were counted after illumination with different wavelengths (491 nm, 642 nm). The results indicate that at 491 nm illumination also other fluorescent compartments of the cell are exited than nanogold particles. This has been avoided at 642 nm illumination.

Illumination wavelength	491 nm			642 nm		
	Number of cells analyzed	Mean value of signals	Standard deviation	Number of cells analyzed	Mean value of signals	Standard deviation
Control without nanogold particles	4	24 990	8740	—	—	—
Specimen with nanogold particles	48	17 236	6110	8	22 285	7569
Specimen with specifically labelled nanogold particles	42	18 972	7260	9	41 122	9888

with super-resolution single molecule microscopy at the same cell but also to use the same specimen of SMLM in electron microscopy as being demonstrated by the CILEM (Contextual Interactive Light and Electron Microscopy) approach (Hildenbrand *et al* 2018) which is going to be further developed (Pilarczyk *et al* unpublished results).

Acknowledgments

The authors thank Dr Felix Bestvater, German Cancer Research Center, Heidelberg, for using the localization microscope setup. The authors also thank Xin Chen, Department of Radiooncology, Universitätsmedizin Mannheim, for providing figure 11.3(b). Furthermore, we thank Jin-Hau Ewwer, Institute of Research Rating and Enhancement (IRRE), Altenburschla, Germany, and Paul I M Prinz Zippl, University of Vienna, Austria, for always finding the right way of haziness in constructive discussions. The work was supported by the Heidelberg University Mobility Grant for International Research Cooperation within the excellence initiative II of the Deutsche Forschungsgemeinschaft (DFG), and by the Mobility project DAAD-19-03 to Michael Hausmann.

References

Bazylewski P, Ezugwu S and Fanchini G 2017 A review of three-dimensional scanning near-field optical microscopy (3D-SNOM) and its applications in nanoscale light management *Appl. Sci.* **7** 973

Boyd P S, Struve N, Bach M, Eberle J P, Gote M, Schock F, Cremer C, Kriegs M and Hausmann M 2016 Clustered localization of EGFRvIII in glioblastoma cells as detected by high precision localization microscopy *Nanoscale* **8** 20037–47

Burger N, Biswas A, Barzan D, Kirchner A, Hosser H, Hausmann M, Hildenbrand G, Herskind C, Wenz F and Veldwijk M R 2014 A method for the efficient cellular uptake and retention of small modified gold nanoparticles for the radiosensitization of cells *Nanomedicine* **10** 1365–73

Cremer C *et al* 2011 Superresolution imaging of biological nanostructures by spectral precision distance microscopy (SPDM) *Rev. Biotech. J.* **6** 1037–51

Eryilmaz M, Schmitt E, Krufczik M, Theda F, Lee J-H, Cremer C, Bestvater F, Schaufler W, Hausmann M and Hildenbrand G 2018 Localization microscopy analyses of MRE11 clusters in 3D-conserved cell nuclei of different cell lines *Cancers* **10** 25

Hausmann M *et al* 2017 Challenges for super-resolution localization microscopy and biomolecular fluorescent nano-probing in cancer research *Int. J. Mol. Sci.* **18** 2066

Hausmann M, Wagner E, Lee J-H, Schrock G, Schaufler W, Krufczik M, Papenfuß F, Port M, Bestvater F and Scherthan H 2018 Super-resolution microscopy of radiation-induced histone H2AX phosphorylation in relation to H3K9-trimethylation in HeLa cells *Nanoscale* **10** 4320–31

Hildenbrand G *et al* 2018 Dose enhancement effects of gold nanoparticles specifically targeting RNA in breast cancer cells *PLoS One* **13** e0190183

Lemmer P, Gunkel M, Baddeley D, Kaufmann R, Urich A, Weiland Y, Reymann J, Müller P, Hausmann M and Cremer C 2008 SPDM—light microscopy with single molecule resolution at the nanoscale *Appl. Phys.* B **93** 1–12

Lemmer P *et al* 2009 Using conventional fluorescent markers for far-field fluorescence localization nanoscopy allows resolution in the 10 nm range *J. Microsc.* **235** 163–71

Lorat Y, Brunner C U, Schanz S, Jacob B, Taucher-Scholz G and Rübe C E 2015 Nanoscale analysis of clustered DNA damage after high-LET irradiation by quantitative electron microscopy—The heavy burden to repair *DNA Repair* **28** 93–106

Moser F *et al* 2016 Cellular uptake of gold nanoparticles and their behavior as labels for localization microscopy *Biophys. J.* **110** 947–53

Ngwa W *et al* 2017 Critical review: Smart radiotherapy biomaterials *Int. J. Radiat. Oncol. Biol. Phys.* **97** 624–37

Pagáčová E *et al* 2018 Challenges and contradictions of metal nano-particle applications for radio-sensitivity enhancement in cancer therapy *Int. J. Mol. Sci.* **20** 588

Pilarczyk G, Nesnidal I, Gunkel M, Bach M, Bestvater F and Hausmann M 2017 Localisation microscopy of breast epithelial ErbB-2 receptors and gap junctions: trafficking after gamma-irradiation, Neuregulin-1b and Herceptin application *Int. J. Mol. Sci.* **18** 362

Rübe C E, Lorat Y, Schuler N, Schanz S, Wennemuth G and Rübe C 2011 DNA repair in the context of chromatin: new molecular insights by the nanoscale detection of DNA repair complexes using trans mission electron microscopy *DNA Repair* **10** 427–37

Seferos D S, Giljohann D A, Hill H D, Prigodich A E and Mirkin C A 2007 Nano-flares: probes for transfection and mRNA detection in living cells *J. Am. Chem. Soc.* **129** 15477–9

Stuhlmüller M, Schwarz-Finsterle J, Fey E, Lux J, Bach M, Cremer C, Hinderhofer K, Hausmann M and Hildenbrand G 2015 *In situ* optical sequencing and nano-structure analysis of a trinucleotide expansion region by localization microscopy after specific COMBO-FISH labelling *Nanoscale* **7** 17938–46

IOP Publishing

Nanoparticle Enhanced Radiation Therapy
Principles, methods and applications
Erno Sajo and Piotr Zygmanski

Chapter 12

X-ray based nanoparticle imaging

Juergen Hesser and Davide Brivio

Nanoparticles are a class of materials with interesting physical properties. In particular, they allow tailoring to a given application via their size distribution and by functionalization of their surface. Their small size allows transport within inter-cellular space and also enables cellular uptake. In particular, this property allows for nanoparticles to act as blood contrast agent but also for functional imaging when they specifically bind to receptors on the cell surface. Different image modalities thereby offer manifold opportunities using nanoparticles. In the following, their role for x-ray imaging technologies is reviewed.

12.1 Computed tomography (CT)

X-ray radiographic imaging and computed tomography (CT) are some of the most frequently used medical imaging modalities. They offer high contrast between soft tissue and bony or calcified structure, yet their ability to differentiate between different soft tissue regions is limited. Hence, contrast agents are intended to provide additional anatomical or functional information. For example, $BaSO_4$ contrast agent is typically used for imaging the alimentary and digestive tract. More relevant to this chapter are blood contrast agents containing molecules that include a high-Z element such as iodine. These agents enable imaging of not only the blood, e.g. for the purposes of diagnosing stenosis in coronary arteries, or bleeding after accidents, but also functional imaging such as perfusion measurements where the in- and out-flow of contrast agent in an organ or tumor is monitored and evaluated.

The imaging mechanics of contrast agents in x-ray projection and CT is via differential x-ray attenuation characteristics of the imaged object. Here, attenuation follows the Lambert–Beer law. X-rays with initial intensity I_0 penetrate the tissue, and are attenuated to intensity $I = I_0 \exp\{-\int_s \mu(x)dx\}$, where I is the measured intensity in a detector, I_0 is the intensity of x-rays incident on the tissue, s is the path through tissue along a ray, and μ is the absorption coefficient at each position on this path. This formula is exact when written for absorption. The absorption coefficient depends on three physical parameters: atomic number Z, energy E and physical density ρ. In particular, often one considers a normalized parameter, $\mu(Z, E, \rho) = \rho \cdot \left(\frac{\mu}{\rho}\right)$, using the specific mass attenuation coefficient $\left(\frac{\mu}{\rho}\right)$.

X-ray imaging relies on the attenuation properties of tissues. The energy of the photons used in diagnostic imaging is in the range of tens of kiloelectronovolts (keV) to over a hundred keV. The energy chosen for a particular imaging task is such that: (a) the radiation can penetrate the tissue and can hence be detected when it emerges from the body (lower energy limit) and (b) the obtained image is highly sensitive to the material composition of the body (upper energy limit). The lower energy limit is typically about 30 kVp for penetration of a few cm of soft tissue (e.g. female breast in mammography) and up to approximately 140 kVp for computed tomography of the pelvis, which contains bone structures that highly absorb radiation.

Technically, x-ray photons are generated by an x-ray source where accelerated electrons hit an anode and generate bremsstrahlung photons of a continuous energy spectrum with a maximum that corresponds to the kinetic energy of the accelerated electrons. For low energies, the generated bremsstrahlung photons are mostly absorbed inside of the anode, giving rise to emission of characteristic x-rays, which appear as peaks over the broad bremsstrahlung spectrum at specific energies due to atomic excitation processes between discrete energies in the electron shell of the corresponding anode material.

The emitted photons are typically hardened by a filter (thin metal plates of e.g. Al or Cu) in order to reduce the width of the photon spectrum, in particular to absorb low-energy photons that would not pass through the body anyway and would contribute to the absorbed dose. Hence, x-ray radiography and CT sources emit a significantly hardened bremsstrahlung spectrum. Although there are developments towards monochromatic x-ray sources that may have a strong impact on image quality, this technology is not sufficiently mature to be considered here [1–3].

Photons emitted by the x-ray source are penetrating the body. In the diagnostic energy range, these photons primarily interact via Rayleigh scatter, photoelectric absorption and Compton scattering, both leading to energy absorption. Compton interaction is an inelastic incoherent scatter mechanism that leads to energy loss in the scattered x-rays. Rayleigh scattering has a high cross-section at low energies, however, it is a coherent scatter that does not result in energy absorption; it only changes the photon direction.

Typically, the mathematical imaging model of x-ray CT considers unscattered photons as the primary contribution to projection images. Scattered photons are considered as the secondary contamination contribution. Hence, CT is using the Lambert–Beer model, we consider $-\log\frac{I}{I_0} = \int_{\Omega} \mu(x)dx$ as the expected image, ignoring noise and scattered radiation. Current detector generations only capture the intensity without energy differentiation so there is no possibility to differentiate between scattered and unscattered radiation on the detector side. For this reason, x-ray radiography uses anti-scatter grids in order to block scattered radiation (at the cost of higher dose to the patient). These grids let pass only photons that are (nearly) unscattered or have the direction of unscattered photons. For CT, scatter grids cannot be applied and hence potential scatter can only be physically removed by collimators (for fan beams) or virtually removed during the reconstruction process (figure 12.1).

Considering absorption, the total mass attenuation coefficient in the energy range of diagnostic x-rays is the sum of the mass attenuation coefficients of the different interactions, the photons may have while passing through tissue, i.e.

$$\left(\frac{\mu}{\rho}\right)_{\text{tot}} = \left(\frac{\mu}{\rho}\right)_{\text{Photoelectric}} + \left(\frac{\mu}{\rho}\right)_{\text{Rayleigh}} + \left(\frac{\mu}{\rho}\right)_{\text{Compton}}.$$

The photoelectric effect leads to complete photon absorption. A photon interacts with an inner electron of the atomic shell where the latter is emitted; the difference between photon energy and the binding energy for this electron manifests as kinetic energy of the electron. The vacancy generated by the released electron is filled by another electron from a neighboring higher energy shell, followed by emissions of either characteristic x-rays or by Auger electrons. For further details, including emission probabilities and photoelectric interaction cross-sections, please consult chapter 1 of this book.

The photoelectric effect is the interaction, which mainly contributes to the quality of the image since it is highly sensitive to the material composition of the body that is in the x-ray beam. For a given material with atomic number Z and a photon energy E, the interaction cross section (or probability of interaction) depends on energy E and atomic number Z. $\sigma_{PE} \sim Z^n/E^m$ where n is in the range of 3.6–5.3 and m is in the range of 2.5–3.5 being largest for low atomic numbers [4]. This means that a slight change in energy or atomic number could have a dramatic effect on the absorption and hence on the image contrast.

Elastically scattered photons on electrons of the atomic shell have an effective cross section $\sigma_{el} \sim Z^\alpha/E^2$, $\alpha = 2$ for low energies and $\sigma_{el} \sim 1/E^2$ for high energies, which is much less sensitive to energy and atomic number. The same is true for the

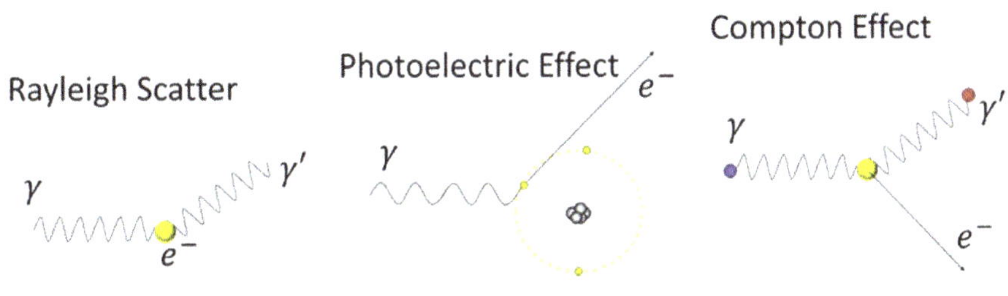

Figure 12.1. Pictorial representation of the three interactions, from left to right, Rayleigh scatter, photoelectric effect, Compton effect. The Rayleigh effect describes an incoming photon γ that is scattered at an electron e^- and yields a scattered photon with unchanged phase and wavelength (coherent). Rayleigh interaction only results in change of photon direction but not in energy transfer. By the photoelectric effect an incoming photon is absorbed and an electron is released. The Compton effect models the incoherent scatter of an incoming photon with a high energy, transfers a part of its energy to an electron (either to free electron or to atomic-shell bound electrons) and a scattered photon with lower energy leaves the interaction.

Compton effect, where electrons from the outer shell may be released for which the cross section is $\sigma_{CE} \sim Z/E^{-0.5}$.

X-ray radiography and computed tomography differ in the way the image is generated. While for x-ray radiography a projection image is acquired that accumulates the absorption coefficients of all the tissues along the rays according to the projection model, CT solves an inverse problem. In the inverse CT problem, the effective absorption coefficient of tissues is computed from a set of measured projections g acquired at different angles with respect to the scanned object. The standard CT reconstruction method is filtered backpropagation (FBP). The basic idea is that an x-ray projection corresponds mathematically to the Radon transform, which, for parallel rays means that slice by slice is imaged in the Fourier space. Each rotated projection generates a rotated slice in the Fourier space such that accumulated slices for all rotations fill the Fourier space with data and the inverse Fourier transform generates the solution as a 3D volume. Yet, before applying the inverse transform, the coordinate system shall be transformed from a cylindrical (r, ϕ, z) (radius, rotation angle, z-direction) to a Euclidian coordinate system (x, y, z), involving a multiplication in the Fourier space with a term $|r|$. A multiplication in the Fourier space corresponds to a convolution in the real space, i.e. a filtering of all projections with the Fourier transform of $|r|$ and then a backprojection of them—hence the name filtered backprojection (figure 12.2).

Due to higher computational power of the underlying workstations and graphics processor units, more recent CT reconstruction methods use iterative strategies (figure 12.3). Hereby, one simulates the x-ray propagation called forward projection $f(x)$, where x denotes the effective absorption coefficient. The deviation between measurement g and simulated projection $f(x)$ is minimized, $\min_x \| f(x) - g \|$ by estimating the corresponding effective absorption coefficients x. In even newer strategies, regularization using *a priori* information of the solution is applied, such as to minimize $\min_x \|f(x) - g\| + \lambda R(x)$, where λ is a regularization parameter and

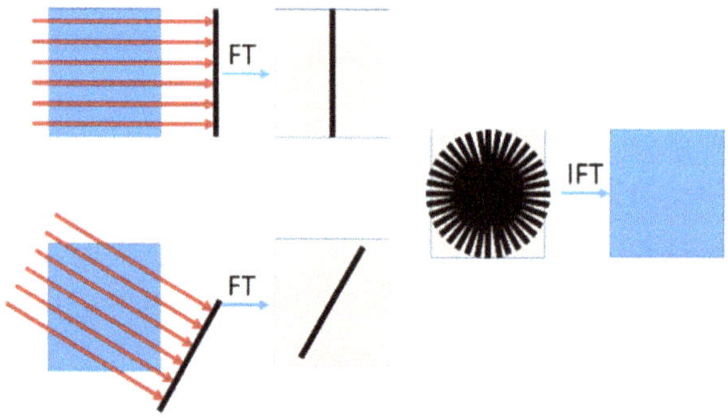

Figure 12.2. (Left) upper: the Fourier transform (FT) of parallel beam projection corresponds to a line in the Fourier space. Lower: a rotation of the beam direction leads to a rotation of the Fourier line. (Right) a complete set of such Fourier lines fills the Fourier space; which again enables one by inverse Fourier transformation (IFT) to obtain the reconstructed image.

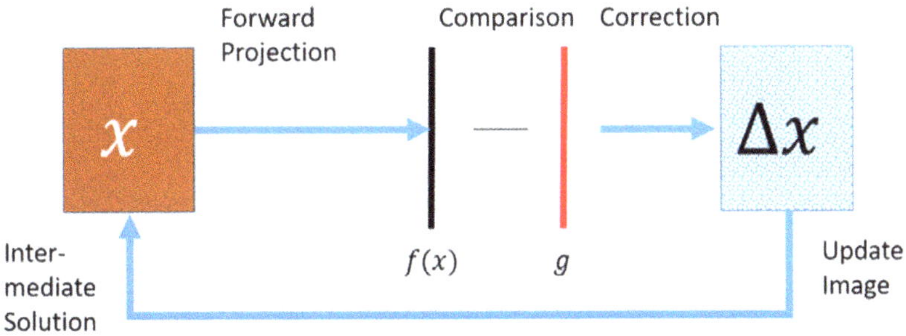

Figure 12.3. Mechanics of iterative reconstruction: given an initial solution, first a simulated x-ray projection is computed (forward projection). This projection is compared with the data and yields an error. A correction scheme (gradient descent) is applied to iteratively refine the model in order to minimize this error.

$R(x)$ is a regularization functional. $R(x)$ is often chosen to enhance smoothness in order to improve image quality further and thereby reduces noise and artifacts.

In order to discuss the relevance of nanoparticles for x-ray radiography and CT, we have to focus on the magnitude of different contributions to the contrast in the reconstructed image. In particular, the contrast depends on the additional attenuation and scatter of x-rays by nanoparticles distributed within the body. The contrast is achieved mostly via the high atomic number Z and only marginally through higher density of high-Z material. Therefore, it makes sense to use only low toxicity nanoparticles with a high atomic number Z elements such as bismuth ($Z = 83$), gold ($Z = 79$), platinum ($Z = 78$), tungsten ($Z = 74$), tantalum ($Z = 73$), hafnium ($Z = 72$), gadolinium ($Z = 64$)[1].

Attenuation enhancement by a mixture of gold with water with respect to pure water is depicted in figure 12.4. The enhancement is computed as the total mass attenuation ratio as a function of x-ray energy based on NIST tables[2]. For small concentrations of gold ($c = 0.5$, 1, 2 mg g^{-1}) seen in figure 12.4 the attenuation enhancement scales linearly with the concentration and it appears that relatively small concentrations of contrast might be detectable provided certain conditions are met. Individual contributions to the total x-ray cross section for gold and oxygen are seen in figure 12.5. Oxygen is the most abundant element in soft tissues due to high water content of the human body, therefore its cross sections are relevant in the following discussion. In real clinical beams, several competing factors are important for signal formation. One of them is the source flux a patient is exposed to and another one is the transmitted flux that can be detected by the detector. The source flux is limited by the dose a patient can receive from the imaging procedure and the transmitted flux depends on the attenuation inside the patient. If the transmitted flux is too low, detection noise is large and signal-to-noise ratio small. Signal-to-noise ratio is important for detection of low contrast regions. Thus, while the data in figures 12.4 and 12.5 appears promising for x-ray detectability of high-Z nanoparticle agents, the reality is much more complex.

[1] https://www.sbir.gov/sbirsearch/detail/400308.
[2] https://physics.nist.gov/PhysRefData/XrayMassCoef/chap2.html.

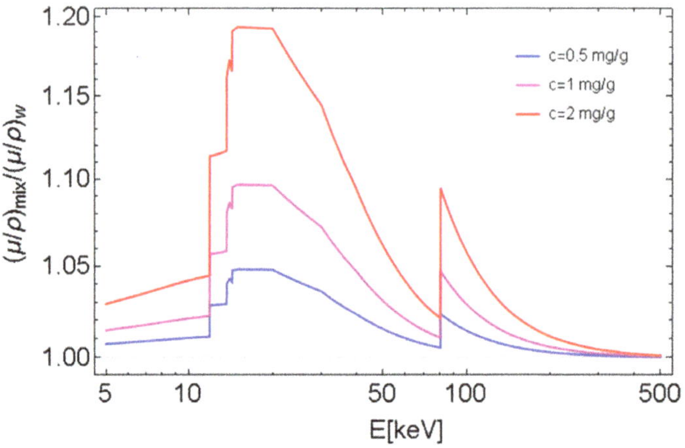

Figure 12.4. A ratio of mass attenuation coefficients for a mixture of gold with water to that of water computed from NIST database for concentrations c = 0.5, 1, 2 mg of gold in 1 g of water.

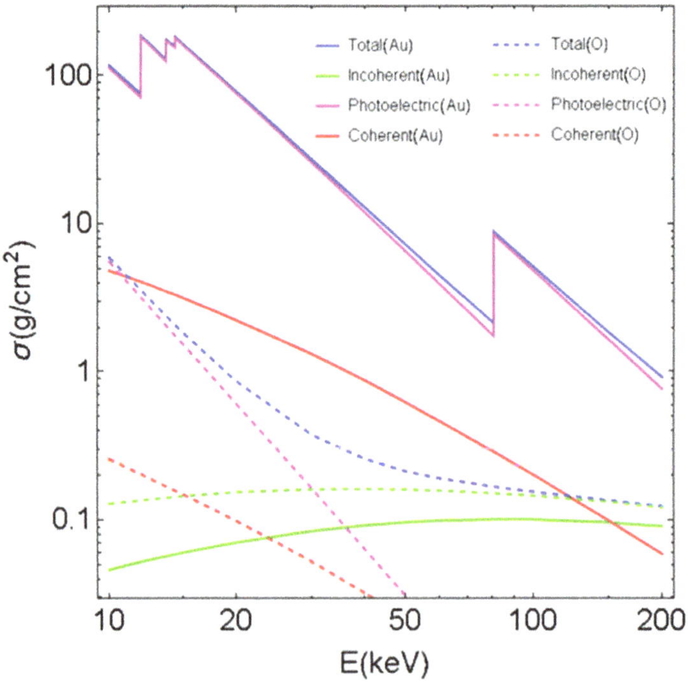

Figure 12.5. X-ray cross sections for gold and oxygen based on XCOM NIST database (https://physics.nist.gov/PhysRefData/Xcom/html/xcom1.html).

Let us have a closer look at figure 12.5, at the energy of 100 keV (0.1 MeV), which is relevant for x-ray and computed tomography (CT). We observe the following: for oxygen, the mass attenuation coefficient, i.e. the probability of an interaction of an incident photon per unit length traveled scaled by the material density, is about

10^{-1} cm^2 g^{-1}, whereas for gold this total mass attenuation coefficient is about 10^1 cm^2 g^{-1}, i.e. 100 times higher.

For high Z values and low-keV x-ray energies, the photoelectric effect is the dominating interaction. Rayleigh scatter reflects photons into a different direction-generating image blur or they even do not reach the detector. This interaction is only significant for very low energy photons. In our two examples, it is by far not the dominating effect. Incoherent or Compton scatter interacts with free and outer shell electrons, which take over part of the photon energy while the scattered photon has now less energy. In addition, the Compton effect contributes to image blur, but in contrast to Rayleigh scatter, is appears mainly at higher keV energies. In our example, it is the dominating effect for 100 keV photons in oxygen.

The photoelectric effect is the interaction that generates the contrast in images. Hence, we have to consider the atomic number Z of the atoms on the one hand and the concentration of high-Z-atoms on the other. For example, the increase of absorption from oxygen ($Z_O = 8$) to gold ($Z_{Au} = 79$) is about 1000 to ~10 000 fold from the photoelectric effect alone, but due to the other interactions, it is effectively smaller since for oxygen, the incoherent scatter dominates (see figure 12.5). This has to be taken into account when estimating the potential for nanoparticles.

In addition, the cross section of the photoelectric effect drops with $\sim E^{-3}$ and is hence prominent for low keV radiation while for higher energies the Compton effect dominates. Hence, we have to take the energy of the imaging system into account as well: the smaller the energy the larger the influence of the photoelectric effect and hence the better the expected contrast. Using nanoparticles as contrast agent hence makes most sense in this low-keV range, where the high sensitivity of high-Z-material versus tissue can be used.

Generally, nanoparticles find their application as pure blood pool contrast agents, with passive targeting (since nanoparticles and other contrast agents accumulate in e.g. tumor tissue), and active targeting (where functionalization of the nanoparticle surface allows binding to receptors [5]).

Let us now consider the gain of using nanoparticles versus conventional contrast agents. In cases where the same application is envisioned, in the standard single energy CT, they are competing head-to-head, while in other situations where additional functionalization of nanoparticles allows for novel applications of functional imaging, or when dual energy or photon counting detector CT are used, we have a completely different situation.

A thorough overview of recent developments for x-ray and CT contrast agents with special focus on nanoparticles was published by Cole *et al* [5] and by Cormodea *et al* [6], which are referred to in the following. Besides being based on barium [7], conventional contrast agents for x-ray/CT were molecules that contain iodine [8] as high-Z-material ($Z_I = 53$). Many recent nanoparticle-based contrast agents, however, rely on gold ($Z_{Au} = 79$) which is an inert metal and has a high specific x-ray absorption. A theoretical gain under equi-concentrations of the high-Z-atoms between iodine and gold should deliver a higher absorption in the range of a factor ~4.6 using the photoelectric effect alone, and hence a comparable dose reduction could be achieved at best. Yet, considering all interactions, the full spectral information and the so-called K-edges of the photoelectric effect, the advantage of gold nanoparticles over conventional contrast agents shrinks in the standard CT. Jackson *et al* [9] find no significant difference for 70–90 kVp, whereas 40–60 kVp or 100–140 kVp offer an option for nanoparticles.

Nanoparticles as contrast agents were developed some decades ago [10]. In many cases, these particles are coated in order to achieve solubility and biocompatibility. *In vivo* studies have demonstrated higher contrast for blood pool and passive targeting [11, 12]. Distribution effects [13] offer an explanation. Compared to classical contrast agents, these nanoparticles can have a long residence or circulation time of up to 15 h [14] compared to a few minutes for classical contrast agents, which is due to their increased size and henceforth slower excretion by the kidney. The effect opens the opportunity to use these nanoparticles for cases where repeated injections are necessary (blood pool contrast agent), where particles are to be tracked or where targeting is relevant (e.g. for protein expression).

Ding *et al* [15] suggested iodinated oil which produced a high contrast in CT for a concentration of 240 mg ml^{-1} and which diffuses into atherosclerotic plaques in rabbits within 2 h. Gold nanoparticles are (since they are inert) per se biocompatible. In a publication of Hainfeld [11, 16], 1.9 nm gold nanoparticles were introduced into rats with a concentration of 2.7 g gold per kg tissue and achieved excellent CT contrast. In 2007 Cai *et al* [14] developed 10 nm gold nanoparticles that were covered with polyethylene glycol. With a ~500 mg gold per kg tissue concentration, a good contrast could be achieved and a circulation time of about 15 h has been reported. Since gold as contrast agent is expensive, targeting helps to concentrate the agent into regions of interest. It was found that for monoenergetic beams a figure of merit consideration yields a factor of about two in favor of gold nanoparticles versus iodine improving to a factor of 3.3 for 80/140 kVp polyenergetic spectra [17].

From the clinical perspective, the main advantage of nanoparticles versus conventional molecular iodine contrast agents is their capability of targeting cancer by accumulating in tumor cells or being entrapped in tumor micro vasculature (both passive or active targeting) [18–20]. From the physics perspective, the advantage of nanoparticle-based versus conventional contrast agents is limited when the standard CT techniques are used. However, when nanoparticle contrast agents are considered either as multimodal agents (fluorescence, photoacoustic, magnetic resonance imaging) or in combination with multi energy CT their role significantly increases. This is especially true when nanoparticles are coated with functional layer for binding in order to obtain functional images or use these contrast agents for tracking purposes.

12.2 Dual- and multi-energy CT (DECT, MECT)

Standard computed tomography uses only one energy, or more precisely, one x-ray tube voltage (kVp) and therefore it can be referred to as single energy CT (SECT). Dual or multi-energy CT (DECT, MECT) uses two or more energy (kVp) levels [21–28]. X-ray tubes inside DECT/MECT scanners may be equipped with custom filters to separate the multiple spectra from each other as much as possible. Alternatively, depending on the type of MECT scanner, detector arrays used in the scanners may also be equipped with additional filters. By proper selection of target filter materials, their thicknesses; and kVp levels DECT(MECT) scanners employ two distinct spectra [23–26], albeit partially overlapping. Based on CT projections obtained for different spectra and based on model of attenuation coefficients for various materials, virtual monoenergetic or 'spectral' CT can be computed in a forward manner by using approximate formulae. The ability to unambiguously determine monoenergetic spectral CT is greater when photon counting detectors (PCD) with energy discrimination are employed. For this reason, MECT equipped with PCD can be referred to as PCD-MECT or spectral CT (SCT) in the true sense of the meaning [28, 29]. The field of DECT/MECT and especially PCD based SCT is in its early stage and its future depends on the development of application specific contrast agents loaded with various high-Z and functional materials as well as improvements in single photon detection [28, 29].

Dual energy computed tomography (DECT) is a CT scanning technique utilizing two energy levels. The standard CT uses a single energy polychromatic x-ray beam with tube voltages stretching from about 70 kVp to 140 kVp. Dual energy CT is realized in various ways by different manufacturers of CT scanners—by obtaining two scans or one scan with fast switching between two tube potentials of 80 kVp and 140 kVp or with a single tube potential of 140 kVp and/or with different detectors and filters. Each design has its own pros and cons in terms of the simultaneity of data acquisition of two images, maximum field of view (FOV), spectral overlapping, single or multiple detectors, cost, etc. The main idea of DECT is to obtain two sets of CT projections for low and high keV energy ranges (partially overlapping) of x-rays and based on this to reconstruct several types of quantities, which cannot be extracted from a single energy level (kVp) scan. Figure 12.6 shows an example of dual energy spectra and differences in the total attenuation coefficients for various materials for the peak energies corresponding to the 80 kVp and 140 kVp spectra. One can observe that the change in attenuation coefficient for the two spectra is material dependent, a fact which is employed in deriving several CT parameters.

Dual energy CT generates several types of virtual image sets (contrast only, no contrast, monochromatic as a function of keV energy, weighted polychromatic images) and it quantifies iodine contrast or calcium content, as well as determining the effective atomic number (Z_{eff}) and density (ρ) of the tissue [21–26].

The ability of DECT to compute monochromatic images as a function of keV energy, and to quantify contrast agent, or other high-Z materials, and the effective atomic number Z_{eff} and density (ρ) makes this modality potentially suitable for computer-aided analysis and for quantitative imaging capable of measuring contrast concentration including the standard iodine contrast agent and high-Z nanoparticle-based contrast agents.

Specifically, DECT has several quantitative metrics at its disposal:

- Hounsfield unit as a function of monochromatic energy keV (HU(x,y,z,keV)) representing the effective linear attenuation coefficient $\mu(E)$ of tissue including x-ray Compton scatter and photoelectric effects;

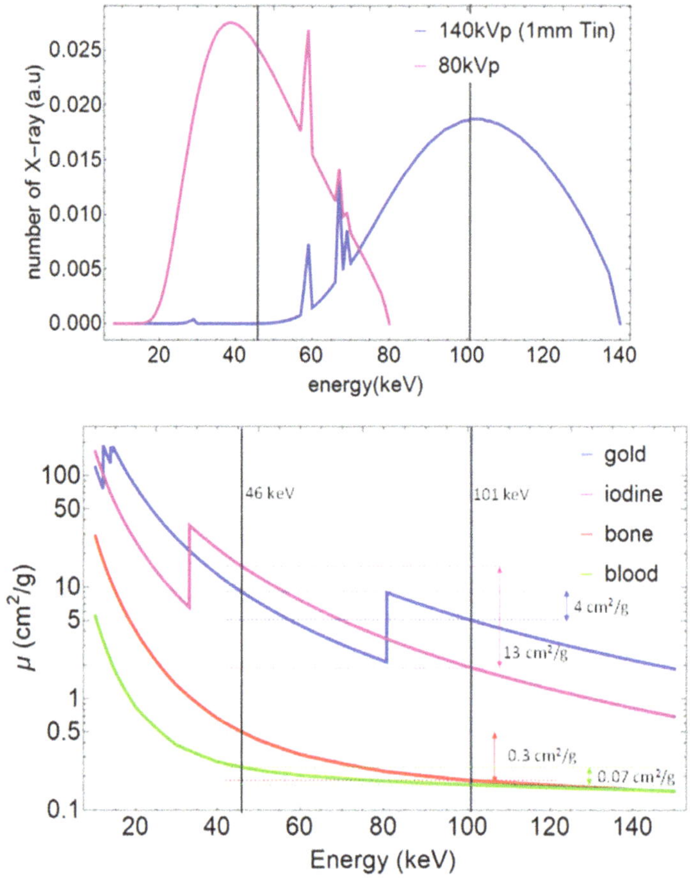

Figure 12.6. Example of dual energy spectra and differences in the total attenuation coefficients for various materials for the peak energies corresponding to the 80 kVp and 140 kVp spectra.

- the effective atomic number ($Z_{eff}(x,y,z)$) signifying the chemical content of tissues;
- the effective density (ρ (x,y,z) (g cm^{-3})) signifying the physical mass of tissues (like in single energy CT);
- concentration of contrast agent ($c(x,z,y)$ mg g^{-1}) signifying the uptake of the contrast by tissues.

The above parameters have to be regarded as effective parameters depending on specific DECT scanner/method used. Moreover, the parameters derived from only two energy levels may lack specificity. In this respect, because MECT and especially PCD MECT (SCT) use more energy ranges, they provide a better basis for specific quantitative imaging [28, 30, 31].

Dependence of (HU, Z_{eff}, ρ, c) quantities on the tissue (lesion, tumor) type and location within tissue may reveal characteristic features (signatures) differentiating them from the neighboring background and from each other. This in turn leads to a challenging goal of multi energy quantitative imaging, which is to determine contrast and specificity of detection for each tissue/contrast type and to automate the analysis by computer assisted or artificial intelligence based decision making in radiology and radiotherapy.

Specific quantitative imaging with the standard iodine contrast agents is inefficient due to low value of K-edge of iodine. Efficient imaging with high-*Z* (HZ) contrast agents depends on the relative value of K-edge of the contrast, attenuation of x-rays in this energy range by tissue and sufficient abundance of K-edge range x-rays in the CT scanner spectrum. Higher K-edge materials such as gold, bismuth, tantalum, hafnium, or ytterbium are required to make proper use of PCD MECT. High atomic number (HZ) nanoparticles are of great interest for development of new contrast agents because of high-load of HZ elements. Moreover, possibility of loading HZ nanoparticles with biomarkers or receptors for specific disease conditions or labeling them with molecules suitable for other imaging modalities (PET, optical, acousto-optical, or MRI imaging), makes them even more attractive. Finally, using multiple contrast agents or mixed contrast agents with different K-edges and different labels or bio-active molecules may lead to greater specificity of detection of various disease and normal conditions or functioning of the body. New contrast HZ nanoparticle-based agents can be potentially used for diseases diagnosis and progression or remission under treatment, for radiotherapy of cancer, as well as imaging pharmacokinetics or biodistribution of specific drugs/agents.

Recent research in this area showed feasibility of MECT imaging with new HZ nanoparticle agents such as: HDL loaded HZ-NP interacting with macrophages, bismuth nanoparticle targeting fibrin, LDL loaded HZ-NP accumulating in tumors that overexpress LDL receptor, low toxicity tantalum oxide nanoparticles [32–35]. One of the problems of nanoparticle imaging and radiotherapy is that large nanoparticles cannot be excreted and pose long term toxicity challenge, and while small nanoparticles can be excreted they do not accumulate sufficiently in a diseased organ or long enough to be imaged or used in therapy. A potential solution to this problem is to use small nanoparticle clusters encapsulated in polymer matrix, which degrades with time and allows release of small nanoparticles and their excretion [36, 37].

In summary, multi-energy CT might open another application for nanoparticles as new contrast agents. Due to the energy dependence of the photoelectric effect, one can detect and quantify the nanoparticle concentration and distribution in tissue directly. With the advent of photon counting detectors, which are energy sensitive, a much better material decomposition compared to conventional SECT is possible, opening the path for using multiple contrast agents. In particular, nanoparticles can be very useful in this context since they could be fabricated from different materials and architectures, yet the discussion of toxicity and rapid renal elimination (in order to overcome potential deposition of these particles and their retention in tissue) are thereby of high relevance.

12.3 X-ray fluorescence computed tomography (XFCT)

X-ray fluorescence CT (XFCT) [38] is an additional interesting imaging modality where nanoparticle contrast agents can find potentially application. It uses the K-photons emitted as a result of the photoelectric effect. These photons have a mean travel distance in tissue only of a few cm. Hence, XFCT mainly makes sense in small animal imaging or shallow tissues, however, it can directly measure the nanoparticle concentration. First studies [39–41] give evidence that such imaging can be realized in animal models.

X-ray fluorescence computed tomography (XFCT) is a technique that can identify, quantify, and locate elements within objects by detecting x-ray fluorescence (characteristic x-rays) stimulated by an excitation source. In figure 12.7(a) a diagram of a typical XFCT setup is shown in 2D. A fan or cone beam x-ray source is used to excite the gold nanoparticles in a small animal. A detector capable of spectral discrimination acquires signal at each plane for several projection angles obtained by rotating the stage with the object to be imaged. At each angle a single detector mounted on a two-axis stage is used for voxel by voxel acquisition of the projection. Detector collimation is necessary to identify the incoming direction of the fluorescence photons. The fluorescence signal is extracted by subtraction of the background from the $K_{\alpha 1,2}$ peaks in the spectra at each voxel/location (as shown in figure 12.7(b)). The image reconstruction is performed in a similar way to CT.

Challenges of this technique include long scanning times, large dose to object, fluorescence attenuation within a few cm of tissue. Note the time inefficiency but also the loss of flux due to three issues: observing x-rays only at right angle with respect to beamline, and collimating them, and finally by rejecting all except the characteristic x-rays from K-line or L-line, which is inefficient in larger objects.

To our knowledge XFCT has not been applied to imaging of high-Z nanoparticles in humans. Determination of nanoparticle distribution in tissues by means

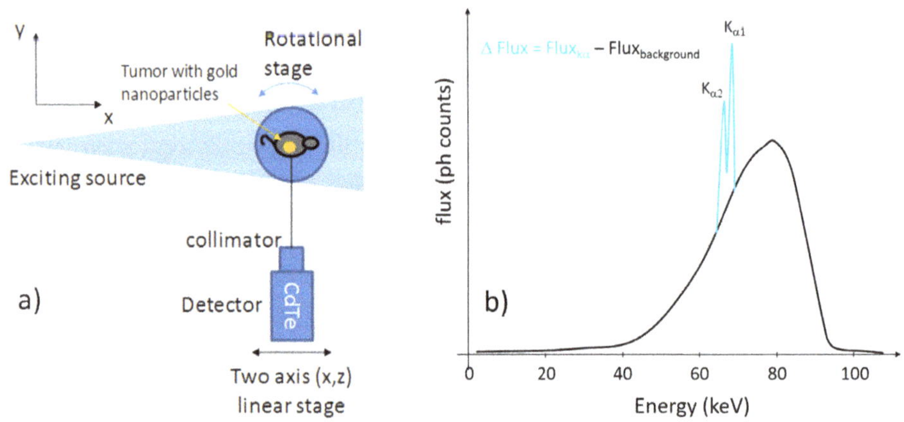

Figure 12.7. (a) Diagram showing a typical scanning geometry in XFCT systems. (b) typical spectra acquired at each detector location. The fluxes from fluorescence photons are obtained by subtracting the background from the $K_{\alpha 1,2}$ peaks (Δ flux).

of XFCT has been demonstrated in mice [40]. Application of this imaging method to larger subjects faces several challenges including large dose from imaging (>70 cGy per slice), large total data acquisition time (>1 h per slice), attenuation and scatter of $K_{\alpha 1,2}$ photons.

In XFCT $K_{\alpha 1}$ (68.80 keV) and $K_{\alpha 2}$ (66.99 keV) photons are emitted by gold atoms (fluorescence yield of 0.964) when an electron in the L-shell decays to fill the K-shell vacancy created after the photoelectric absorption of a photon with energy larger than the K-edge of gold (80.72 keV). Therefore, the larger the portion of the exciting x-ray spectra above the K-edge of gold the larger is the fluorescence production. Filtration of kVp beams with lead and tin filters have been investigated to improve the signal-to-background ratio [42]. Nevertheless, the absorption of $K_{\alpha 1}$ photons in 15 cm of tissue is about 95%, therefore, the use of XFCT for imaging is limited to small animal models or shallow tissues.

In figure 12.8 we show the flux of $K_{\alpha 1}$ photons as a function of depth *x* in the phantom after background subtraction generated from gold nanoparticles of different concentrations placed in a 5 cm slab centered in a 35 cm water phantom. The larger the energy of the exciting x-rays and the larger the nanoparticle concentration, the larger is the fluorescence production, both upstream and downstream. Larger concentrations also show more attenuation of the $K_{\alpha 1}$ photons inside the nanoparticle region.

Despite relatively large number of photons/cGy per cm^2 generated in the nanoparticle region, their detectability outside of the phantom is challenging because of attenuation within the phantom.

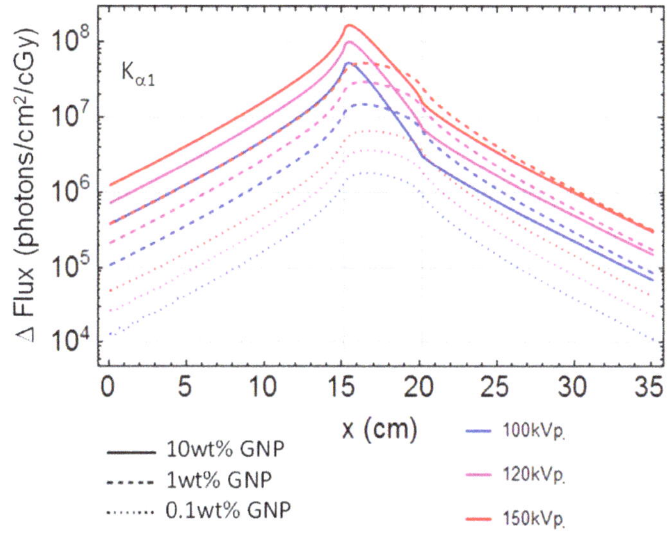

Figure 12.8. CEPXS/ONDANT [43] simulation showing $K_{\alpha 1}$ Δ flux, i.e. the flux of $K_{\alpha 1}$ photons after background subtraction, as a function of depth for water and AuNP for three concentrations (10 wt%, 1 wt%, 0.1 wt%) and three spectra used to excite the nanoparticles (100 kVp, 120 kVp and 150 kVp). Data are normalized to the total dose in water at depth between 15 cm and 20 cm, where AuNPs are placed.

In summary, imaging nanoparticles using XFCT is feasible in small animal models (or shallow locations) with some limitations due to long scanning times and large delivered doses.

12.4 SPECT/PET

While x-ray or CT are able (so far) to image morphology, single photon emission computed tomography (SPECT) or positron emission tomography (PET) can directly image the metabolism, and give rise to functional imaging (figure 12.9). SPECT hereby relies on a gamma emitter (radiotracer) such as ^{123}I, ^{99m}Tc, ^{133}Xe [44]. The radiotracer ideally enriches in tumor tissue but also in eliminating organs e.g. the kidney. The tracer emits gamma photons in all directions. Using collimators in front of single photon detectors (scintillators coupled with photo multipliers (PMTs)) allows selecting only those photons that come from a desired direction. An x-ray transmission image of the source can be measured for many views from which a reconstruction of source activity inside patient is possible. The reconstructed image shows the concentration of the contrast agent only with no anatomical features; however, the latter can be superimposed based on CT.

PET is based on a positron emitter bound to a molecule such as fluorine-18 to glucose replacing an OH-group (FDG), for example (figure 12.10). Typical tracer isotopes are hereby ^{68}Ga, ^{76}Br, ^{94m}Tc, ^{11}C, ^{13}N, ^{15}O, ^{18}F, ^{64}Cu [44]. The tracer is injected into the body and in the case of FDG, the tracer is metabolized in tissues with high energy demand such as brain, inflammation or tumor tissues. The positron emitter decays in the tissue. It emits a positron that is diffusing a few mm before annihilating with an electron in two oppositely emitted photons of 511 keV each.

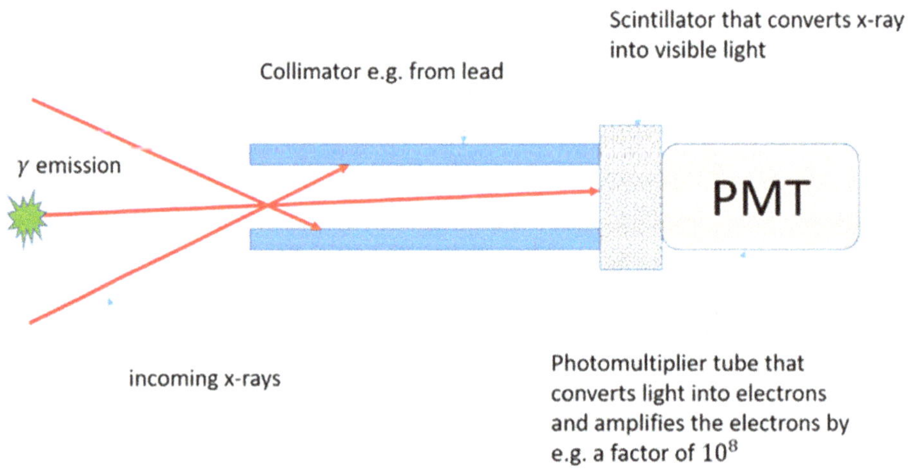

Figure 12.9. Sketch of the imaging principle of SPECT: An activated nucleus emits a photon (γ-process), from all incident γ-photons only those pass the collimator (and are not absorbed by the collimator wall) that are essentially parallel to the collimation. The passed photons reach a scintillator where the photon is converted into visible light. This is converted into an electron in a photomultiplier tube (PMT). The amount of electrons is then multiplied by a high factor such as 10^8, producing a high current pulse that can be measured.

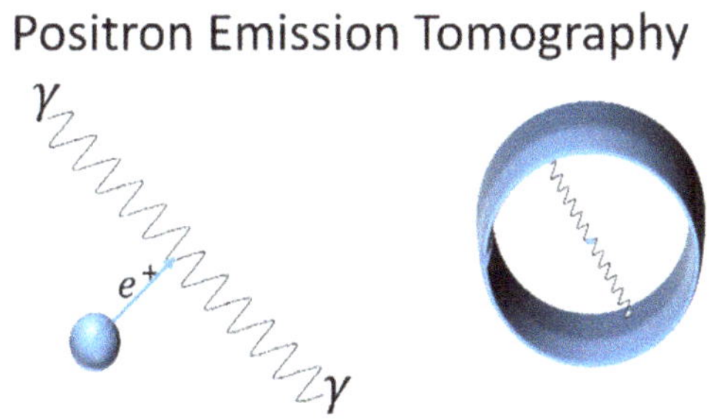

Figure 12.10. Positron emission tomography: (left) A β^+-emitter in the patient body emits a positron, which together with a nearby electron decays into two diametrically emitted photons. These photons are detected coincidentally in a ring detector. This defines that on the line of emission, a decay took place and hence reconstruction algorithms similar to those for computed tomography reconstruct the amount of β^+-decays per volume element.

A correlated detection of these two photons with a photon-counting detector allows determining the trajectory of both photons and again with a similar technique like for CT one can reconstruct the positron emitter concentration in 3D.

There are different kind of nanoparticles that can be used for this purpose, as described in the reviews of Zhao [45] and Xing [46], such as liposomes, micelles, nanopolymers, or dendrimers. Following the excellent review of Thomas *et al* for dual-modality SPECT developments [47], ^{111}In [48], and ^{99m}Tc [49, 50] are generally chosen as isotopes. PET radionuclide conjugated with an MRI agent such as superparamagnetic iron oxide nanoparticles offers the option of both MRI and PET imaging at the same time. The paper of Thomas *et al* also gives an excellent overview of recent dual-modality developments [47]. In particular, Yang [51], Lee [52] and Rosales [53] use a ^{64}Cu isotope as tracer.

References

[1] Bech M, Bunk O, David C, Ruth R, Rifkin J, Loewen R, Feidenhans'l R and Pfeiffer F 2009 Hard x-ray phase-contrast imaging with the Compact Light Source based on inverse Compton X-rays *J. Synchrotron Radiat.* **16** 43–7

[2] Achterhold K, Bech M, Schleede S, Potdevin G, Ruth R, Loewen R and Pfeiffer F 2013 Monochromatic computed tomography with a compact laser-driven x-ray source *Sci. Rep.* **3** 1313

[3] Serafini L *et al* 2019 MariX, an advanced MHz-class repetition rate X-ray source for linear regime time-resolved spectroscopy and photon scattering *Nucl. Instrum. Methods Phys. Res. Sect. A Accel. Spectrom. Detect. Assoc. Equip.* **930** 167–72

[4] International Atomic Energy Agency 2014 *Diagnostic Radiology Physics* (Vienna: IAEA)

[5] Cole L E, Ross R D, Tilley J M R, Vargo-Gogola T and Roeder R K 2015 Gold nanoparticles as contrast agents in x-ray imaging and computed tomography *Nanomedicine* **10** 321–41

[6] Cormodea D P, Naha P C and Fayad Z A 2014 Nanoparticle contrast agents for computed tomography: a focus on micelles *Contrast Media Mol. Imaging* **9** 37–52

[7] Yu S-B and Watson A D 1999 Metal-based x-ray contrast media *Chem. Rev.* **99** 2353–77

[8] Lusic H and Grinstaff M W 2013 X-ray-computed tomography contrast agents *Chem. Rev.* **113** 1641–66
[9] Jackson P A, Rahman W N W A, Wong C J, Ackerly T and Geso M 2010 Potential dependent superiority of gold nanoparticles in comparison to iodinated contrast agents *Eur. J. Radiol.* **75** 104–9
[10] Sugarbaker P H, Vermess M, Doppman J L, Miller D L and Simon R 1984 Improved detection of focal lesions with computerized tomographic examination of the liver using ethiodized oil emulaion (EOE-13) liver contrast *Cancer* **54** 1489–95
[11] Hainfeld J F, Slatkin D N, Focella T M and Smilowitz H M 2006 Gold nanoparticles: a new x-ray contrast agent *Br. J. Radiol.* **79** 248–53
[12] Wang H *et al* 2012 Dendrimer-entrapped gold nanoparticles as potential CT contrast agents for blood pool imaging *Nanoscale Res. Lett.* **7** 190
[13] Moghimi S M, Hunter A C and Murray J C 2001 Long-circulating and target specific nanoparticles: theory to practice *Pharmacol. Rev.* **53** 283–318
[14] Cai Q-Y *et al* 2007 Colloidal gold nanoparticles as a blood-pool contrast agent for x-ray computed tomography in mice *Invest. Radiol.* **42** 797–806
[15] Ding J *et al* 2013 CT/fluorescence dual-modal nanoemulsion platform for investigating atherosclerotic plaques *Biomaterials* **34** 209–16
[16] Hainfeld J F, Slatkin D N and Smilowitz H M 2004 The use of gold nanoparticles to enhance radiotherapy in mice *Phys. Med. Biol.* **49** N309–15
[17] Ducote J L, Alivov Y and Molloi S 2011 Imaging of nanoparticles with dual-energy computed tomography *Phys. Med. Biol.* **56** 2031–44
[18] Perrault S D and Chan W C W 2010 *In vivo* assembly of nanoparticle components to improve targeted cancer imaging *Proc. Natl Acad. Sci. USA* **107** 11194–9
[19] Wang M and Thanou M 2010 Targeting nanoparticles to cancer *Pharmacol. Res.* **62** 90–9
[20] Hainfeld J F, Smilowitz H M, O'Connor M J, Dilmanian F A and Slatkin D N 2013 Gold nanoparticle imaging and radiotherapy of brain tumors in mice *Nanomedicine* **8** 1601–9
[21] Chawla A, Srinivasan S, Lim T C, Pulickal G G, Shenoy J and Peh W C G 2017 Dual-energy CT applications in salivary gland lesions *Br. J. Radiol.* **90** 20160859
[22] De Cecco C N, Laghi A, Schoepf U J and Meinel F G (ed) 2015 *Dual Energy CT in Oncology* (Berlin: Springer)
[23] Lam S, Gupta R, Kelly H, Curtin H D and Forghani R 2015 Multiparametric evaluation of head and neck squamous cell carcinoma using a single-source dual-energy CT with fast kVp switching: state of the art *Cancers* **7** 2201–16
[24] Roele E D, Timmer V C M L, Vaassen L A A, van Kroonenburgh A M J L and Postma A A 2017 Dual-energy CT in head and neck imaging *Curr. Radiol. Rep.* **5** 19
[25] McCollough C H, Leng S, Yu L and Fletcher J G 2015 Dual- and multi-energy CT: principles, technical approaches, and clinical applications *Radiology* **276** 637–53
[26] Ashton J R, Castle K D, Qi Y, Kirsch D G, West J L and Badea C T 2018 Dual-energy CT imaging of tumor liposome delivery after gold nanoparticle-augmented radiation therapy *Theranostics* **8** 1782–97
[27] Ashton J R, Clark D P, Moding E J, Ghaghada K, Kirsch D G, West J L and Badea C T 2014 Dual-energy micro-CT functional imaging of primary lung cancer in mice using gold and iodine nanoparticle contrast agents: a validation study *PLoS One* **9** e88129
[28] Taguchi K and Iwanczyk J S 2013 Vision 20/20: Single photon counting x-ray detectors in medical imaging *Med. Phys.* **40** 100901

[29] Camrode D 2018 *AAPM Annual Meeting—Session: Multi-Energy and Multi-Contrast CT Imaging, Novel contrast agents for multi-energyCT imaging, AAPM 2018* http://amos3.aapm.org/abstracts/pdf/137-41529-446581-142224.pdf
[30] Tacguchi K 2018 *AAPM Annual Meeting—Session: Multi-Energy and Multi-Contrast CT Imaging* http://amos3.aapm.org/abstracts/pdf/137-41528-446581-142225.pdf
[31] Steadman R, Herrmann C and Livne A 2017 ChromAIX2: A large area, high count-rate energy-resolving photon counting ASIC for a Spectral CT Prototype *Nucl. Instrum. Methods Phys. Res. Sect.* A **862** 18–24
[32] Cormode D P *et al* 2017 Multicolor spectral photon-counting computed tomography: *in vivo* dual contrast imaging with a high count rate scanner *Sci. Rep.* **7** 4784
[33] Pan D *et al* 2010 Computed tomography in color: Nanok-enhanced spectral CT molecular imaging *Angew. Chem. Int. Ed.* **49** 9635–9
[34] Allijn I E *et al* 2013 Gold nanocrystal labeling allows low-density lipoprotein imaging from the subcellular to macroscopic level *ACS Nano* **7** 9761–70
[35] Symons R *et al* 2017 Photon-counting CT for simultaneous imaging of multiple contrast agents in the abdomen: an *in vivo* study *Med. Phys.* **44** 5120–7
[36] Torres A S *et al* 2012 Biological performance of a size-fractionated core–shell tantalum oxide nanoparticle x-ray contrast agent *Invest. Radiol.* **47** 578–87
[37] Cheheltani R *et al* 2016 Tunable, biodegradable gold nanoparticles as contrast agents for computed tomography and photoacoustic imaging *Biomaterials* **102** 87–97
[38] Cong W, Shen H, Cao G, Liu H and Wang G 2013 X-ray fluorescence tomographic system design and image reconstruction *J. X-Ray Sci. Technol.* **21** 1–8
[39] Jones B L, Manohar N, Rynoso F, Karellas A and Cho S H 2012 Experimental demonstration of benchtop x-ray fluorescence computed tomography (XFCT) of gold nanoparticle-loaded objects using lead- and tin-filtered polychromatic cone-beams *Phys. Med. Biol.* **57** N457–67
[40] Manohar N, Reynoso F J, Diagaradjane P, Krishnan S and Cho S H Quantitative imaging of gold nanoparticle distribution in a tumor-bearing mouse using benchtop x-ray fluorescence computed tomography *Nat. Sci. Rep.* **6** 22079
[41] Ren L, Wu D and Li Y 2014 Three-dimensional x-ray fluorescence mapping of a gold nanoparticle-loaded phantom *Med. Phys.* **41** 031902ff
[42] Manohar N, Jones B L and Cho S H 2014 Improving x-ray fluorescence signal for benchtop polychromatic cone-beam x-ray fluorescence computed tomography by incident x-ray spectrum optimization: a Monte Carlo study *Med. Phys.* **41** 101906-1–10
[43] Lorence L J J and Morel J E 1992 *CEPXS/ONELD: A One-dimensional Coupled Electron-photon Discrete Ordinates Code Package*
[44] Cassidy P J and Radda G K 2005 Molecular imaging perspectives *J. R. Soc. Interface R. Soc.* **2** 133–44
[45] Zhao L, Zhu M, Li Y, Xing Y and Zhao J 2017 Radiolabeled dendrimers for nuclear medicine applications *Molecules* **22** 1350
[46] Xing Y, Zhao J, Conti P S and Chen K 2014 Radiolabeled nanoparticles for multimodality tumor imaging *Theranostics* **4** 290ff
[47] Thomas R, Park I-K and Jeong Y Y 2013 Magnetic iron oxide nanoparticles for multimodal imaging and therapy of cancer *Int. J. Mol. Sci.* **14** 15910–30

[48] Misri R, Meier D, Yung A C, Kozlowski P and Hafeli U O 2012 Development and evaluation of a dual-modality (mri/spect) molecular imaging bioprobe *Nanomed. Nanotechnol. Biol. Med.* **8** 1007–16

[49] Torres Martin de Rosales R, Tavare R, Glaria A, Varma G, Protti A and Blower P J 2011 (^{99}m)tc-bisphosphonate-iron oxide nanoparticle conjugates for dual-modality biomedical imaging *Bioconjug. Chem.* **22** 455–65

[50] Madru R *et al* 2012 99mtc-labeled superparamagnetic iron oxide nanoparticles for multi-modality spect/mri of sentinel lymph nodes *J. Nucl. Med.* **53** 459–63

[51] Yang X *et al* 2011 Crgd-functionalized, dox-conjugated, and ^{64}Cu-labeled superparamagnetic iron oxide nanoparticles for targeted anticancer drug delivery and pet/Mr imaging *Biomaterials* **32** 4151–60

[52] Lee H Y, Li Z, Chen K, Hsu A R, Xu C, Xie J, Sun S and Chen X 2008 Pet/mri dual-modality tumor imaging using arginine-glycine-aspartic (rgd)-conjugated radiolabeled iron oxide nanoparticles *J. Nucl. Med.* **49** 1371–9

[53] Torres Martin de Rosales R, Tavare R, Paul R L, Jauregui-Osoro M, Protti A, Glaria A, Varma G, Szanda I and Blower P J 2011 Synthesis of ^{64}Cu(ii)-bis(dithiocarbamatebisphosphonate) and its conjugation with superparamagnetic iron oxide nanoparticles: *In vivo* evaluation as dual-modality pet-MRI agent *Angew. Chem. Int. Ed. Engl.* **50** 5509–13

IOP Publishing

Nanoparticle Enhanced Radiation Therapy
Principles, methods and applications
Erno Sajo and Piotr Zygmanski

Chapter 13

MRI based nanoparticle imaging

Frank G Zöllner

Magnetic resonance imaging (MRI) is widely used e.g. in cardiovascular, neurological and oncological diagnostics. Imaging is based on tissue-specific contrasts generated by nuclear magnetic properties (relaxation times) of the protons within the respective tissues. Contrast agents comprising nanoparticle-based ones are used to enhance this contrast locally to derive further morphological and physiological information on the tissue of interest. Over the last 25 years, various MR contrast agents have been investigated and several formulations have been approved for clinical use. These contrast agents are based on either transition or lanthanide metals or on iron oxide nanoparticles. Recently, ferrite nanoparticles have been studied, too. Applications range from measuring the perfusion in tissue towards tissue characterization and tumor staging and therapy monitoring.

To understand the contrast formation, at first briefly the signal and contrast mechanism of MRI are explained. For a more detailed description of the physical principles of MRI the reader is referred to respective textbooks [1–3]. After the basic MRI concepts, different types of MRI nanoparticles and their applications are outlined.

MRI is based on a physical property of each atom's nucleus, namely the magnetic spin. It results from the inner structure of the nuclei, the protons and neutrons. Nuclei that have an odd number of protons and/or neutrons exhibit a net spin and an associated magnetic moment and therefore can be used for MRI [1]. The most common nucleus used in MRI is the proton. It has a very high natural abundance in the human body and it possess a very high gyromagnetic ratio, i.e. a high proportion between spin and the respective magnetic moment, of all nuclei. But also other nuclei can be used for imaging such as sodium or fluorine [4].

In an external magnetic field $B0$ given by the MR scanner, the magnetic moment and the $B0$ field interact. Thereby, the nuclear spin of a proton can occupy two energy states. The energy states correspond to either parallel or antiparallel orientation with respect to $B0$ and thus, split up into two distinct energy level

doi:10.1088/978-0-7503-2396-3ch13

(Zeeman effect) [5]. For a larger number of protons in the probe a macroscopic magnetization is formed. For conducting an MRI experiment, it is necessary to flip the magnetization into the transversal plane. This can be achieved by exciting the spin system using an additionally oscillating magnetic field, i.e. by applying a radio frequency (RF-) pulse. After excitation the magnetization vector starts rotating in the transversal plane and the change of magnetization can be measured as it induces a voltage in a receive coil. Furthermore, the magnetization vector starts aligning with the $B0$ field after the RF-pulse is switched off. This process is called relaxation and can be divided into the spin-lattice relaxation, also called T_1 or longitudinal relaxation, and spin–spin relaxation, called T_2 or transverse relaxation, respectively. The T_1 relaxation time is defined as the time an ensemble of spins needs to rebuild 63% of its net longitudinal magnetization after excitation by a 90° RF pulse. The T_2 relaxation time describes the degree of dephasing the spins acquire. Both times highly depend on the tissue and therefore can be used to generate contrast in MR images.

In theory, a homogeneous magnetic field is assumed, however, in reality the local magnetic field is disturbed by various factors. This leads to an additional dephasing of the transversal magnetization and thus, to a reduction in the relaxation time, called T_2^*. The relaxation times T_1, T_2 and T_2^* can be measured by specialized MR sequences and are used among others for tissue characterization [6–8].

Nanoparticles used in MRI can be termed endogenous tracers (or contrast agents) and have para- or ferromagnetic properties [9]. After injection, they interact with the surrounding protons, cause local field inhomogeneities and susceptibility artifacts. This affects the relaxation of the proton spins, i.e. the relaxation time and the obtained signal is altered. Most contrast agents shorten T_1 and T_2/T_2^* [10]. A contrast agent with relatively high relaxivity may be detected at lower concentrations, which in turn allows the imaging of subtle changes at the molecular level. The relaxivity is highly dependent on a dipolar mechanism of the ion–nuclear distance to the inverse 6th power. Therefore, metal ions with a large spin number, are highly desired for MR contrast agents. The relaxivity r reflects how the relaxation rates ($R_1 = 1/T_1$, $R_2 = 1/T_2$) of a CA solution changes with respect to its concentration

$$\frac{1}{\Delta T_1} = r_1[C] \quad \frac{1}{\Delta T_2} = r_2[C],$$

with $\Delta T_{1,2}$ the changes in T_1/T_2 for different concentrations of CAs, i.e. $r_{1,2}$ are the respective slopes of this function. Figure 13.1 depicts T_1 and T_2 relaxation times for different concentrations of GD and manganese contrast agent. In table 13.1, relaxivities for several contrast agents are depicted. Since relaxivities are dependent on $B0$, data for field strengths other than 1.5 T can be found in [11].

The most prominent application of such endogenous tracer is called dynamic contrast enhanced (DCE) MRI where the tracer is injected as a bolus [12]. Combining it with fast repeated imaging of the same field of view (slices or volume), the passage of a contrast agent within the field of view can be recorded, i.e. the dynamics of the tracer within the tissue can be observed and hemodynamic

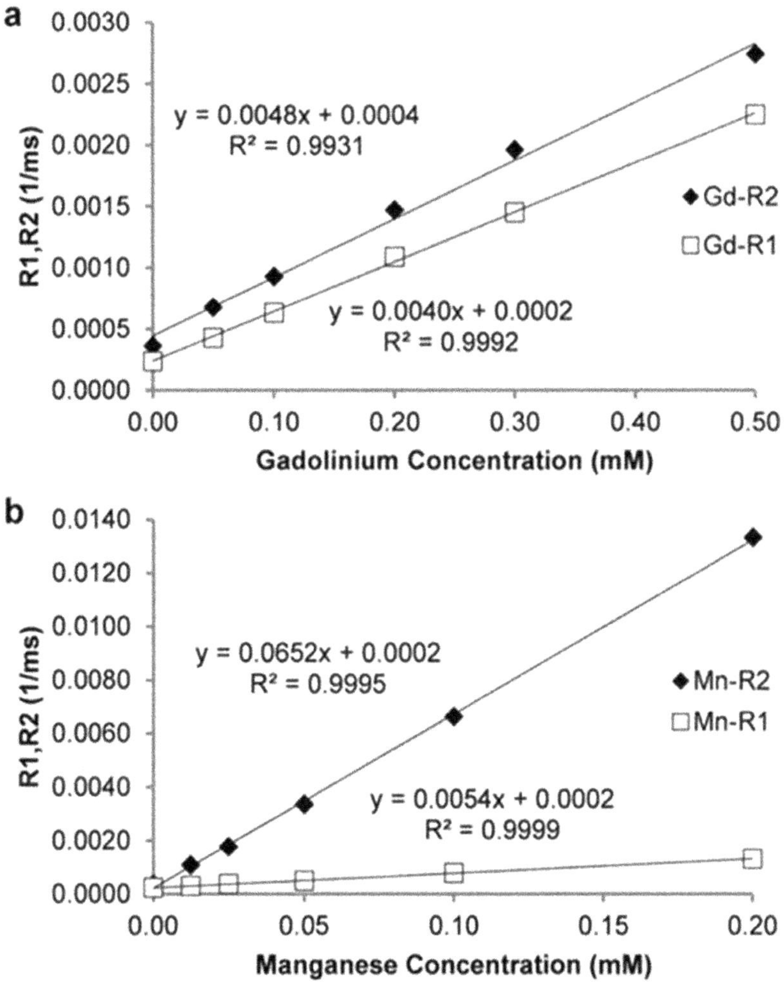

Figure 13.1. Relaxivity assessments for (a) gadolinium (Gd) and (b) manganese (Mn) contrast agents from a 60 MHz relaxometer using phantoms containing varying concentrations of a single contrast agent. Slopes of the fitted lines of R_1, R_2 versus agent concentration ($n = 6$ for each agent) were used to determine the relaxivities (r_1 and r_2) of the two agents. Pearson correlations resulted in significant correlations of concentration versus R_1 and R_2 for both contrast agents ($R_2 > 0.993$, two-tailed probability $p < 0.0001$). $R_1 = 1/T_1$, $R_2 = 1/T_2$. Reproduced from [10], copyright the authors 2017, CC BY 4.0.

parameters like blood flow, blood volume, transit times or exchange rates between blood pool and interstitial space can be quantified [13] (figure 13.2).

Tracers used for DCE-MRI are mostly based on Gadolinium (Gd^{3+}) coated with a chelate (e.g. diethylene-triamine-pentaacetic acid (DTPA)) to eliminate biotoxicity [14]. Recently, discussions have arisen about the safety of these contrast agents [15] and alternative techniques likes arterial spin labeling are gaining more and more attention [16]. Gd based contrast agents alter the T_1 relaxation and produce hyperintense signals in T_1 weighted images (figure 13.3).

Table 13.1. Relaxivities r_1 and r_2 for different contrast agents. Relaxivities were measured at 1.5 T and at 37° in blood. Data from [11].

Contrast agent			r_1 [L mmol^{-1} s^{-1}]	r_2 [L mmol^{-1} s^{-1}]
Short name	Generic name	Trade Name		
Gd-DTPA	Gadopentetate dimeglumine	MAGNEVIST	4.3 (4.0–4.6)	4.4 (3.6–5.2)
Gd-DO3A-butrol	Gadobutrol	GADOVIST	5.3 (5.0–5.6)	5.4 (4.6–6.2)
Gd-HP-DO3A	Gadoteridol	PROHANCE	4.4 (4.1–4.7)	5.5 (5.0–6.0)
Gd-BOPTA	Gadobenate dimeglumine	MULTIHANCE	6.7 (6.3–7.1)	8.9 (7.9–9.9)
Gadoterate	Meglumine	DOTAREM	4.2 (3.9–4.5)	6.7 (6.0–7.4)
Gd-DTPA-BMA	Gadodiamide	OMNISCAN	4.6 (4.3–4.9)	6.9 (5.5–8.3)
Mn-DPDP	Mangafodipir trisodium	TESLASCAN	5.2 (4.9–5.5)	8.9 (8.2–9.6)
Gd-DTPA-BMEA	Gadoversetamide	OPTIMARK	5.2 (4.9–5.5)	6.0 (5.4–6.6)
SHU555A	Ferucarbotran	RESOVIST	8.0 (7.5–8.5)	77 (71–83)
AMI-25	Ferumoxide	FERIDEX/ ENDOREM	7.0 (6.6–7.4)	66 (61–71)
SHL643A (Gadomer)	Gadodenterate	—	17 (16–18)	22 (21–23)
MS-325 trisodium	Gadofosveset	—	19 (18–20)	37 (35–39)
Gd-EOB-DTPA	Gadoxetic acid, disodium	PRIMOVIST	7.3 (6.9–7.7)	9.1 (8.2–10.0)
SH U 555 C	Ferucarbotran	—	14 (13–15)	90 (82–98)

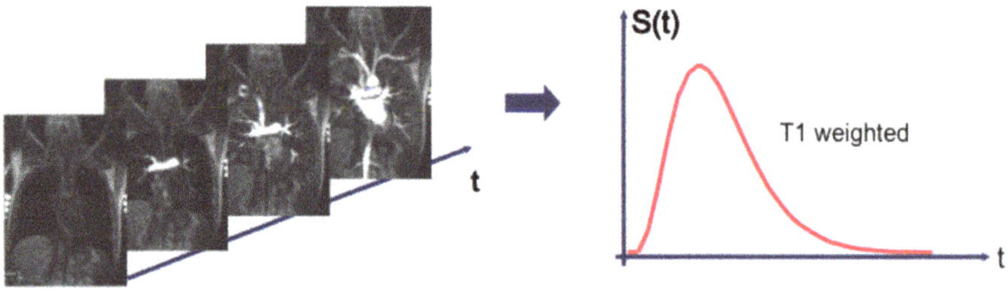

Figure 13.2. Illustration of DCE-MRI. From the dynamic image series, for each voxel a time intensity curve can be derived showing the passage of the contrast agent. Signal intensity values and curve shapes are arbitrary and just for illustrative purpose.

DCE-MRI is nowadays applied in nearly any organ in pre-clinical and in clinical research. The applications of DCE-MRI comprise diagnostics (e.g. characterization of tissue function via perfusion parameters) [17], cancer staging [18, 19], therapy monitoring [20, 21] or outcome [22] or survival predictions [23, 24].

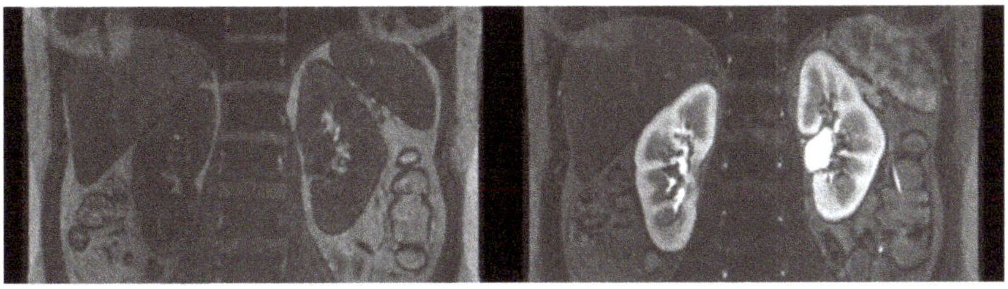

Figure 13.3. Example of a pre (left) and post contrast (right) image of the human abdomen. Images were acquired using a T_1 weighted 3D FLASH sequence. Tissue enhancement is clearly seen in the vessels, the kidneys, and the spleen. As contrast agent, GD-DTPA was used.

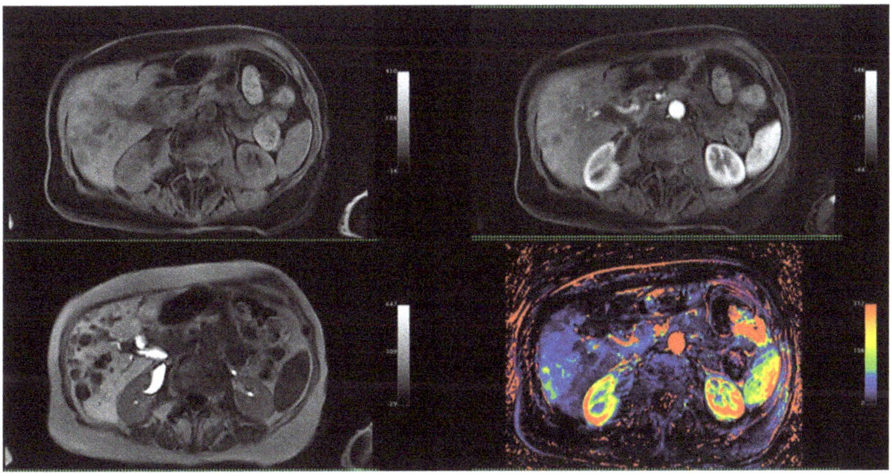

Figure 13.4. Example of a liver perfusion showing three phases, pre-contrast, first pass, late enhancement and map of blood flow quantified from the DCE-MRI in a patient with hepatic metastasis of mama CA.

Gadolinium ethoxybenzyl diethylene-triamine pentaacetic acid (Gd-EOB-DTPA) or gadobenate dimeglumine (Gd-BOPTA), both liver-specific Gd based contrast agent, were developed to improve the detection and characterization of focal liver lesions at MRI since common GD contrast agents were too unspecific [25] (figure 13.4).

Superparamagnetic iron oxides (SPIO) are contrast agents composed of nano-sized iron oxide crystals coated with dextran or carboxydextran [26]. Five types of superparamagnetic iron oxide (SPIO), i.e. Ferumoxides (Feridex® IV, Berlex Laboratories), Ferucarbotran (Resovist®, Bayer Healthcare), Ferumoxtran-10 (AMI-227/Code-7227, Combidex®, AMAG Pharma; Sinerem®, Guerbet), NC100150 (Clariscan®, Nycomed), and (VSOP C184, Ferropharm) have been clinically tested as MR contrast agents. However, except for Resovist®, which is currently available in only a few countries, all other agents have been stopped for further development or withdrawn from the market. Another SPIO agent called Ferumoxytol (Feraheme®) is approved for the treatment of iron deficiency in adult chronic kidney disease patients. It is comprised of iron oxide particles surrounded by a carbohydrate coat, and it is being explored as a potential imaging approach for evaluating lymph nodes and certain liver tumors [26].

Ultrasmall superparamagnetic iron oxide (USPIO) includes several chemically and pharmacologically distinct materials selected for a specific use. Some USPIO particles (median diameter < 50 nm) were used as MRI contrast agents (e.g. Sinerem®, Combidex®) to differentiate metastatic from inflammatory lymph nodes. However, as for the SPIOs, these two substances have been withdrawn from the market [27]. USPIO showed also potential for providing important information about angiogenesis in cancer tumors and could have possibly complemented MRI helping physicians to identify dangerous arteriosclerosis plaques. Because of the disadvantageous large T_2^*/T_1 ratio, USPIOs were found less suitable for contrast enhanced MR angiography than GD complexes [28]. Furthermore, the tiny USPIOs do not accumulate in the RES system as fast as larger particles, which results in a long plasma half-life. USPIO particles, with a small median diameter (<10 nm), will accumulate in lymph nodes after an intravenous injection by e.g. direct trans-capillary passage through endothelial venules or taken up from the interstitium by lymphatic vessels and transported to regional lymph nodes (see figure 13.5).

A lymph node with normal function shows a reduction of the signal intensity caused by T_2 shortening effects and magnetic susceptibility as it takes up a considerable amount of these particles while metastatic lymph nodes appear with less signal reduction due to its small uptake and thus, permit the differentiation of healthy lymph nodes from normal-sized, metastatic nodes [27].

Ferritin is a protein-based iron oxide nanoparticle. It has been proposed as a useful natural nanoparticle CA because of its uniform size (8–13 nm, 424 kDa), biocompatibility [30] and ease of functionalization [31–33]. Because the ferritin nanoparticle has an iron oxide core, its accumulation creates a signal reduction in T_2^*-weighted MRI. Ferritin can be detected by MRI in several forms, including the native form [31] or in a modified form with a core of high metal content [32, 33].

Cationized ferritin has been mainly used in pre-clinical studies, e.g. to detect the glomerular number and size in rodent kidney [34, 35] or to detect microstructural changes in a rat model of non-alcoholic steatohepatitis [36].

The non-lanthanide metal manganese (Mn) represents one of the early reported examples of paramagnetic contrast agents for MRI. In its bivalent state, the metal carries five unpaired electrons to produce efficient positive contrast enhancement [37]. The intrinsic properties of manganese include high spin number, long electronic relaxation time and labile water exchange. When used as a contrast agent, manganese ion (Mn^{2+}) works similarly to other paramagnetic ions, like gadolinium (Gd^{3+}), which is capable of shortening the T_1 of water protons, therefore increasing the signal intensity of T_1 weighted MR images. Additionally, Mn also has a minor T_2 effect, which reduces the signal intensity to produce dark signals. At cellular level, manganese is involved in mitochondrial function. The mitochondria density in the cell is therefore directly correlated to higher levels of Mn uptake. Mitochondria are also a rich component of hepatocytes. Taking its physical properties and the uptake into mitochondria together, manganese is an excellent contrast agent for MR

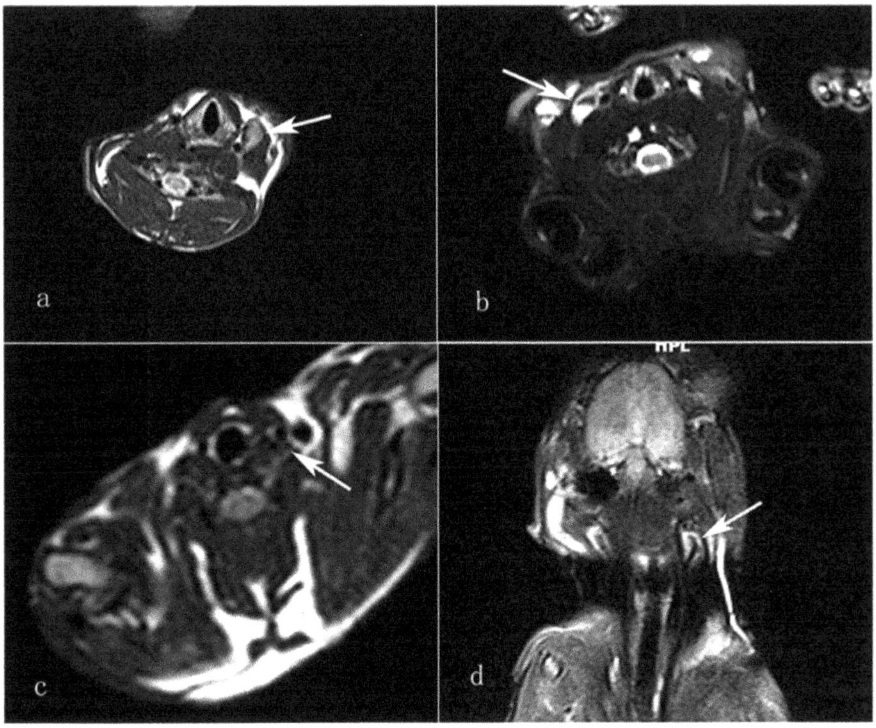

Figure 13.5. (a) T_2-weighted image of the neck shows a metastatic lymph node with partial high signal intensity, significantly higher than that of muscle tissue (white arrow). (b) T2-weighted image of the neck shows the metastatic lymph nodes that had irregular signal reduced intensity (white arrow). (c) The inflammatory lymph nodes showed homogeneous signal falls on T2-weighted image (white arrow). (d) The metastatic lymph nodes also had irregular signal reduced intensity on coronal view (white arrow). Reproduced from [29], copyright 2014 Shen *et al*, CC BY 4.0.

imaging of the liver, the pancreas and the kidneys [38]. Two Mn(II)-based agents, the liver-specific Mn-dipyridoxal diphosphate (DPDP) (Teslascan™) and an oral contrast containing Mn(II) chloride (LumenHance™), are available clinically for human use. Spath *et al* reported also a few Mn contrast agents for cardiac MRI [39] recently available, see table 13.2.

Moreover, a huge variety of possible chelates that can be linked to Mn exist. A detailed overview can be found in Pan *et al* [38]. Over the last 10 years, Mn^{2+} has been used as a contrast agent in various manganese-enhanced MRI (MEMRI) applications [40]. Applications in neuroscience can be grouped in three major classes: neuronal tract tracing, morphological, and functional imaging. For neuronal tract-tracing studies manganese is directly injected into a specific brain region while in other applications, it is administered either systemically into the bloodstream or directly into the cerebrospinal fluid (CSF). Another application for Mn MRI has been reported in cardiac MRI for T_1 mapping [39]. Figure 13.6 shows an example of T_1 maps of the human heart generated by manganese-enhanced MRI.

Table 13.2. Status of manganese contrast agents with clinical experience in myocardial imaging. Data from [39].

Contrast agent	Proposed clinical dose (μmol kg^{-1})	Clinical trial/ licensing status	Commercial availability	Barriers to clinical application	Currently recruiting or yet-to-report cardiac clinical trials
Chelated manganese: MnDPDP	5	Previously licensed in EU Phase III clinical trials complete	Previously available as Teslascan[a], withdrawn due to lack of demand	No current clinical production	Manganese-enhanced MRI (MEMRI) of the myocardium (NCT03607669)
Non-chelated manganese:					
$MnCl_2$[b]	5	Not licensed or undergoing clinical trial	Not available	Significant cardiotoxic potential in cardiac patients	None
EVP1001–1	1–10	Phase II clinical trials complete	Not available	Currently undergoing further clinical trial Toxicity profile in cardiac patients not well established	Clinical Trial of MEMRI to assess peri-infarct Injury (NCT02933034) Efficacy of EVP1001–1 (see more) in the Assessment of myocardial viability in patients With cardiovascular disease (NCT01989195)

[a] Marketing authorisation holder: GE Healthcare AS.
[b] No current plans for routine clinical use at time of writing due to toxicity profile.
EU, European Union; EVP1001–1, Eagle Vision Pharmaceutical; $MnCl_2$, manganese chloride; MnDPDP, manganese dipyridoxyl diphosphate.

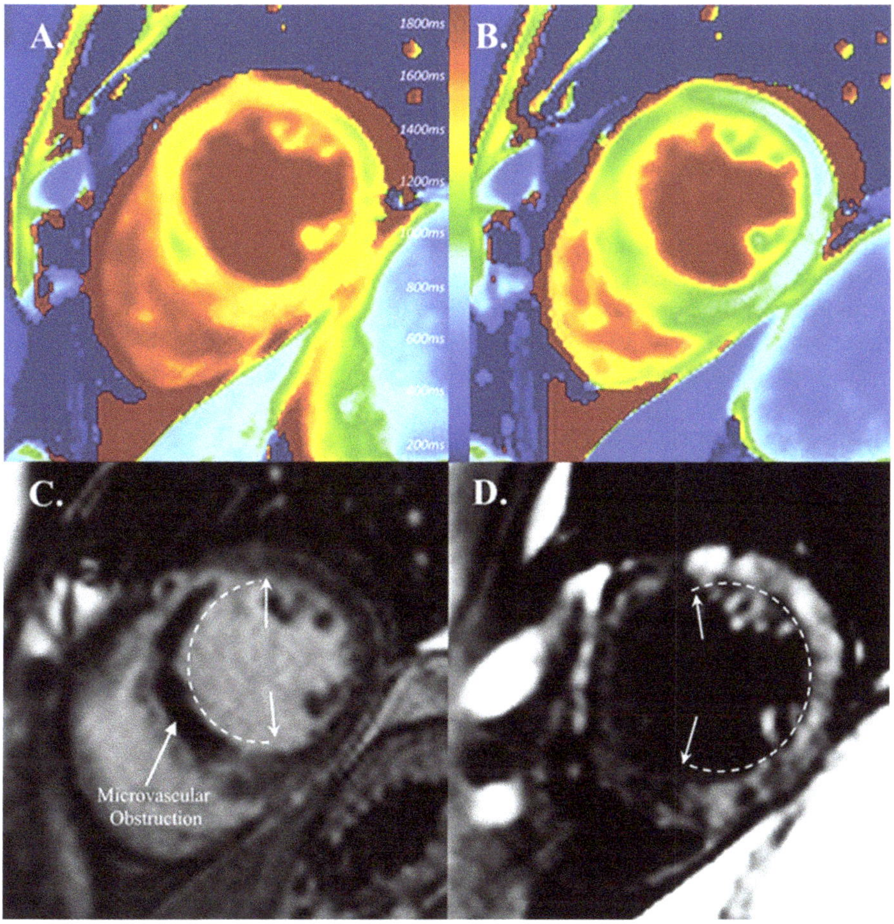

Figure 13.6. Clinical manganese-enhanced MRI (MEMRI) in a patient with myocardial infarction. Clinical tissue characterisation acutely post-myocardial infarction with native T_1 mapping (A), MEMRI T_1 mapping (B), gadolinium delayed-enhanced MRI (C) and manganese enhancement (D). Note shortened T_1 in remote myocardium on MEMRI compared with native T_1 mapping (A, B). Inversion recovery images demonstrate shortening in infarct with gadolinium (C) and in remote myocardium with manganese (D) (extent of enhancement indicated by arrows and dashed lines). Reproduced from [39], copyright 2019, CC BY 4.0.

References

[1] Vlaardingerbroek M and den Boer J 2003 *Magnetic Resonance Imaging. Theory and Practice* 3rd edn (Berlin: Springer)

[2] Haacke E *et al* 1999 *Magnetic Resonance Imaging: Physical Principles and Sequence Design* (New York: Wiley)

[3] Liang Z and Lauterbur P 2000 *Principles of Magnetic Resonance Imaging: A Signal Processing Perspective. IEEE Press Series in Biomedical Engineering* (Bellingham, WA: SPIE Optical Engineering Press)

[4] Konstandin S and Schad L R 2014 30 Years of sodium/X-nuclei magnetic resonance imaging *MAGMA* **27** 1–4

[5] Zeeman P 1897 The effect of magnetisation on the nature of light emitted by a substance *Nature* **55** 347
[6] de Bazelaire C *et al* 2004 MR imaging relaxation times of abdominal and pelvic tissues measured *in vivo* at 3.0 T: preliminary results *Radiology* **230** 652–9
[7] Rieger B *et al* 2018 Time efficient whole-brain coverage with MR Fingerprinting using slice-interleaved echo-planar-imaging *Sci. Rep.* **8** 6667
[8] Messner N M *et al* 2018 Saturation-recovery myocardial T1-mapping during systole: accurate and robust quantification in the presence of arrhythmia *Sci. Rep.* **8** 5251
[9] Geraldes C F and Laurent S 2009 Classification and basic properties of contrast agents for magnetic resonance imaging *Contrast Media Mol. Imaging* **4** 1–23
[10] Anderson C E *et al* 2017 Dual contrast - magnetic resonance fingerprinting (DC-MRF): a platform for simultaneous quantification of multiple mri contrast agents *Sci. Rep.* **7** 8431
[11] Rohrer M *et al* 2005 Comparison of magnetic properties of MRI contrast media solutions at different magnetic field strengths *Invest. Radiol.* **40** 715–24
[12] Rosen B R *et al* 1990 Perfusion imaging with NMR contrast agents *Magn. Reson. Med.* **14** 249–65
[13] Zöllner F G *et al* 2016 Quantitative Perfusionsbildgebung in der Magnetresonanztomographie *Radiologe* **56** 113–23
[14] Caravan P *et al* 1999 Gadolinium(III) chelates as MRI contrast agents: Structure, dynamics, and applications *Chem. Rev.* **99** 2293–352
[15] Rogosnitzky M and Branch S 2016 Gadolinium-based contrast agent toxicity: a review of known and proposed mechanisms *Biometals* **29** 365–76
[16] Alsop D C *et al* 2015 Recommended implementation of arterial spin-labeled perfusion MRI for clinical applications: a consensus of the ISMRM perfusion study group and the European consortium for ASL in dementia *Magn. Reson. Med.* **73** 102–16
[17] Riffel P *et al* 2016 One-stop shop: free-breathing dynamic contrast-enhanced MRI of the kidney using iterative reconstruction and continuous golden-angle radial sampling *Invest. Radiol.* **51** 714–9
[18] Zöllner F G, Emblem K E and Schad L R 2012 SVM-based glioma grading: Optimization by feature reduction analysis *Z. Med. Phys.* **22** 205–14
[19] Schoenberg S and Zöllner F G 2017 Technische Grundlagen der Prostata-MRT *MR- und PET-Bildgebung der Prostata* ed U Attenberger, U Ritter and F Wenz (Heidelberg: Springer) pp 1–18
[20] Libicher M *et al* 2013 Dynamic contrast-enhanced MRI for monitoring bisphosphonate therapy in Paget's disease of bone *Skeletal Radiol.* **42** 225–30
[21] Sterzik A *et al* 2015 DCE-MRI biomarkers for monitoring an anti-angiogenic triple combination therapy in experimental hypopharynx carcinoma xenografts with immunohistochemical validation *Acta Radiol.* **56** 294–303
[22] Weis M *et al* 2016 MR lung perfusion in 2-year old children after congenital diaphragmatic hernia repair–comparison of children after ECMO therapy and children without ECMO requirement *Am. J. Roentgenol.* **206** 1–6
[23] Emblem K E *et al* 2015 A generic support vector machine model for preoperative glioma survival associations *Radiology* **275** 228–34
[24] Emblem K E *et al* 2014 Machine learning in preoperative glioma MRI: survival associations by perfusion-based support vector machine outperforms traditional MRI *J. Magn. Reson. Imaging* **40** 47–54

[25] Caraiani C N *et al* 2015 Description of focal liver lesions with Gd-EOB-DTPA enhanced MRI *Clujul Med.* **88** 438–48

[26] Wang Y X 2011 Superparamagnetic iron oxide based MRI contrast agents: Current status of clinical application *Quant. Imaging Med Surg* **1** 35–40

[27] Fortuin A S *et al* 2018 Ultra-small superparamagnetic iron oxides for metastatic lymph node detection: back on the block *Wiley Interdiscip. Rev. Nanomed. Nanobiotechnol.* **10** e1471

[28] Varallyay P *et al* 2002 Comparison of two superparamagnetic viral-sized iron oxide particles ferumoxides and ferumoxtran-10 with a gadolinium chelate in imaging intracranial tumors *Am. J. Neuroradiol.* **23** 510–9

[29] Shen N *et al* 2014 Indirect magnetic resonance imaging lymphography identifies lymph node metastasis in rabbit pyriform sinus VX2 carcinoma using ultra-small super-paramagnetic iron oxide *PLoS One* **9** e94876

[30] Beeman S C, Georges J F and Bennett K M 2013 Toxicity, biodistribution, and *ex vivo* MRI detection of intravenously injected cationized ferritin *Magn. Reson. Med.* **69** 853–61

[31] Bulte J W *et al* 1995 Initial assessment of magnetoferritin biokinetics and proton relaxation enhancement in rats *Acad. Radiol.* **2** 871–8

[32] Bennett K M *et al* 2008 Controlled aggregation of ferritin to modulate MRI relaxivity *Biophys. J.* **95** 342–51

[33] Uchida M *et al* 2008 A human ferritin iron oxide nano-composite magnetic resonance contrast agent *Magn. Reson. Med.* **60** 1073–81

[34] Heilmann M *et al* 2012 Quantification of glomerular number and size distribution in normal rat kidneys using magnetic resonance imaging *Nephrol. Dial. Transplant.* **27** 100–7

[35] Chacon-Caldera J *et al* 2016 Fast glomerular quantification of whole *ex vivo* mouse kidneys using Magnetic Resonance Imaging at 9.4 Tesla *Z. Med. Phys.* **26** 54–62

[36] Beeman S C *et al* 2013 Cationized ferritin as a magnetic resonance imaging probe to detect microstructural changes in a rat model of non-alcoholic steatohepatitis *Magn. Reson. Med.* **70** 1728–38

[37] Wendland M F 2004 Applications of manganese-enhanced magnetic resonance imaging (MEMRI) to imaging of the heart *NMR Biomed.* **17** 581–94

[38] Pan D P J *et al* 2011 Manganese-based MRI contrast agents: past, present, and future *Tetrahedron* **67** 8431–44

[39] Spath N B *et al* 2019 Manganese-enhanced MRI of the myocardium *Heart* **105** 1695–700

[40] Malheiros J M *et al* 2015 Manganese-enhanced MRI: biological applications in neuroscience *Front. Neurol.* **6** 161

Chapter 14

Nanoparticle detection using photoacoustic imaging (PAI)

Romy Mueller, Wilfred Ngwa and Juergen Hesser

Photoacoustic imaging (PAI) is a biomedical imaging modality allowing for the detection of hemoglobin [1], superficial vasculature [2], and cancer [3] by combining both functional and molecular information [4]. Hemoglobin is a 5 nm sized spherical iron-containing protein responsible for transporting oxygen in the blood from the lung to tissue [5]. Its detectability using PAI allows differentiation between soft tissue and blood vessels and is hence an important tool for imaging tumor vasculature [6].

PAI uses the photoacoustic effect, where absorbed light leads to the formation of a sound wave [7] that is recorded as image: the sample is illuminated with visible or near-infrared intense light. This light energy is absorbed by chemical compounds in tissue and transferred to heat, causing thermoelastic expansion [4]; the concomitant pressure is detected by an ultrasound transducer, as illustrated in figure 14.1.

Two different modes of PAI are distinguished, PA tomography (PAT) and PA microscopy (PAM). In PAT, the tissue surface is irradiated with full field illumination using a large diameter pulsed laser beam. The generated acoustic waves are detected in arrays of transducers receiving the time-variant signal, which can be reconstructed to obtain the initial 3D pressure distribution as described in more detail below. In PAM, a spherically focused ultrasound transducer or focused laser beam are used to measure the time of arrivals of the acoustic waves to obtain a depth-resolved 1D image (A-line). While scanning the sample, generating 3D images is possible without the need of reconstruction [8].

For both modalities, the thermal expansion needs to be time-variant for generating acoustic waves [7]. This can be achieved using continuous wave lasers with intensity-modulation at constant or variable frequency [9, 10]. This is an uninterrupted beam with stable output power, whose wavelength is determined by the laser medium. However, pulsed lasers are more commonly employed compared to continuous intensity-modulated lasers due to their higher signal-to-noise ratio [11] and difference in time-of-flight reducing signal cluttering [9]. These laser pulses are in

doi:10.1088/978-0-7503-2396-3ch14

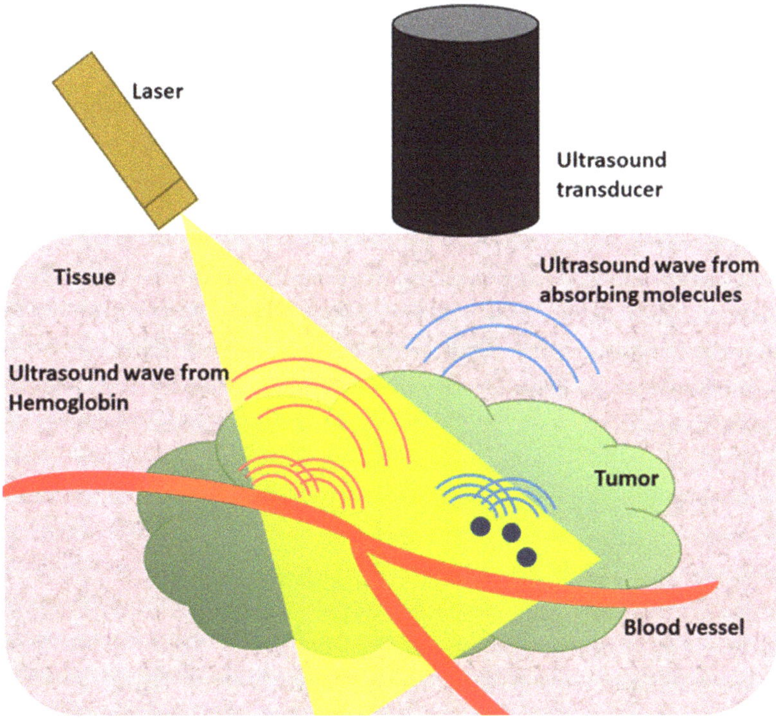

Figure 14.1. Incident laser light (yellow beam) is absorbed by different molecules such as hemoglobin in blood (red) or nanoparticles (blue). The concomitant thermoelastic expansion is measured as a pressure wave by an ultrasound transducer.

the order of a few nanoseconds to fulfill thermal confinement and acoustic stress confinement, i.e. that thermal diffusion and volume expansion during the illumination period are negligible. Lasers are operated in a wavelength between 550 nm and 900 nm generating low-amplitude (less than 10 kPa) acoustic waves representing a technological challenge to the transducer design [12, 13]. For PAT, this is a multi-element transducer array picking up the signal at different locations. For PAM this is a single-element ultrasonic transducer.

Heat conversion from the incident laser creates an initial pressure distribution p_0, which, for laser pulses less than the acoustic confinement time (< 10 ns) [14], is proportional to the absorbed optical energy $H(r)$ at location r. The absorbed optical energy $H(r)$ depends on various parameters, for which many can be assumed to be invariant to biological tissues. In biomedical applications, the initial pressure distribution and hence image contrast depend on the scatter in tissue and on optical absorption [12]. These two factors as well as wavelength dependency limit the penetration depth of PA signal to a few centimeters in biological tissues. In this respect, detection up to 4 cm depth has been demonstrated *in vivo* in the human breast [15]. Optical absorption of various tissues and molecules is shown in figure 14.2, demonstrating that hemoglobin is one of the most relevant absorbers, rendering PAI a useful tool for vasculature detection [6]. Deeper penetration can be

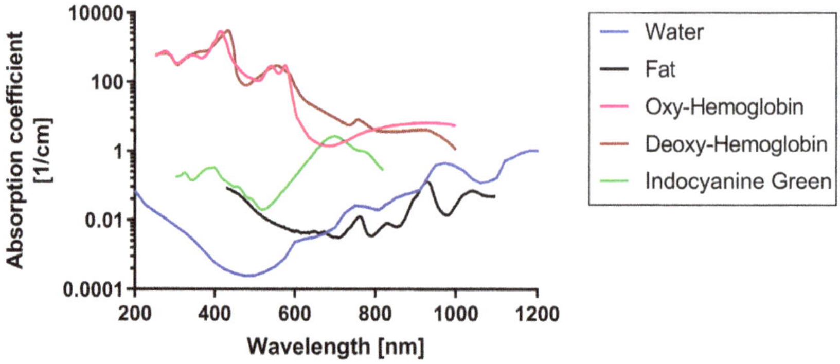

Figure 14.2. Absorption spectra of various tissues and molecules. Data taken from https://omlc.org/spectra/, last accessed on 02/04/2020; [17, 18]; W B Gratzer, Medical Research Council Labs, Holly Hill, London; N Kollias, Wellman Laboratories, Harvard Medical School, Boston.

achieved by avoiding hemoglobin absorption using wavelength in the infrared regimen where absorption by fat and water become more dominant. The use of appropriate contrast agents such as nanoparticles (NPs) at these long wavelengths increased the contrast in murine tissue *in vivo* [16]. Spatial resolution is dependent of the used ultrasound receiver, which again is dictated by the requested depth for imaging due to ultrasound absorption. For penetration within a few centimeters, resolution in the sub-millimeter range is achievable and it further improves with shorter depth [12].

In PAT, image formation corresponds to the recovery of the initial pressure distribution p_0 from the time-dependent ultrasound signal. The reconstruction algorithm employed further determines the image quality. Early reconstruction methods were based on analytical methods such as filtered back-projection [19] or deconvolution reconstruction [20]. A major limitation is the contrast decrease with increasing depth. In about 2002 iterative reconstruction methods were established to improve performance [21]. Modern optimization-based approaches achieved significant reduction in sample number by using e.g. compressed sensing models [22], facilitating reconstruction when geometrical constraints such as body shape limit the number of scans. Recent developments have focused also on deep learning regularization-based reconstruction [23]. Detailed descriptions of reconstruction methods and approaches are available [24, 25].

Besides different endogenous chemical compounds such as hemoglobin, melanin, and water in tissue, exogenous contrast agents are used in research. These include dyes such as fluorescent molecules and NPs [26]. In particular, NPs can be divided into two classes according to their mechanism of light absorption [27]: dye-containing NPs or metallic/metal-coated, so called plasmonic NPs, as shown in figure 14.3. The optical absorption of dye-containing NPs can be modified by utilizing different payloads of near-infrared dyes, such as the Food and Drug Administration (FDA)-approved indocyanine green (ICG) [28]. Plasmonic NPs benefit from a tunable light absorption resulting from surface plasmon resonance (SPR) [4], in which free electrons undergo collective oscillation. For this, free

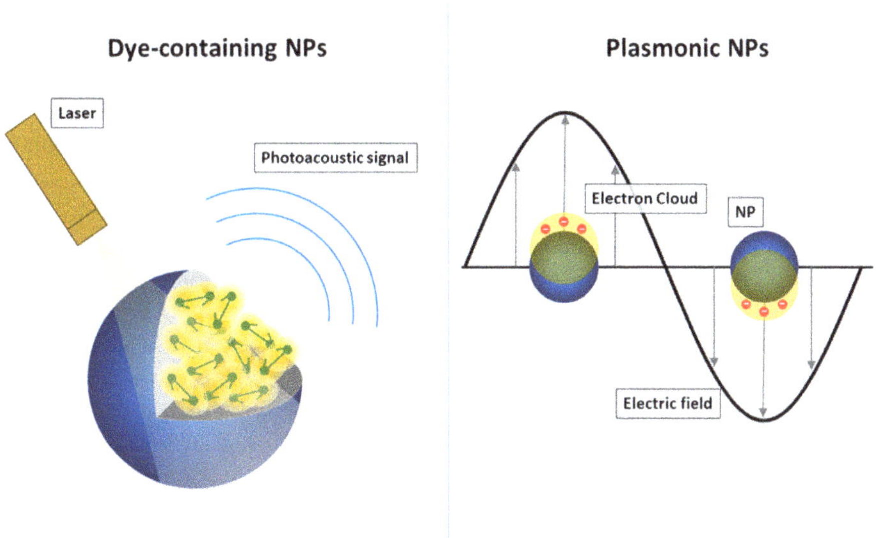

Figure 14.3. Dye-containing versus plasmonic NPs. Dye-based NPs emit photoacoustic signal by absorption of the incident light by fluorescent molecules. For plasmonic NPs, the incident electromagnetic wave forms electron clouds oscillating over the NP with the same frequency. NP = nanoparticle.

electrons of the metallic NPs deflect in the electromagnetic field. The attractive Coulomb force between electron cloud and metal NP leads to oscillation of electrons in a frequency, which depends on electron density, effective electron mass, and charge distribution [29]. The fluctuation, called plasmon, corresponds to a dipole antenna formed on the NP surface and radiates an electric field, which will be measured in the ultrasound transducer.

Light absorption of plasmonic gold nanospheres (80 nm in size) was shown to have light scattering five orders of magnitude higher than for fluorescent dyes [30]. However, size and shape of NPs have a significant impact on their PAI detectability. For nanospheres, the surface plasmon extinction maximum increases to longer wavelength with increasing nanosphere diameter [30], making the photoacoustic signal prone to be affected by NP clusters which will appear with lower signal when illuminated with the same laser wavelength. In addition, different composition of nanoshells [31] as well as the NP shape [32] has an impact on the extinction spectra. For example, nanorods show a splitting of SPR into two modes, identified in the spectra as two maxima compared to one maximum for nanospheres. These two modes correspond to transverse and longitudinal direction with respect to the long axis of the rod. When increasing the rod's aspect ratio while maintaining their width, the transverse mode experienced only a slight wavelength change, whereas the longitudinal mode shifts [32]. These characteristics must be considered when choosing the ideal wavelength for absorption depending on absorber type (endogenous or exogenous), size, and shape.

These properties further influence the sensitivity of photoacoustic imaging. Single-walled carbon nanotubes, enhanced with ICG, showed in an *in vivo* model

300 times higher photoacoustic contrast compared to previously reported single-walled carbon nanotubes [33]. Extrapolation of their signal-concentration curve forecasts a concentration detection limit of 170 pM [33]. The minimum required concentration of gold NPs for detection using multi-wavelength PAI was determined as 3×10^7 NPs ml^{-1} [34]. Accordingly, non-invasive detection of cells containing NPs is achievable if a sufficient number of NPs are present, as shown for gold nanocages detected in sentinel lymph nodes *in vivo* [35].

NPs cannot be used as contrast agents only but can be quantified as well since, assuming a constant laser fluence, PA amplitude is proportional to the absorber concentration [34]; leading to an estimate of the local laser fluence. This has been used in various studies *in vitro* and *in vivo*, including tracking transport kinetics of gold nanocages in a lymphatic system [36]. Hence, PAI allows studying NP excretion mechanisms in the body; a crucial step for clinical implementation of NPs. Further studies have focused on eliminating the need of knowing the local fluence, but rather knowing the relative change in fluence, for NP quantification [37], allowing for better quantitative assessment of NP biodistribution.

Functionalization of NPs allows further applications as tumor microenvironment detection. One application is imaging of reactive oxygen species (ROS) by near-infrared absorbing semi-conducting polymer NPs [38]. Their high structural flexibility together with strong resistance to photodegradation and oxidation allows for real-time imaging of ROS down to a detection limit of 50 nM. In contrast, the ability of hemoglobin/oxygen detection using PAI offers *in vivo* oxygen sensing with potential better radiotherapy planning and treatment efficacy monitoring [39, 40].

The field of PAI in biomedical research is extending from imaging superficial vasculature and monitoring hemodynamics. One emerging field of PAM is functional imaging at the cell and sub-cellular level at depths exceeding the capability of competing microscopic approaches [41]. Recent technological advances on transducer design will allow further improvements as long laser pulse induced dual photoacoustic (LDPA), in which two photoacoustic signals are produced by one excitation [42]. By not satisfying stress confinement, two signals are produced following the positive and negative edge of the long laser pulse, leading to improved image contrast [42] and suspected improved axial resolution [43]. PAI is further moving towards cancer screening and observation due to the ability of observing tumor perfusion and the use of NPs. These do not only act as contrast agents allowing deeper tissue penetration, but allow in addition targeting of different structures, making them an important tool for cancer diagnostics. Together with the amplified cell kill during radiotherapy for high atomic number NPs as gold, these NPs not only serve as contrast enhancer during PAI but also possess the ability of promoting the field of theranostics.

References

[1] Wang X, Xie X, Ku G, Wang L V and Stoica G 2006 Noninvasive imaging of hemoglobin concentration and oxygenation in the rat brain using high-resolution photoacoustic tomography *J. Biomed. Opt.* **11** 024015

[2] Zhang E Z, Laufer J G, Pedley R B and Beard P C 2009 *In vivo* high-resolution 3D photoacoustic imaging of superficial vascular anatomy *Phys. Med. Biol.* **54** 1035

[3] Manohar S, Vaartjes S E, van Hespen J C, Klaase J M, van den Engh F M, Steenbergen W and Van Leeuwen T G 2007 Initial results of *in vivo* non-invasive cancer imaging in the human breast using near-infrared photoacoustics *Opt. Express* **15** 12277–85

[4] Luke G P, Yeager D and Emelianov S Y 2012 Biomedical applications of photoacoustic imaging with exogenous contrast agents *Ann. Biomed. Eng.* **40** 422–37

[5] Schechter A N 2008 Hemoglobin research and the origins of molecular medicine *Blood* **112** 3927–38

[6] Laufer J G, Zhang E Z, Treeby B E, Cox B T, Beard P C, Johnson P and Pedley B 2012 *In vivo* preclinical photoacoustic imaging of tumor vasculature development and therapy *J. Biomed. Opt.* **17** 056016

[7] Xia J, Yao J and Wang L V 2014 Photoacoustic tomography: principles and advances *Prog. Electromagn. Res.* **147** 1

[8] Kim C, Favazza C and Wang L V 2010 *In vivo* photoacoustic tomography of chemicals: high-resolution functional and molecular optical imaging at new depths *Chem. Rev.* **110** 2756–82

[9] Maslov K I and Wang L V 2008 Photoacoustic imaging of biological tissue with intensity-modulated continuous-wave laser *J. Biomed. Opt.* **13** 024006

[10] Lashkari B and Mandelis A 2010 Photoacoustic radar imaging signal-to-noise ratio, contrast, and resolution enhancement using nonlinear chirp modulation *Opt. Lett.* **35** 1623–5

[11] Lashkari B and Mandelis A 2011 Comparison between pulsed laser and frequency-domain photoacoustic modalities: Signal-to-noise ratio, contrast, resolution, and maximum depth detectivity *Rev. Sci. Instrum.* **82** 094903

[12] Beard P 2011 Biomedical photoacoustic imaging *Interface Focus* **1** 602–31

[13] Omar M, Schwarz M, Soliman D, Symvoulidis P and Ntziachristos V 2015 Pushing the optical imaging limits of cancer with multi-frequency-band raster-scan optoacoustic mesoscopy (RSOM) *Neoplasia* **17** 208–14

[14] Meiburger K M 2016 *Quantitative Ultrasound and Photoacoustic Imaging for the Assessment of Vascular Parameters* (Berlin: Springer)

[15] Kruger R A, Lam R B, Reinecke D R, Del Rio S P and Doyle R P 2010 Photoacoustic angiography of the breast *Med. Phys.* **37** 6096–100

[16] Homan K, Kim S, Chen Y S, Wang B, Mallidi S and Emelianov S 2010 Prospects of molecular photoacoustic imaging at 1064 nm wavelength *Opt. Lett.* **35** 2663–5

[17] Hale G M and Querry M R 1973 Optical constants of water in the 200 nm to 200 micron wavelength region *Appl. Opt.* **12** 555–63

[18] van Veen R L P, Sterenborg H J C M, Pifferi A, Torricelli A and Cubbedu R 2004 Determination of VIS–NIR absorption coefficients of mammalian fat, with time- and spatially resolved diffuse reflectance and transmission spectroscopy *OSA Annual BIOMED Topical Meeting, 2004*

[19] Xu M, Xu Y and Wang L V 2003 Time-domain reconstruction algorithms and numerical simulations for thermoacoustic tomography in various geometries *IEEE Trans. Biomed. Eng.* **50** 1086–99

[20] Zhang C and Wang Y 2008 Deconvolution reconstruction of full-view and limited-view photoacoustic tomography: a simulation study *J. Opt. Soc. Am.* A **25** 2436–43

[21] Paltauf G, Viator J A, Prahl S A and Jacques S L 2002 Iterative reconstruction algorithm for optoacoustic imaging *J. Acoust. Soc. Am.* **112** 1536–44
[22] Haltmeier M, Berer T, moon S and Burgholzer P 2016 Compressed sensing and sparsity in photoacoustic tomography *J. Opt.* **18** 114004
[23] Hauptmann A, Lucka F, Betcke M, Huynh N, Adler J, Cox B, Beard P, Ourselin S and Arridge S 2018 Model-based learning for accelerated, limited-view 3-d photoacoustic tomography *IEEE Trans. Med. Imaging* **37** 1382–93
[24] Lutzweiler C and Razansky D 2013 Optoacoustic imaging and tomography: reconstruction approaches and outstanding challenges in image performance and quantification *Sensors* **13** 7345–84
[25] Wang J and Wang Y 2018 Photoacoustic imaging reconstruction using combined nonlocal patch and total-variation regularization for straight-line scanning *Biomed. Eng. Online* **17** 105
[26] Wu D, Huang L, Jiang M S and Jiang H 2014 Contrast agents for photoacoustic and thermoacoustic imaging: a review *Int. J. Mol. Sci.* **15** 23616–39
[27] Yang X, Stein E W, Ashkenazi S and Wang L V 2009 Nanoparticles for photoacoustic imaging *Wiley Interdisc. Rev.: Nanomed. Nanobiotechnol.* **1** 360–8
[28] Yang X, Skrabalak S, Stein E, Wu B, Wei X, Xia Y and Wang L V 2008 Photoacoustic tomography with novel optical contrast agents based on gold nanocages or nanoparticles containing near-infrared dyes *Photons Plus Ultrasound: Imaging and Sensing 2008: The Ninth Conf. on Biomedical Thermoacoustics, Optoacoustics, and Acousto-optics* vol 6856 (Bellingham, WA: Int. Society for Optics and Photonics) p 68560I
[29] Kelly K L, Coronado E, Zhao L L and Schatz G C 2003 The optical properties of metal nanoparticles: the influence of size, shape, and dielectric environment *J. Phys. Chem.* B **107** 668–77
[30] Jain P K, Lee K S, El-Sayed I H and El-Sayed M A 2006 Calculated absorption and scattering properties of gold nanoparticles of different size, shape, and composition: applications in biological imaging and biomedicine *J. Phys. Chem.* B **110** 7238–48
[31] Li W and Chen X 2015 Gold nanoparticles for photoacoustic imaging *Nanomedicine* **10** 299–320
[32] El-Brolossy T A, Abdallah T, Mohamed M B, Abdallah S, Easawi K, Negm S and Talaat H 2008 Shape and size dependence of the surface plasmon resonance of gold nanoparticles studied by photoacoustic technique *Eur. Phys. J.: Spec. Top.* **153** 361–4
[33] Zerda A D, Liu Z, Bodapati S, Teed R, Vaithilingam S, Khuri-Yakub B T, Chen X, Dai H and Gambhir S S 2010 Ultrahigh sensitivity carbon nanotube agents for photoacoustic molecular imaging in living mice *Nano Lett.* **10** 2168–72
[34] Mallidi S, Larson T, Tam J, Joshi P P, Karpiouk A, Sokolov K and Emelianov S 2009 Multiwavelength photoacoustic imaging and plasmon resonance coupling of gold nanoparticles for selective detection of cancer *Nano Lett.* **9** 2825–31
[35] Song K H, Kim C, Cobley C M, Xia Y and Wang L V 2008 Near-infrared gold nanocages as a new class of tracers for photoacoustic sentinel lymph node mapping on a rat model *Nano Lett.* **9** 183–8
[36] Cai X, Li W, Kim C H, Yuan Y, Wang L V and Xia Y 2011 *In vivo* quantitative evaluation of the transport kinetics of gold nanocages in a lymphatic system by noninvasive photoacoustic tomography *ACS Nano* **5** 9658–67
[37] Cook J R, Frey W and Emelianov S 2013 Quantitative photoacoustic imaging of nanoparticles in cells and tissues *ACS Nano* **7** 1272–80

[38] Pu K, Shuhendler A J, Jokerst J V, Mei J, Gambhir S S, Bao Z and Rao J 2014 Semiconducting polymer nanoparticles as photoacoustic molecular imaging probes in living mice *Nat. Nanotechnol.* **9** 233

[39] Ashkenazi S, Huang S W, Horvath T, Koo Y E and Kopelman R 2008 Oxygen sensing for *in vivo* imaging by photoacoustic lifetime probing *Photons Plus Ultrasound: Imaging and Sensing 2008: The Ninth Conf. on Biomedical Thermoacoustics, Optoacoustics, and Acousto-optics* vol 6856 (Bellingham, WA: Int. Society for Optics and Photonics) p 68560D

[40] Shao Q, Morgounova E, Jiang C, Choi J H, Bischof J C and Ashkenazi S 2013 *In vivo* photoacoustic lifetime imaging of tumor hypoxia in small animals *J. Biomed. Opt.* **18** 076019

[41] Liu Y, Nie L and Chen X 2016 Photoacoustic molecular imaging: from multiscale biomedical applications towards early-stage theranostics *Trends Biotechnol.* **34** 420–33

[42] Gao F, Feng X, Zhang R, Liu S, Ding R, Kishor R and Zheng Y 2017 Single laser pulse generates dual photoacoustic signals for differential contrast photoacoustic imaging *Sci. Rep.* **7** 1–2

[43] Wang L, Zhang C and Wang L V 2014 Grueneisen relaxation photoacoustic microscopy *Phys. Rev. Lett.* **113** 174301

Part III

Applications

IOP Publishing

Nanoparticle Enhanced Radiation Therapy
Principles, methods and applications
Erno Sajo and Piotr Zygmanski

Chapter 15

Radiotherapy application with *in situ* dose-painting (RAiD) via inhalation delivery

Yao Hao

15.1 Introduction

Lung cancer is one of the most common cancers in both men and women, and is by far the leading cause of cancer deaths. The five-year overall survival rate is 16% for men and slightly higher, 22%, for women (American Cancer Society 2019). Radiation is one of the most common treatments for lung cancer. By boosting radiation dose, survival for lung cancer patients could be significantly increased (Keall *et al* 2006, Machtay *et al* 2012). Clinical studies indicated that a 1 Gy boost in biologically effective dose is statistically significantly associated with 4% relative improvement in survival (Machtay *et al* 2010). However, radiation boosting is compromised for the sake of normal tissue toxicity, especially with impact of respiratory motion (Keall *et al* 2006). Concomitant chemoradiotherapy (CCRT) provides improved survival and local control compared to radiation alone or sequential chemotherapy and radiation with higher overlap toxicity (Furuse *et al* 1999). New chemotherapy drug delivery strategies, radiation treatment strategies (Keall *et al* 2006), optimal chemotherapy regimen or radiation therapy dose fractionation are being investigated to improve the balance between complications and cure.

In recent years, nanoparticle-aided radiotherapy has emerged as a promising modality to enhance radiation therapy via the radiosensitizing action of high atomic number (Z) nanoparticles (NPs), such as gold nanoparticles (GNPs). These particles can be employed during external beam radiotherapy (EBRT) or brachytherapy, and have the potential to boost target radiation dose with minimal normal tissue toxicities (Ngwa *et al* 2014). For clinical megavoltage radiotherapy, however, many studies stated that radiation boosting from high-Z NPs would not be clinically significant, partly due to the limited concentration of high-Z NPs in tumor (Rousseau *et al* 2010).

doi:10.1088/978-0-7503-2396-3ch15

For intravenous (IV) administration route, studies show that only up to 5% of NPs reach the lung (Taratula *et al* 2011). Significant efforts have been made to increase the concentrations of nanoparticles inside the tumor, and thus reduce the amount received by healthy tissue. But delivery of sufficiently high concentrations of NPs to the tumor remains a challenge (Ngwa *et al* 2014).

Taratula *et al* recently developed a special drug delivery system (DDS) to achieve higher concentrations of NPs in lung tumors via inhalation. Their animal experimental results showed that the inhalation route (IR) delivery could provide 3.5–14.6 times higher NP concentrations compared to IV (Taratula *et al* 2011, 2013). Their NP delivery system showed excellent normal tissue sparing compared to IV injection. Many studies studied aerosol delivery of chemotherapy agents in animal models, and Phase I/II human studies (Zarogoulidis *et al* 2012). These studies included chemotherapy particles like cisplatin, which have a high-*Z* platinum component.

In this study, it is hypothesized that sufficiently potent concentrations of platinum-based chemotherapy drugs can be delivered to the tumor by NP inhalation/instillation. The administration of FDA approved platinum-based chemotherapy drugs, cisplatin and carboplatin, will allow significant dose enhancement via photoelectric mechanism during external beam radiotherapy (EBRT). GNPs were used for comparison.

15.2 Materials and methods

An analytic method (Ngwa *et al* 2010, Berbeco *et al* 2011, Sinha *et al* 2015, Altundal *et al* 2015) was used to estimate the dose enhancement to lung tumors due to radiation-induced photoelectrons from the localized NPs. Monte Carlo-generated megavoltage energy spectra (Liu and Verhaegen 2002, Parsons *et al* 2014) was employed to compare the dose enhancement from NPs administrated via IR versus via IV.

A tumor voxel is modeled with dimensions 10 μm cube (figure 15.1). NPs are assumed to be distributed uniformly over the tumor voxel. FDA-approved concentrations of 100 mg m^{-2} cisplatin (Boulikas 2009) and 300 mg carboplatin (FDA n.d.) were used to determine the maximum concentrations of NPs. Here, the unit mg m^{-2} represents mg of human body per human body surface area, which corresponds to 1.79 m^2 for the average human body. In this way, the maximum FDA approved concentrations of cisplatin and carboplatin are calculated as 43 mg g^{-1} and 72 mg g^{-1}, respectively. Here, mg in the unit refers to the mass of drug while g is the mass of tumor. The high-*Z* component, platinum contained in cisplatin and carboplatin, is the major contributor to the dose enhancement. Based on the mass fraction of platinum, platinum concentration can be further determined for the dose enhancement factor (DEF) calculation. 5% of either cisplatin nanoparticles (CNPs), carboplatin nanoparticles (CBNPs), or GNPs are assumed to reach the tumor via IV administration. While, IR administration can lead to 3.5–14.6 times higher concentrations than IV (Taratula *et al* 2011, 2013). 3.5 and 14.6 are used as lower side (IR1) and higher side (IR2) scenarios.

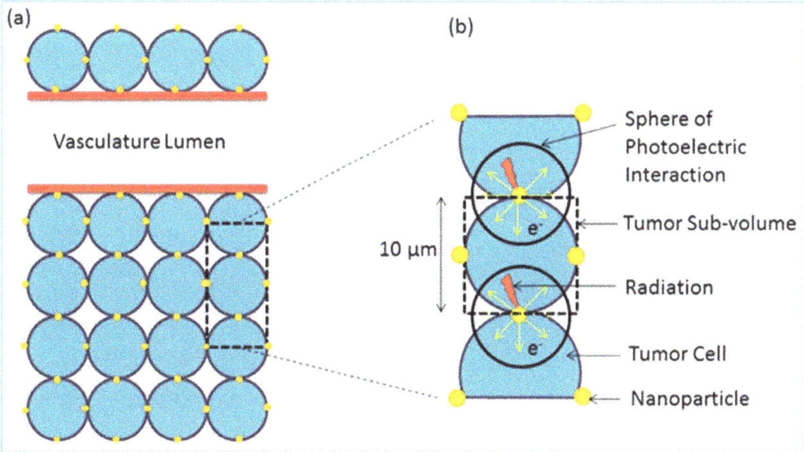

Figure 15.1. Illustration of the sphere of photoelectric energy deposition within the tumor sub-volume.

During radiation, photons interact with the atomic orbital electrons of high-Z atoms to produce photoelectrons as well as Auger electrons with a defined yield. The energy of the photoelectron is the difference between the energy of the incident photons and the electron's binding energy. Detailed explanation of the analytical calculations for the dose enhancement factor (DEF) in the tumor voxel is provided by Ngwa and others (Ngwa *et al* 2010, Berbeco *et al* 2011, Altundal *et al* 2015).

In this work, the DEF is defined as,

$$\mathrm{DEF} = \frac{\text{Dose with nanoparticles}}{\text{Dose without nanoparticles}}, \tag{15.1}$$

The absorbed dose is found by dividing the total energy deposited to a volume by its mass. For a tumor sub-volume with NPs, the total deposited energy via the photoelectric effect was calculated by taking the sum of all the deposited energies by photoelectrons to the tumor voxel. For each NP, the number of emitted photoelectrons is the product of the number of incident photons and the probability of photoelectric interaction. Most photoelectrons have very short range and will deposit their kinetic energy nearly locally. In this work, the photoelectrons' distribution is assumed isotropic and their energy is deposited in the spherical volume surrounding the NPs within a radius equivalent to the range of these photoelectrons (R_{tot}) (figure 15.1). Cole *et al* derived a relation between the deposited kinetic energy (E) and the photoelectron's residual range (R) (Cole 1969),

$$\frac{dE}{dR} = 3.316(R + 0.007)^{-0.435} - 0.0055R^{0.33}, \tag{15.2}$$

E and R have the units of keV and µm, respectively. For each photoelectron, the total deposited energy inside of the tumor sub-volume can be calculated by integrating equation (15.2), from the surface (R_n) of the NP to the distal side of the tumor voxel ($R_n + D_E$).

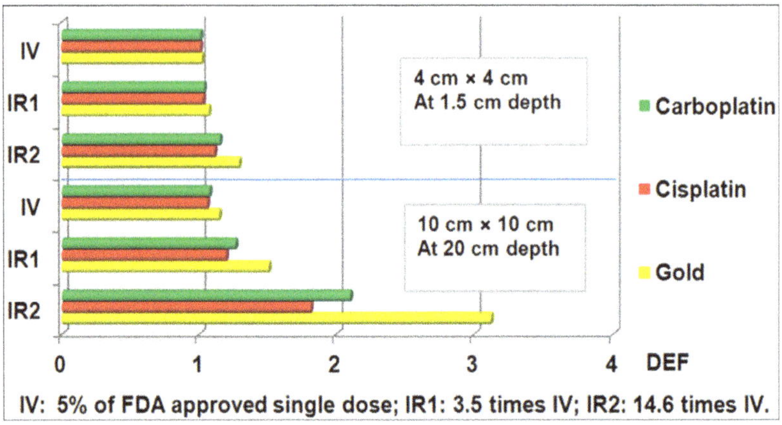

Figure 15.2. DEFs for gold, cisplatin and carboplatin-based NPs (GNPs, CNPs, CBNPs, respectively) irradiated at different phantom depths and field sizes using 6 MV x-rays. Copyright 2015 IOP Publishing Ltd. Reproduced with permission from Hao *et al* (2015). All rights reserved.

$$E_{\text{voxel}} = 2\int_{R_n}^{R_n+D_E} \frac{A_{\text{hemisphere}}}{A_{\text{entire sphere}}}\frac{dE}{dr}dr, \tag{15.3}$$

$A_{\text{hemisphere}}$ is the hemisphere surface area, and $A_{\text{entire sphere}}$ is the surface area of the whole sphere, and r (= $R_{\text{tot}} - R$) is photoelectron traveling distance. The factor of 2 is used to account for the contribution of the NP on the other side of the tumor sub-volume.

The effects of two different spectral photon beams were investigated in this work. One is a 6 MV linac beam whose spectra was generated using the EGS4 Monte Carlo code transported to a depth at 1.5 cm (4 cm × 4 cm field size) and depth at 20 cm (10 cm × 10 cm field size) (Liu and Verhaegen 2002). The second spectrum was a 2.35 MV 2100EX Clinac beam, whose energy distribution was obtained via Monte Carlo simulation using the BEAMnrc computer code (Parsons *et al* 2014). DEF was calculated for a nanoparticle diameter of 2 nm in a range of concentrations for both IR and IV administration. Tumor size was chosen as 2 cm diameter as default dimension. Dose enhancement for a serial of tumor sizes was investigated.

15.3 Results

DEFs for single therapy cycle of GNPs, CNPs and CBNPs when irradiated using 6 MV x-rays are shown in figure 15.2. Since gold is less toxic compared to NPs made of other materials, DEFs of GNPs were calculated at the same concentrations as those of CBNPs. IV concentrations of each type of NPs are calculated based on 5% of FDA concentration. IR1 is 3.5 times of IV, and IR2 is 14.6 times of IV. In this way, the single cycle tumor concentrations of GNPs, CNPs and CBNPs are 3.6 mg g^{-1}, 2.2 mg g^{-1}, and 3.6 mg g^{-1}, respectively, for IV administration. These factors are applied for IR1 and IR2 administration for all the NPs. The results suggest that substantial dose enhancement can be achieved for NPs administrated via inhalation, especially with higher translocation efficiency (IR2).

DEF as a function of CNPs concentration for 6 MV beam is shown in figure 15.3. The maximum concentration of CNPs is the FDA-approved cumulative concentration. Red solid line and blue dashed line represent calculations for 1.5 cm and 20 cm depths, respectively. DEF at any depth between those two is expected to fall into the shaded region.

This work also looked at the tumor size dependence of DEF (figure 15.4). Increasing the tumor size while keeping the NP load constant reduces the DEF due to the decreasing NP concentration in the tumor. The NP load is expressed as concentrations, which were calculated in a default tumor size (2 cm in diameter) using FDA-allowed maximum concentrations. Each NP is applied in two concentrations representing FDA-allowed single concentration administrated via inhalation at different efficiencies (IR1 and IR2). For instance, 7.5 mg g^{-1} is at lower efficiency IR1, while 31.4 mg g^{-1} is at higher efficiency IR2.

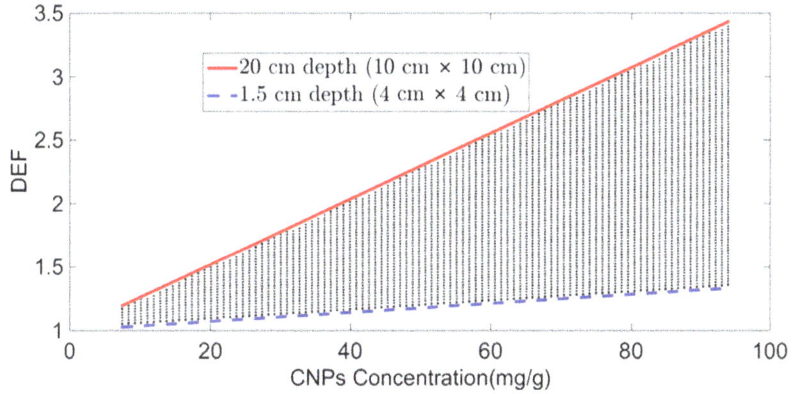

Figure 15.3. The expected range of DEFs for CNPs exposed to 6 MV x-rays between 1.5 cm depth with 4 × 4 cm^2 field size and 20 cm depth with 10 × 10 cm^2 field size. Copyright 2015 IOP Publishing Ltd. Reproduced with permission from Hao *et al* (2015). All rights reserved.

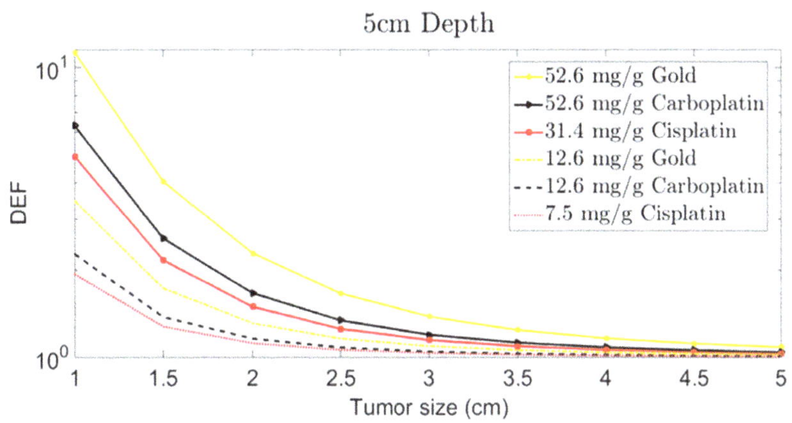

Figure 15.4. Variation of DEF with tumor size at 5 cm depth. The indicated NP load is expressed as concentrations in a default tumor size (2 cm in diameter) using FDA-allowed maximum values. Copyright 2015 IOP Publishing Ltd. Reproduced with permission from Hao *et al* (2015). All rights reserved.

15.4 Discussion

Since the work by Hainfeld and others (Hainfeld *et al* 2004), there has been considerable interest in the use of high-Z NPs to boost the dose to tumors. However, many studies have stated that radiation dose enhancement from gold or other high-Z NPs would not be clinically significant for clinical megavoltage radiotherapy beams (Rousseau *et al* 2010). One of the main reasons is the limited concentrations of NPs accumulating in tumor for intravenous NP administration. Recently, Berbeco *et al* (2011) demonstrated that radiation dose to the tumor vasculature can be boosted by administrating GNPs intravenously. Instead of targeting the whole tumor, their innovative approach proposed to focus on the tumor vasculature. In this way, even a small number of IV-administrated NPs may lead to sufficient concentration in the tumor vasculature to result in a significant dose enhancement.

This work investigated the dose enhancement potential of high-Z NPs administrated by IR. The results suggest that IR can be a very promising route to deliver sufficient concentrations of the NPs locally for dose boosting of tumors/tumor vasculature. Platinum-based chemotherapy NPs, like cisplatin NPs or carboplatin particles, delivered via IR could also boost the tumor dose significantly via the photoelectric effect. Considering that CCRT is a common treatment for lung cancer, this highly localized dose boosting approach can potentially reduce the overlap toxicity from chemotherapy and radiotherapy.

Compared to IV, IR can be optimal because of the large lung surface area, thin alveolar epithelium, rapid absorption, lack of first-pass metabolism, and high capacity to absorb large quantities of drug. Once the NPs are inhaled by the patient, they may deposit in any part of the respiratory tract. For tumors located inside the respiratory tract, IR can be efficient to delivery sufficient concentration locally. Kumar *et al* showed that PEGylated NPs, with sufficient mass, suitable size and other relative characteristics, can help with the NPs' translocation efficiency (Kumar *et al* 2013). Due to high NP concentration in the lung region, those particles can also reach a deeper seated tumor via diffusion.

Lung cancer cells can invade nearby healthy tissues and are more likely to spread to nearby lymph nodes before metastasizing to other regions of the body. Studies have shown that noncationic NPs, with sizes between 6 nm and 34 nm, are able to travel rapidly from the lung to mediastinal lymph nodes (Choi *et al* 2010). The third generation GNP platforms developed by Kumar *et al* can provide higher efficiency of NP administration to lymph nodes and boost radiotherapy treatment of lung tumor metastases (Kumar *et al* 2013).

Comparing to IV administration, this work demonstrates that IR administrated gold and platinum-based NPs can provide a significant dose enhancement. In the calculation, it was assumed that NPs distribute homogeneously inside the tumor. In reality, NPs will likely have a non-uniform distribution via inhalation administration. That being said, some parts of the tumor may have higher DEF than others. Since IR can provide much higher concentration locally, the NPs' nonisotropic distribution may not be that important. Also theoretical and experimental *in vitro* studies have shown that sufficient concentrations could still lead to major dose enhancement during external beam RT (Berbeco *et al* 2011, 2012).

In addition to the concentration of high-*Z* NPs, the beam quality also plays an important role in dose enhancement. Tsiamas *et al* investigated the dose enhancement effect of flattening filter free (FFF) beams (Tsiamas *et al* 2013, Berbeco *et al* 2012). Owing to the rapid drop in the photoelectric cross-section with increasing photon energy, low-energy photons contribute more to the dose enhancement than higher energy photons. 6 MV FFF beam has more low-energy photons compared to a 6 MV standard beam, and is commonly used for stereotactic body radiation therapy (SBRT) in treating lung cancer. While normal tissue toxicity for medically inoperable early-stage non-small cell lung cancer patients with central lesions is significant when using SBRT (Timmerman *et al* 2006, Song *et al* 2009), the IR delivery approach can be used to boost tumor dose with minimal normal tissue toxicity, which can be especially beneficial for those patients.

In addition, such high-*Z* NPs can be expanded to smart radiation therapy material combining RT with immunotherapy or chemotherapy (Ngwa *et al* 2017, Hao *et al* 2016). The clinical benefits of such an expansion includes major improvement in cancer treatment, substantially reduced systemic toxicity, systemic tumor rejection, as well as shorter treatment time.

15.5 Conclusion

Results from this study suggest that IR-administrated GNPs, CNPs and CBNPs can be used to provide a substantial dose enhancement to lung tumors during EBRT. The proposed approach would benefit patients who undergo concomitant chemoradiotherapy. An optimal inhalation delivery approach for NP-aided radiotherapy needs to be developed for lung cancer treatment.

Acknowledgments

This study was supported by National Institutes of Health National Cancer Institute grant 1 K01 CA172478–01.

References

American Cancer Society 2019 *Cancer Facts & Figures* Atlanta: American Cancer Society; 2019. Online: https://cancer.org/content/dam/cancer-org/research/cancer-facts-and-statistics/annual-cancer-facts-and-figures/2019/cancer-facts-and-figures-2019.pdf

Altundal Y, Cifter G, Detappe A, Sajo E, Tsiamas P, Zygmanski P, Berbeco R, Cormack R A, Makrigiorgos M and Ngwa W 2015 New potential for enhancing concomitant chemoradiotherapy with FDA approved concentrations of cisplatin via the photoelectric effect *Phys. Medica* **31** 25–30

Berbeco R I, Korideck H, Ngwa W, Kumar R, Patel J, Sridhar S, Johnson S, Price B D, Kimmelman A and Makrigiorgos G M 2012 DNA damage enhancement from gold nanoparticles for clinical MV photon beams *Radiat. Res.* **178** 604–8

Berbeco R I, Ngwa W and Makrigiorgos G M 2011 Localized dose enhancement to tumor blood vessel endothelial cells via megavoltage X-rays and targeted gold nanoparticles: new potential for external beam radiotherapy *Int. J. Radiat. Oncol. Biol. Phys.* **81** 270–6

Boulikas T 2009 Clinical overview on Lipoplatin: a successful liposomal formulation of cisplatin *Expert Opin. Invest. Drugs* **18** 1197–218

Choi H S, Ashitate Y, Lee J H, Kim S H, Matsui A, Insin N, Bawendi M G, Semmler-Behnke M, Frangioni J V and Tsuda A 2010 Rapid translocation of nanoparticles from the lung airspaces to the body *Nat. Biotechnol.* **28** 1300–3

Cole A 1969 Absorption of 20-eV to 50,000-eV electron beams in air and plastic *Radiat. Res.* **38** 7–33

FDA About the Center for Drug Evaluation and Research—Carboplatin Dosing Online http://fda.gov/AboutFDA/CentersOffices/OfficeofMedicalProductsandTobacco/CDER/ucm228974.htm

Furuse K, Fukuoka M, Kawahara M, Nishikawa H, Takada Y, Kudoh S, Katagami N and Arivoshi Y 1999 Phase III study of concurrent versus sequential thoracic radiotherapy in combination with mitomycin, vindesine, and cisplatin in unresectable stage III non-small cell lung cancer *J. Clin. Oncol.* **17** 2692–9

Hainfeld J F, Slatkin D N and Smilowitz H M 2004 The use of gold nanoparticles to enhance radiotherapy in mice *Phys. Med. Biol.* **49** N309–15

Hao Y, Altundal Y, Moreau M, Sajo E, Kumar R and Ngwa W 2015 Potential for enhancing external beam radiotherapy for lung cancer using high-Z nanoparticles administered via inhalation *Phys. Med. Biol.* **60** 7035

Hao Y, Yasmin-Karim S, Moreau M, Sinha N, Sajo E and Ngwa W 2016 Enhancing radiotherapy for lung cancer using immunoadjuvants delivered *in situ* from new design radiotherapy biomaterials: a preclinical study *Phys. Med. Biol.* **61** N697–707

Keall P J *et al* 2006 The management of respiratory motion in radiation oncology report of AAPM Task Group 76 *Med. Phys.* **33** 3874–900

Kumar R, Korideck H, Ngwa W, Berbeco R I, Makrigiorgos G M and Sridhar S 2013 Third generation gold nanoplatform optimized for radiation therapy *Transl. Cancer Res.* **2** 228–39

Liu H H and Verhaegen F 2002 An investigation of energy spectrum and lineal energy variations in mega-voltage photon beams used for radiotherapy *Radiat. Prot. Dosimetry* **99** 425–7

Machtay M, Bae K, Movsas B and Paulus R 2012 Higher biologically effective dose of radiotherapy is associated with improved outcomes for locally advanced non-small cell lung carcinoma treated with chemoradiation: an analysis of the Radiation Therapy Oncology Group *Int. J. Radiat. Oncol. Biol. Phys.* **82** 425–34

Machtay M, Bae K, Movsas B, Paulus R, Gore E M, Komaki R, Albain K, Sause W T and Curran W J 2012 Higher biologically effective dose of radiotherapy is associated with improved outcomes for locally advanced non-small cell lung carcinoma treated with chemoradiation: an analysis of the Radiation Therapy Oncology Group *Int. J. Radiat. Oncol. Biol. Phys.* **82** 425–34

Ngwa W *et al* 2017 Smart radiation therapy biomaterials *Int. J. Radiat. Oncol. Phys.* **97** 624–37

Ngwa W, Kumar R, Sridhar S, Korideck H, Zygmanski P, Cormack R A, Berbeco R and Makrigiorgos G M 2014 Targeted radiotherapy with gold nanoparticles: current status and future perspectives *Nanomedicine* **9** 1063–82

Ngwa W, Makrigiorgos G M and Berbeco R I 2010 Applying gold nanoparticles as tumor-vascular disrupting agents during brachytherapy: estimation of endothelial dose enhancement *Phys. Med. Biol.* **55** 6533–48

Parsons D, Robar J L and Sawkey D 2014 A Monte Carlo investigation of low-Z target image quality generated in a linear accelerator using Varian's VirtuaLinac *Med. Phys.* **41** 021719

Rousseau J, Barth R F, Fernandez M, Adam J F, Balosso J, Estève F and Elleaume H 2010 Efficacy of intracerebral delivery of cisplatin in combination with photon irradiation for treatment of brain tumors *J. Neurooncol.* **98** 287–95

Sinha N, Cifter G, Sajo E, Kumar R, Sridhar S, Nguyen P L, Cormack R A, Makrigiorgos G M and Ngwa W 2015 Brachytherapy application with *in situ* dose painting administered by gold nanoparticle eluters *Int. J. Radiat. Oncol.* **91** 385–92

Song S Y, Choi W, Shin S S, Lee S w, Ahn S D, Kim J H, Je H U, Il P C, Lee J S and Choi E K 2009 Fractionated stereotactic body radiation therapy for medically inoperable stage I lung cancer adjacent to central large bronchus *Lung Cancer* **66** 89–93

Taratula O, Garbuzenko O B, Chen A M and Minko T 2011 Innovative strategy for treatment of lung cancer: targeted nanotechnology-based inhalation co-delivery of anticancer drugs and siRNA *J. Drug Target.* **19** 900–14

Taratula O, Kuzmov A, Shah M, Garbuzenko O B and Minko T 2013 Nanostructured lipid carriers as multifunctional nanomedicine platform for pulmonary co-delivery of anticancer drugs and siRNA *J. Control. Release* **171** 349–57

Timmerman R *et al* 2006 Excessive toxicity when treating central tumors in a phase II study of stereotactic body radiation therapy for medically inoperable early-stage lung cancer *J. Clin. Oncol.* **24** 4833–9

Tsiamas P *et al* 2013 Impact of beam quality on megavoltage radiotherapy treatment techniques utilizing gold nanoparticles for dose enhancement *Phys. Med. Biol.* **58** 451–64

Zarogoulidis P, Chatzaki E, Porpodis K, Domvri K, Hohenforst-Schmidt W, Goldberg E P, Karamanos N and Zarogoulidis K 2012 Inhaled chemotherapy in lung cancer: future concept of nanomedicine *Int. J. Nanomed.* **7** 1551–72

IOP Publishing

Nanoparticle Enhanced Radiation Therapy
Principles, methods and applications
Erno Sajo and Piotr Zygmanski

Chapter 16

High-*Z* ORAYA therapy for wet AMD and ocular cancers

Yucel Altundal and Wilfred Ngwa

16.1 Introduction

Age-related macular degeneration (AMD) and intraocular malignancies tend to cause blindness both in adults and children [1–5]. Plaque therapy is a common treatment option for medium-sized eye tumors (2.5–10 mm thick and 16 mm diameter at most) such as choroidal melanoma (CM) [6]. However, the undesirable radiation to the optic nerve and retina may cause loss of vision in months [7, 8]. Chemotherapy is the first option for children with retinoblastoma. Platinum-based chemotherapy agents (e.g. carboplatin), however, have side effects, such as kidney dysfunctions and hearing loss [1, 9]. For AMD, external beam radiotherapy with low-energy x-ray source is an alternative treatment modality. The Oraya IRay radiotherapy system (Oraya Therapeutics Inc., Carl Zeiss Meditec) delivers highly targeted low-energy x-rays, and specifically targets the choroidal neovasculature to treat wet AMD with a potential of preserving the vision by reducing the number of anti-vascular endothelial growth factor (anti-VEGF) injections [10].

The Oraya IRay radiotherapy system includes an external kV source and an eye tracking system. The device delivers up to 24 Gy of dose to radiosensitive choroidal neovasculature to treat wet AMD in a 5 min single session via three external beams [11–13]. These beams enter the eye from different locations on the sclera and precisely target the rapidly proliferating neovascular endothelial cells (EC). One of the new treatment modalities proposed to reduce the toxicities is using high atomic number (high-*Z*) nanoparticles (NPs) with low-energy radiation therapy. High-*Z* NPs such as gold NPs (AuNPs) or carboplatin NPs (CbNPs) enhance the radiation dose to ocular tumor cells and endothelial cells (EC) locally.

doi:10.1088/978-0-7503-2396-3ch16

16.2 Materials and methods

Figure 16.1 shows the diseased EC model (2 μm × 10 μm × 10 μm) and the tumor sub-volume or voxel (10 μm × 10 μm × 10 μm) away from the tumor vasculature, with the targeted NPs attached to the exterior [14]. In this model, the NPs are distributed homogenously outside the tumor sub-volume and on one side of endothelial cells. The interaction of ionizing radiation with the high-Z NPs generates short-ranged photoelectrons and Auger electrons via the photoelectric effect, which is described in detail elsewhere in this book.

Table 16.1 shows the emitted photon energies and relative intensities of typical low-energy plaque brachytherapy sources (Pd-103 and I-125) [15, 16]. Figure 16.2

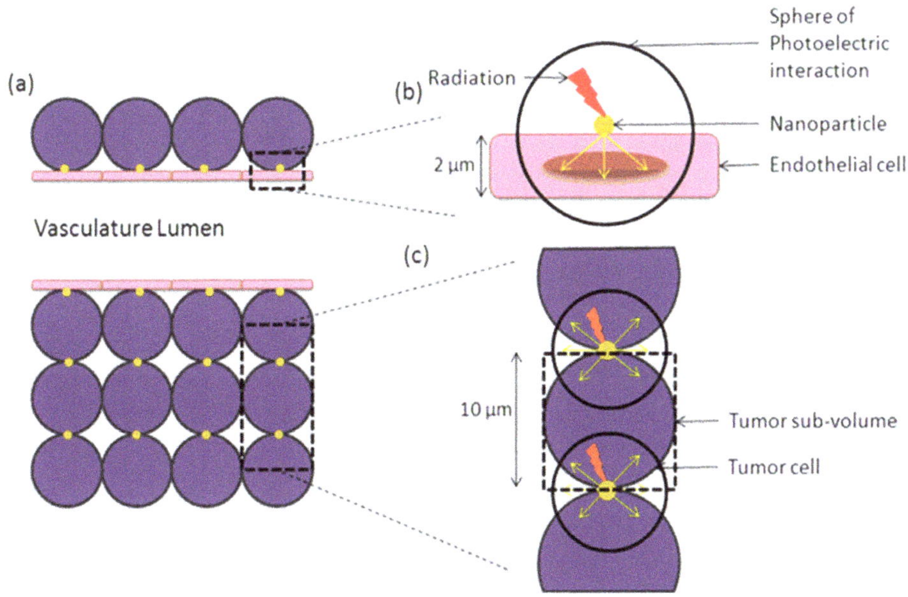

Figure 16.1. (a) NP distribution outside the tumor cell and endothelial cells. (b) Endothelial cell model. (c) High-risk tumor sub-volume model. Reprinted by permission from Springer [21], copyright 2015.

Table 16.1. Brachytherapy source spectra.

Isotope	Energy (keV)	Relative intensity
Pd-103	20.1	0.656
	23.0	0.125
I-125	22.1	0.25
	25.2	0.07
	27.4	1.00
	31.4	0.25
	35.5	0.06

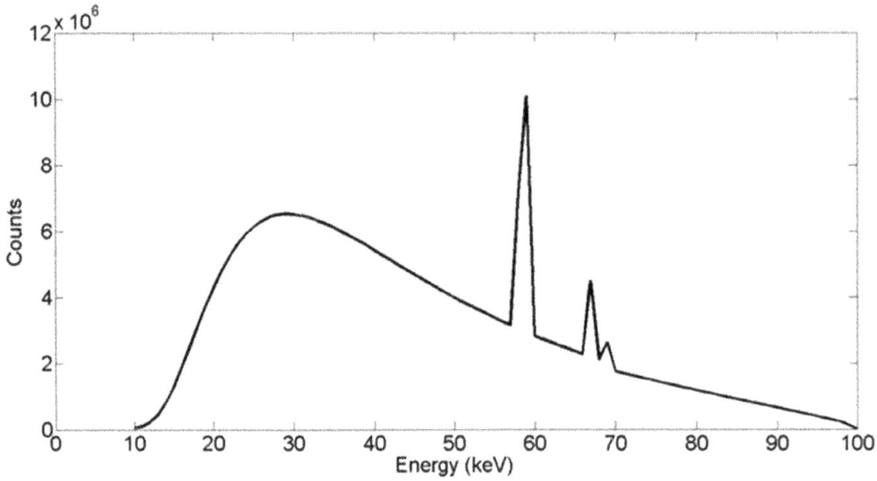

Figure 16.2. 100 kVp x-ray source spectrum (tungsten target, anode angle of 12, 0.75 mm Al and 0.8 mm Be). Generated by the SpekCalc software [17].

shows 100 kVp external photon energy spectrum generated with the SpekCalc software [17]. The Auger electron spectrum may be obtained from the Evaluated Nuclear Data Library, ENDL97 [18], and it is shown in a different chapter of this book.

The photoelectron's kinetic energy is the difference between the incident photon energy and the electron's binding energy in the NPs high-Z component (gold or platinum). The fluence (Φ) of the incident photons may be determined from an arbitrary delivered dose (D_w) to tissue without the presence of NPs, assuming charged particle equilibrium:

$$D_w = \sum_E \Phi E_P \left(\frac{\mu_{en}}{\rho}\right)_E, \tag{16.1}$$

where Φ is photon fluence (photon/cm^2), E_p is energy per photon (J), and $(\mu_{en}/\rho)_E$ is mass energy absorption coefficient of water (cm^2 g^{-1}) at energy E_p. The number of incident photons on the NP (N_{ph}) may be estimated as the product of this fluence by the cross sectional area of the NP (πr_{NP}^2), where r_{NP} is the radius of the NP.

The number of emitted photoelectrons (N_{PE}) is the product of the photoelectric interaction probability (P) by the number of incident source photons (N_0). Equation (16.2) shows the approximate calculation of the interaction probability:

$$P = \frac{N}{N_0} = 1 - \exp\left\{-\left(\frac{\mu_{PE}}{\rho}\right)_E \rho_{NP} d_{NP}\right\} \approx \left(\frac{\mu_{PE}}{\rho}\right) \rho_{NP} d_{NP}, \tag{16.2}$$

where N is the number of photons that interact via the PE in the NP, N_0 is the number of photons incident on the NP, $(\mu_{PE}/\rho)_E$ is the photoelectric mass absorption coefficient of gold and/or platinum at the given energy E, ρ_{NP} is density of the NP material, and $d_{NP} = 4r_{NP}/3$ is the average distance traversed by photons through a spherical NP. The approximation in equation (16.2) is permitted because the exponent is very small.

The number of NPs (N_{NP}) that are attached to the endothelial cell and tumor sub-volume surface is related to the NP concentration:

$$N_{NP} = \frac{m_{H_2O} \times [NP \text{ concentration (mg g}^{-1})]}{m_{NP}} = \frac{V_{EC \text{ or voxel}}\rho_{H_2O} \times [NP \text{ concentration (mg g}^{-1})]}{\frac{4}{3}\pi r_{NP}^3 \rho_{NP}}, \tag{16.3}$$

where m_{H_2O} is the mass of water, V_{EC} (2×10^{-10}cm^3) is the volume of an endothelial cell, V_{voxel}(10×10^{-10}cm^3) is the volume of a voxel inside a tumor cell, and $\rho_{\text{H}_2\text{O}}$ is the density of water, while ρ_{NP} is the density of NP. Multiplying the number of NPs (N_{NP}) by the number of emitted photoelectrons per NP (N_{PE}) gives the total number of emitted photoelectrons in the EC ($N_{PE\ \text{total}} = N_{NP} \times N_{PE}$).

Photoelectrons and Auger electrons deposit their energy locally around the NPs in a hypothetical sphere, which is the sphere of photo/Auger electron interactions (figure 16.1). The rate of kinetic energy loss, a.k.a. the linear energy transfer, $\frac{dE}{dr}$ (keV μm^{-1}), of 20 eV–20 MeV electrons and their residual range R (μm) was derived experimentally by Cole for unit density materials [19]:

$$\frac{dE}{dR} = 3.316(R + 0.007)^{-0.435} - 0.0055R^{0.33}. \tag{16.4}$$

To calculate the deposited energy of a single electron in the EC, equation (16.4) must be integrated from the NP surface (R_n) to the distal side of the EC ($R_n + D_E$) [20]:

$$E_{EC} = \int_{R_n}^{R_n+D_E} \frac{\text{Shell}_{\text{hemisphere}} - \text{Shell}_{\text{spherical cap beyond the EC}}}{\text{Shell}_{\text{entire sphere}}} \frac{dE}{dr} dr, \tag{16.5}$$

where $\text{Shell}_{\text{hemisphere}}$ represents the surface area of a hemisphere, $\text{Shell}_{\text{spherical cap beyond } EC}$ represents the area of the spherical cap beyond the EC, and $\text{Shell}_{\text{entire sphere}}$ represents the surface area of the whole sphere. The total energy deposited to one EC is the sum of all E_{EC} from each photo- and Auger electrons. The total absorbed dose is the ratio of the total energy deposited to EC by the mass of the EC.

The integral to calculate dose enhancement in the voxel or tumor sub-volume is multiplied by a factor of 2 to include the electron contribution from the other side of the voxel. The modified integral is expressed as:

$$E_{\text{voxel}} = 2\int_{R_n}^{R_n+D_E} \frac{\text{Shell}_{\text{hemisphere}}}{\text{Shell}_{\text{entire sphere}}} \frac{dE}{dr} dr, \tag{16.6}$$

where E_{voxel} is the kinetic energy deposited in the voxel. The total absorbed dose is the ratio of the total energy deposited to tumor sub-volume by the mass of the voxel. The calculations are independent of the NPs locations since the NPs distribution is assumed to be uniform. The dose enhancement factor (DEF) is defined as:

$$DEF = \frac{\text{Dose delivered with nanoparticles}}{\text{Dose delivered without nanoparticles}}, \tag{16.7}$$

where the dose delivered without NPs is the previously defined arbitrary dose (D_w) to tissue without the presence of NPs. The dose delivered with NPs is the total delivered dose by photons, photoelectrons and Auger electrons to EC or the voxel. The above calculations are the same for both photoelectrons and Auger electrons, however the total energy delivered by Auger electron is normalized by its yield.

16.3 Results

Figure 16.3(a) shows the endothelial DEF (EDEF) versus 2 nm gold (AuNPs) and carboplatin (CbNPs) NP concentration for external beam sources (90 kVp and 100 kVp) and brachytherapy sources (Pd-103 and I-125) [21]. The data is plotted up to 31 mg g^{-1} NP concentration since this concentration has shown minimal systemic toxicity of a retinoblastoma mice study with carboplatin NPs [22].

By definition, the dose enhancement is equal to 1 for zero NP concentration, and increases linearly with concentration based on the analytical calculations. This increase is higher for AuNPs compared to carboplatin NPs since only 52% of carboplatin contain platinum. Also platinum has a lower photoelectric interaction cross-section compared to gold. The dose enhancement in the endothelial cells is lower than that in the microscopic tumor sub-volumes or voxels (vDEF) because the homogenous NPs distribution is assumed only on one side of the ECs (figure 16.3(b)). Brachytherapy sources I-125 and Pd-103 with AuNPs provide the highest dose enhancement for vDEF and EDEF. The reason is that the emitted electrons due to photoelectric interactions of I-125 have higher energies compared to Pd-103 and they deposit a substantial amount of their energy beyond the endothelial cells. For external beams, both EDEF and vDEF values are slightly higher for 90 kVp than 100 kVp beams since the photoelectric interaction cross sections is higher at lower energies.

Figure 16.4 shows the vDEF as a function of tumor size for 31 mg g^{-1} NP concentration [21]. As expected, increasing the tumor volume decreases the dose enhancement because for a fixed concentration the number of NPs per cell decreases. Tumor sizes of up to 0.553 c.c. and 0.674 c.c. irradiated with 100 kVp and I-125, respectively, the vDEF is greater than 1.20 when CbNPs are used. In the case of AuNPs, the same enhancement is obtained for tumor sizes of up to 1.124 c.c. and 1.364 c.c. when irradiated with 100 kVp and I-125, respectively.

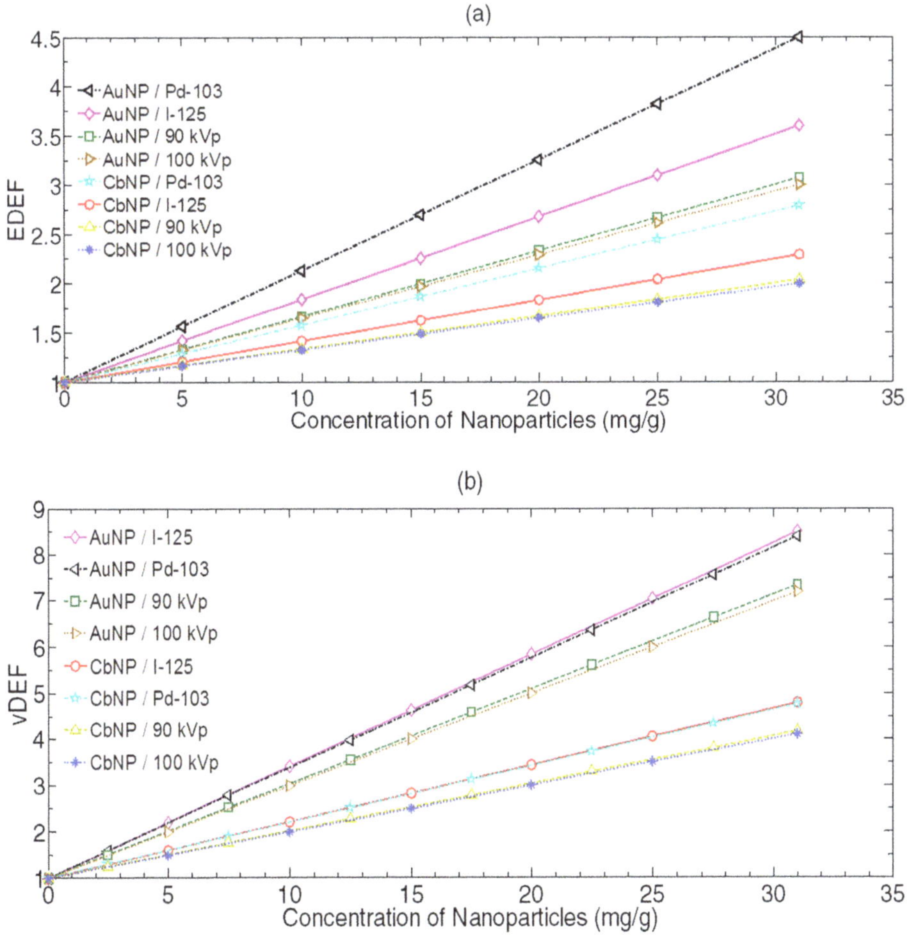

Figure 16.3. (a) EDEF versus NP concentration using gold and carboplatin NPs in combination with various photon sources. (b) Dose enhancement in tumor voxels (vDEF) versus NP concentration using gold and carboplatin NPs in combination with various photon sources. Reprinted by permission from Springer [21], copyright 2015.

16.4 Discussion

The most popular method to bring drugs to the posterior segment of the eye is via intravitreal delivery where the drug is injected into the vitreous humor [23]. The advantage of this direct administration is that the drug can reach the proximity of the retina. However, intravitreal delivery is inadequate to carry the drug to the choroid due to tissue barriers [24]. Another method is the periocular route injection to the exterior surface of the sclera, which is considered less invasive and more feasible to deliver the drug into the choroid [25]. Functionalized NPs targeting molecular epitopes on the tumor cells could be beneficial for both delivery methods by attaching the NPs to the diseased cells. Active targeting to specific tumor cells could be achieved with NPs for both delivery methods. That active targeting would allow NPs to be attached to diseased cells and cleared out from normal cells [26].

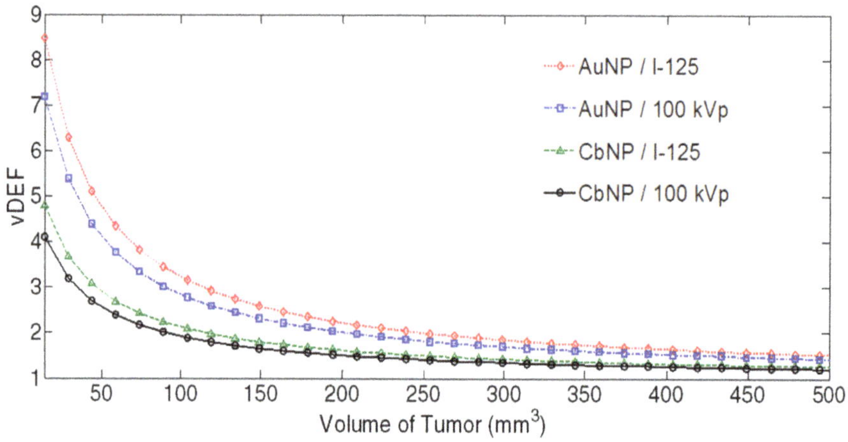

Figure 16.4. vDEF as a function of different tumor volumes for 31 mg g^{-1} gold and carboplatin NPs concentration. Reprinted by permission from Springer [21], copyright 2015.

NPs 2 nm in size have advantages by allowing clearing out from untargeted normal tissues and providing more dose enhancement to the target. Auger electrons can better escape from small NPs compared to large size NPs and result in more dose enhancement [27]. To damage more the DNA of diseased cells, NPs should be as close as possible to the nucleus of the cell [28]. Therefore, nuclear targeting of NPs would increase the effectiveness of NP aided radiotherapy.

100 kVp Oraya therapy yields slightly lower dose enhancement to tumor sub-volumes and to endothelial cells compared to brachytherapy (BT) sources, since BT sources have higher fractions of photon energies close to the L-edge of gold and platinum. However, the external sources have an advantage of being non-invasive. The device could be adapted as an alternative to eye plaques to treat ocular cancers in conjunction with the NPs. NP-aided radiotherapy can improve radiotherapy treatment for ocular cancers by increasing the radiation dose within the tumors and neovascular endothelial cells in micrometer ranges and sparing the surrounding normal tissues, such as the optical nerve.

References

[1] Abramson D H 2014 Retinoblastoma: saving life with vision *Annu. Rev. Med.* **65** 171–84

[2] Damato B 2004 Developments in the management of uveal melanoma *Clin. Exp. Ophthalmol.* **32** 639–47

[3] Stannard C, Sauerwein W, Maree G and Lecuona K 2013 Radiotherapy for ocular tumours *Eye* **27** 119–27

[4] Urban S Personal (Web)

[5] Takeda A *et al* 2009 CCR3 is a target for age-related macular degeneration diagnosis and therapy *Nature* **465** 225–30

[6] Rice J C, Stannard C, Cook C, Lecuona K, Myer L and Scholtz R P 2014 Brachytherapy and endoresection for choroidal melanoma: a cohort study *Br. J. Ophthalmol.* **98** 86–91

[7] Garretson B R, Robertson D M and Earle J D 1987 Choroidal melanoma treatment with iodine 125 brachytherapy *Arch. Ophthalmol.* **105** 1394–7
[8] Hawkins B S 2001 The COMS randomized trial of iodine 125 brachytherapy for choroidal melanoma, III: Initial mortality findings: COMS report no. 18 *Arch. Ophthalmol.* **124** 1684–93
[9] Tscherning C *et al* 1994 Recurrent renal salt wasting in a child treated with carboplatin and etoposide *Cancer* **73** 1761–3
[10] Ngwa W, Makrigiorgos G M and Berbeco R I 2012 Gold nanoparticle enhancement of stereotactic radiosurgery for neovascular age-related macular degeneration *Phys. Med. Biol.* **57** 6371–80
[11] Hanlon J *et al* 2009 Kilovoltage stereotactic radiosurgery for age-related macular degeneration: assessment of optic nerve dose and patient effective dose *Med. Phys.* **36** 3671–81
[12] Hanlon J, Firpo M, Chell E, Moshfeghi D M and Bolch W E 2011 Stereotactic radiosurgery for AMD: A monte carlo-based assessment of patient-specific tissue doses *Invest. Ophthalmol. Vis. Sci.* **52** 2334–42
[13] Cantley J L, Hanlon J, Chell E, Lee C, Smith W C and Bolch W E 2013 Influence of eye size and beam entry angle on dose to non-targeted tissues of the eye during stereotactic x-ray radiosurgery of AMD *Phys. Med. Biol.* **58** 6887–96
[14] Altundal Y *et al* 2015 New potential for enhancing concomitant chemoradiotherapy with FDA approved concentrations of cisplatin via the photoelectric effect *Phys. Medica* **31** 25–30
[15] Cho S H, Jones B L and Krishnan S 2009 The dosimetric feasibility of gold nanoparticle-aided radiation therapy (GNRT) via brachytherapy using low-energy gamma-/x-ray sources *Phys. Med. Biol.* **54** 4889–905
[16] Roeske J C, Nuñez L, Hoggarth M, Labay E and Weichselbaum R R 2007 Characterization of the theorectical radiation dose enhancement from nanoparticles *Technol. Cancer Res. Treat.* **6** 394–401
[17] Poludniowski G, Landry G, Deblois F, Evans P M and Verhaegen F 2009 SpekCalc: a program to calculate photon spectra from tungsten anode x-ray tubes *Phys. Med. Biol.* **54** N433
[18] Perkins S T and Cullen D E 1994 ENDL type formats for the LLNL Evaluated Atomic Data Library, EADL, for the Evaluated Electron Data Library, EEDL, and for the Evaluated Photon Data Library, EPDL *Technical Report*
[19] Cole A 1969 Absorption of 20-eV to 50,000-eV electron beams in air and plastic *Radiat. Res.* **38** 7–33
[20] Ngwa W, Makrigiorgos G M and Berbeco R I 2010 Applying gold nanoparticles as tumor-vascular disrupting agents during brachytherapy: estimation of endothelial dose enhancement *Phys. Med. Biol.* **55** 6533–48
[21] Altundal Y, Sajo E, Makrigiorgos G M, Berbeco R I and Ngwa W 2015 Nanoparticle-aided radiotherapy for retinoblastoma and choroidal melanoma *World Congress on Medical Physics and Biomedical Engineering, June 7-12, 2015, Toronto, Canada (Cham: Springer) pp 907–10*
[22] Kang S J, Durairaj C, Kompella U B, O'Brien J M and Grossniklaus H E 2009 Subconjunctival nanoparticle carboplatin in the treatment of murine retinoblastoma *Arch. Ophthalmol.* **127** 1043–7
[23] Thrimawithana T R, Young S, Bunt C R, Green C R and Alany R G 2011 Drug delivery to the posterior segment of the eye: challenges and opportunities *Drug Deliv. Lett.* **1** 40–4

[24] Diebold Y and Calonge M 2010 Applications of nanoparticles in ophthalmology *Prog. Retinal Eye Res.* **29** 596–609
[25] Bourges J L *et al* 2003 Ocular drug delivery targeting the retina and retinal pigment epithelium using polylactide nanoparticles *Invest. Ophthalmol. Vis. Sci.* **44** 3562–9
[26] Avgoustakis K, Beletsi A, Panagi Z, Klepetsanis P, Karydas A G and Ithakissios D S 2002 PLGA-mPEG nanoparticles of cisplatin: *in vitro* nanoparticle degradation, *in vitro* drug release and *in vivo* drug residence in blood properties *J. Control. Release* **79** 123–35
[27] Pignol J P and Lechtman E 2012 Reply to Comment on 'Implications on clinical scenario of gold nanoparticle radiosensitization in regards to photon energy, nanoparticle size, concentration and location' *Phys. Med. Biol.* **57** 291
[28] Zygmanski P *et al* 2013 A stochastic model of cell survival for high-Z nanoparticle radiotherapy *Med. Phys.* **40** 024102

Chapter 17

Cerium oxide and titanium dioxide

Zi Ouyang and Wilfred Ngwa

17.1 Introduction

Ionizing radiation causes cellular damage by direct and indirect effects. Along the energy deposition track, radiation causes ionization and excitation of molecules, including DNA, protein, lipid, and other essential components of a cell [1]. The direct effect mostly requires the electrons to deliver energy large enough directly to the DNA and lead to single strand break (SSB) and/or double strand break (DSB). While the DNA repair mechanism is not fully understood, it is widely accepted that DSBs are proportional to cell deaths, including apoptosis and mitotic catastrophe [2]. Radiation also interacts with other molecules, like water, and produces reactive oxygen species (ROS). The products, such as hydroxyl, superoxide, hydroperoxide, are highly reactive and oxidizing, and may further interact with DNA and other key targets and lead to cell deaths indirectly. Linear energy transfer (LET) is defined as the energy deposition to the medium per unit length of the charged particle track. For low LET radiation, cell damage is primarily contributed by indirect action [1].

Unfortunately, radiotherapy not only kills cancer cells, it also inflicts damage to surrounding normal tissue and causes side effects. How to maximize the damage to cancer cells while protecting normal tissue has been the key to improvement of radiotherapy in recent decades and remains as an important question today. The practice of radiotherapy has shifted from three-dimensional conformal radiotherapy (3DCRT) to intensity modulated radiotherapy (IMRT) and volumetric modulated arc therapy (VMAT) [3]. The improved radiation dose distribution—better conformality and homogeneity, and sharper dose fall-off outside the target—allows higher dose to be delivered to the tumor and spares the surrounding normal tissue. A newer technique, stereotactic body radiotherapy (SBRT), relies on the machine precision and image guidance and improves the dose distribution even more [4]. Other techniques, such as brachytherapy, intra-operative radiotherapy, non-coplanar external beam radiotherapy, fall in the same category—improving dose distribution. Furthermore, different doses and fractionations have been explored

doi:10.1088/978-0-7503-2396-3ch17

based on the four Rs of radiobiology: repair, redistribution, repopulation, and reoxygenation [2]. Results from clinical trials have helped establish site-specific radiation treatments that allow better tumor control and normal tissue tolerance [5–7].

In order to kill cancer cells selectively, other methods have been investigated by researchers [8–12], including radiation enhancement, normal tissue protection, targeted radiation delivery, etc. One way to achieve the desired effects of radiation enhancement or protection is by manipulating the cellular micro-environment. By changing how ROS are generated and the follow-up events, one can change the outcome of radiation therapy. Nanoparticle (NP) aided radiotherapy is of interest to cancer researchers with promising applications ranging from targeted dose enhancement to selective radioprotection. In this chapter, the mechanisms, applications, and current research status of ROS modulation of cerium oxide NPs (CONPs) and titanium dioxide NPs (TONPs) are discussed.

17.2 CONP mediated ROS scavenging

CONPs are confirmed to be a viable candidate for radiation protection of normal cells in preclinical studies [10, 11, 13]. It is shown that CONPs remove superoxide and hydroxyl radicals via its intrinsic biomimetic catalytic properties [14, 15], which are due to the rapid, reversible transformation of the oxidation state between Ce^{3+} and Ce^{4+}. Cerium oxide, in NP forms, has significantly lower oxygen vacancy formation energy, compared to its bulk counterpart. ROS modulation is achieved by oxygen exchange between adsorbed species and the CONP surface.

The ROS scavenging of CONPs is studied to various extents. Coumarin-3-carboxylic acid (3-CCA) is a chemical dosimeter, which reacts with hydroxyl radicals and produces hydroxylated 3-CCA. The dosimetry is measured by the fluorescence of hydroxylated 3-CCA with an excitation wavelength 350 nm or 395 nm and an emission wavelength 450 nm. By irradiating suspensions containing a pH buffer, 3-CCA, and CONPs, a concentration dependent scavenging activity was observed. Up to 20% of radiation generated hydroxyl radicals were scavenged by the CONPs at a concentration of 0.1 mg ml^{-1} in a HEPES buffer with pH 7.4. The 5 nm sized CONPs were also shown to have higher scavenging capacity compared to the 25 nm CONPs [16].

CONPs were studied as an injectable, radio-protectant material *in vivo* in protecting germ cells. As reported by Das *et al*, 100 nM and 100 μM CONP delivered via weekly tail vein injection protected male mice from irradiation to the scrotal region [17]. Tissues from mice treated with CONPs showed about 13% decreased damage over controls at up to 5 Gy radiation. *In vivo* studies also showed that CONPs protected against radiation induced pneumonitis [18].

The applications of CONPs in cancer treatment is especially interesting due to its potential in selective protection. Nourmohammadi *et al* published an *in vitro* study of anticancer effects of CONPs on mouse fibrosarcoma cell line [19]. Selective damage to cancer cells was observed in viability assays, while normal cells tolerated CONPs at above 250 μg ml^{-1}. CONPs also significantly increased the Bax expression in cancer cells. An *in vitro* model of human prostate cancer cells (PC-3) also showed that CONPs did not protect PC-3 cells against radiation [16]. The selectivity of CONPs are possibly due to the different pH values of normal and cancer micro-environment; previous work has demonstrated that CONP protection decreases in an acidic environment [11]. The intracellular localization plays an important role in the cytotoxicity of CONPs; for example, experiments showed that negatively charged CONPs exhibited cytotoxicity after entering lung cancer cells (A549) and localizing in the lysosomes [10]. CONPs may be designed for simultaneous protection of normal cells and damage of cancer cells.

17.3 TONP aided radiation sensitization

Cherenkov radiation (CR) is light emission when charged particles travel faster than the phase speed of light in a dielectric medium [20]. Electrons polarize the surrounding dielectric medium as they travel through it. The net electromagnetic field is zero when the electrons travel slower than the phase speed of light, as the polarizations are symmetric. However, when the electrons are faster than the phase speed of light, nonzero net field, CR, is produced due to the asymmetric polarizations. Radiation therapy beams, such as photons and electrons, have high energy and produce CR when interacting with tissue or water. The produced CR wavelength ranges from ultraviolet to infrared.

Titanium dioxide is a semiconductor with a bandgap 3 eV [21] and has high absorbance to ultraviolet light. Upon excitation, electron–hole pairs are produced inside TONPs, and ROS are formed on the surfaces [22]. The CR produced by radiation therapy excites TONPs and creates electron–hole pairs; surrounding dissolved oxygen molecules accept electrons and form superoxide radicals; water molecules and hydroxide ions donate electrons and form hydroxyl radicals

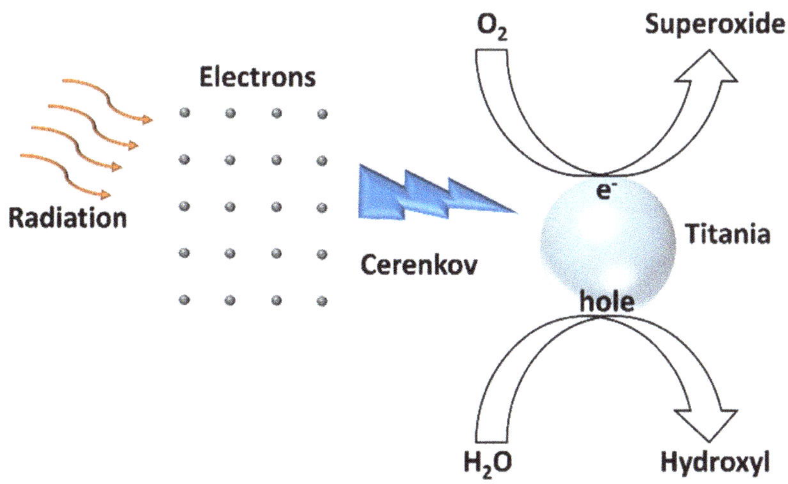

Figure 17.1. Production of CR in radiation therapy, followed by production of hydroxyl and superoxide radicals on the surface of TONP excited by CR. Reprinted from [23], copyright 2016 with permission from Associazione Italiana di Fisica Medica

(figure 17.1). The newly formed superoxide and hydroxyl radicals are capable of causing further oxidation and cell damage, and dose enhancement is therefore achieved.

To confirm the above theory, *in silico* and *in vitro* study was conducted. First, Monte Carlo simulations showed that 6 MV therapeutic radiation produced CR and up to 68% of the emitted CR could be absorbed by 5 $\mu g\ g^{-1}$ TONPs [16]. Second, TONP toxicity was tested on normal human umbilical vein endothelial cells and determined that 1 $\mu g\ g^{-1}$ of TONPs did not have significant impact on normal cell viability [16]. Last, irradiation to cancer cells (human lung and prostate cancers) treated with or without TONPs were performed, and the efficacy of increased cancer cell killing was confirmed using cell viability assays and clonogenic assays. 1 $\mu g\ g^{-1}$ of TONPs increased cancer cell killing by at least 20% for 6 MV radiations [23].

The application of TONPs is not limited to megavoltage external beams. Kotagiri *et al* reported more than three times in cancer cell killing *in vitro*, and complete tumor shrinkage *in vivo* due to the interactions of TONP and the CR generated by radionuclides (F-18) used in imaging [24]. This also indicates that TONPs may be used in conjunction with other radionuclides such as Ir-192 to enhance brachytherapy efficacy.

A detailed mathematical model was published by Kavadiya and Biswas [25] that integrated Cherenkov physics, light scattering, and photocatalytic reaction engineering to simulate ROS production in the presence of radionuclides and TONPs. It was shown that ROS production was dependent on particle size, concentration, light absorption, scattering efficiencies, and charge separation/recombination.

It is known that CR production depends on the charged particle energy—charged particles with higher energy yield more CR [23]. Although experiments with clinical electron beam therapy is not reported, the feasibility of CR enhancement with clinical electron beams is predicted, for its monoenergetic spectrum and higher effective energy compared to x-ray with the same energy peak.

17.4 Discussion

Because of the special physicochemical properties and biological applications, NPs are investigated for their uses in radiation therapy to increase tumor radiosensitization and normal tissue protection [12, 26]. Metal oxide NPs, such as CONPs and TONPs, are interesting for applications in radiation therapy because of the flexibility in oxidation states and catalyzing activities.

Translating preclinical results to clinical applications is challenging. One of the challenges is that preclinical experiments in radiation therapy are often performed with kilovoltage beams which are not for clinical treatment due to the lack of penetration. While ionizing radiations with different energies share many common properties, photon interaction cross-sections are energy dependent. Standardization in radiation dosimetry for *in vivo* and *in vitro* experiments is also necessary [27, 28]. Based on published results, NP size, concentration, and exposure time may affect the final outcome. The differences reported in the literature indicate that a unique optimal treatment may exist for a specific model. To further decide the best disease-specific treatment in preclinical models is urgent in NP aided radiation therapy research.

Monte Carlo simulation in radiation transport is a great tool for validation, dose calculation, and experiment design. However, unlike for ionizing radiation, data in experimentally determined optical photon transport properties in tissue and NP interactions are rare and not standardized. To generalize simulation methods in NP and photocatalysis related studies, much collaborated effort is needed to build an experiment-based database.

As demonstrated by numerous studies, NPs play important roles in ROS modulation and radiation therapy enhancement. The mechanism, although not fully understood, may be categorized into photocatalysis, biomimetic catalysis, NP-mediated radiolysis, etc. Although the categorization is neither perfect nor complete, it provides insights for further study in ROS modulated radiation therapy. Understanding the mechanism in ROS modulation in radiation therapy is essential to the application of NPs in cancer treatment. In conclusion, both CONPs and TONPs have great potential in achieving better treatment outcome and customizability in radiation therapy. Additionally, the low cost and wide availability of NPs may provide further benefits in lowering the cost of radiation therapy.

References

[1] Hall E and Giaccia A 2006 *Radiobiology for the Radiologist* (Philadelphia, PA: Lippincott Williams & Wilkins))

[2] Joiner M and Van der Kogel A 2009 *Basic Clinical Radiobiology* (London: Hodder Arnold)

[3] Khan F and Gibbons J 2014 *Khan's the Physics of Radiation Therapy* (Philadelphia, PA: Lippincott Williams & Wilkins)

[4] Chang B and Timmerman R 2007 Stereotactic body radiation therapy: a comprehensive review *Am. J. Clin. Oncol.* **30** 637–44

[5] Fu K, Pajak T, Trotti A, Jones C, Spencer S, Phillips T, Garden A, Ridge J, Cooper J and Ang K 2000 A Radiation Therapy Oncology Group (RTOG) phase III randomized study to compare hyperfractionation and two variants of accelerated fractionation to standard fractionation radiotherapy for head and neck squamous cell carcinomas: first report of RTOG 9003 *Int. J. Radiat. Oncol. Biol. Phys.* **48** 7–16

[6] Brenner D and Hall E 1999 Fractionation and protraction for radiotherapy of prostate carcinoma *Int. J. Radiat. Oncol. Biol. Phys.* **43** 1095–101

[7] Uematsu M, Shioda A, Tahara K, Fukui T, Yamamoto F, Tsumatori G, Ozeki Y, Aoki T, Watanabe M and Kusano S 1998 Focal, high dose, and fractionated modified stereotactic radiation therapy for lung carcinoma patients: a preliminary experience *Cancer* **82** 1062–70

[8] Hainfeld J, Dilmanian F, Slatkin D and Smilowitz H 2008 Radiotherapy enhancement with gold nanoparticles *J. Pharm. Pharmacol.* **60** 977–85

[9] Su X, Liu P, Wu H and Gu N 2014 Enhancement of radiosensitization by metal-based nanoparticles in cancer radiation therapy *Cancer Biol. Med.* **11** 86

[10] Asati A, Santra S, Kaittanis C and Perez J 2010 Surface-charge-dependent cell localization and cytotoxicity of cerium oxide nanoparticles *ACS Nano* **4** 5321–31

[11] Perez J, Asati A, Nath S and Kaittanis C 2008 Synthesis of biocompatible dextran-coated nanoceria with pH-dependent antioxidant properties *Small* **4** 552–6

[12] Ngwa W *et al* 2017 Smart radiation therapy biomaterials *Int. J. Radiat. Oncol. Biol. Phys.* **97** 624–37
[13] Ouyang Z, Mainali M, Sinha N, Strack G, Altundal Y, Hao Y, Winningham T, Sajo E, Celli J and Ngwa W 2016 Potential of using cerium oxide nanoparticles for protecting healthy tissue during accelerated partial breast irradiation (APBI) *Physica Med.* **32** 631–5
[14] Mullins D 2015 The surface chemistry of cerium oxide *Surf. Sci. Rep.* **70** 42–85
[15] Celardo I, De Nicola M, Mandoli C, Pedersen J, Traversa E and Ghibelli L 2011 Ce^{3+} ions determine redox-dependent anti-apoptotic effect of cerium oxide nanoparticles *ACS Nano* **5** 4537–49
[16] Ouyang Z 2017 Reactive oxygen species modulated radiation therapy *ProQuest* 10643714
[17] Das S, Neal C, Ortiz J and Seal S 2018 Engineered nanoceria cytoprotection *in vivo*: mitigation of reactive oxygen species and double-stranded DNA breakage due to radiation exposure *Nanoscale* **10** 21069–75
[18] Colon J, Herrera L, Smith J, Patil S, Komanski C, Kupelian P, Seal S, Jenkins D and Baker C 2009 Protection from radiation-induced pneumonitis using cerium oxide nanoparticles *Nanomed. Nanotechnol. Biol. Med.* **vol. 5** 225–31
[19] Nourmohammadi E, Khoshdel-sarkarizi H, Nedaeinia R, Sadeghnia H, Hasanzadeh L, Darroudi M and Kazemi Oskuee R 2019 Evaluation of anticancer effects of cerium oxide nanoparticles on mouse fibrosarcoma cell line *J. Cell. Physiol.* **234** 4987–96
[20] Jelley J 1958 *Cherenkov Radiation and its Applications* (London: Pergamon)
[21] Srikant V and Clarke D 1998 On the optical band gap of zinc oxide *J. Appl. Phys.* **83** 5447–51
[22] Morrison S and Freund T 1967 Chemical role of holes and electrons in ZnO photocatalysis *J. Chem. Phys.* **47** 1543–51
[23] Ouyang Z, Liu B, Yasmin-Karim S, Sajo E and Ngwa W 2016 Nanoparticle-aided external beam radiotherapy leveraging the Čerenkov effect *Physica Med.* **32** 944–7
[24] Kotagiri N, Sudlow G, Akers W and Achilefu S 2015 Breaking the depth dependency of phototherapy with Cerenkov radiation and low-radiance-responsive nanophotosensitizers *Nat. Nanotechnol.* **10** 370
[25] Kavadiya S and Biswas P 2018 Design of Cerenkov-assisted photoactivation of TiO_2 nanoparticles and reactive oxygen species generation for cancer treatment *J. Nucl. Med* **60** 702–9
[26] Ngwa W, Kumar R, Sridhar S, Korideck H, Zygmanski P, Cormack R, Berbeco R and Makrigiorgos G 2014 Targeted radiotherapy with gold nanoparticles: current status and future perspectives *Nanomedicine* **9** 1063–82
[27] Ngwa W, Korideck H, Chin L, Makrigiorgos G and Berbeco R 2011 MOSFET assessment of radiation dose delivered to mice using the Small Animal Radiation Research Platform (SARRP) *Radiat. Res.* **176** 816–20
[28] Jermoumi M, Korideck H, Bhagwat M, Zygmanski P, Makrigiogos G, Berbeco R, Cormack R and Ngwa W 2015 Comprehensive quality assurance phantom for the small animal radiation research platform (SARRP) *Physica Med.* **31** 529–35

Chapter 18

Accelerated Partial Breast Irradiation (APBI)

Gizem Cifter and Wilfred Ngwa

Breast cancer is a group of cancer cells that starts in the cells of the breast [1]. These cells can then invade surrounding tissues or spread (metastasize) to other areas of the body. According to the National Breast Cancer Foundation, one in eight women will be diagnosed with breast cancer in their lifetime, making breast cancer the second leading cause of death among women in the United States. The standard care of treatment for breast cancer usually includes surgery, chemotherapy, radiotherapy or combinations of these treatments, depending on the staging of the disease. Breast conserving surgery, or BCS, is often performed on patients who are diagnosed with early stage breast cancer [2]. Following breast conserving surgery, usually radiotherapy is given to patients in order to treat micro-scale disease that is invisible at the time of surgery. The motivation for this approach comes from recent studies, which revealed that the majority of breast cancer recurrences arise at or near the lumpectomy cavity [3, 4]; therefore radiotherapy is administered after BCS in order to kill any remaining cancerous cells around this cavity, which is the primary tumor site [5]. This understanding has led to the development and increasing use of Accelerated Partial Breast Irradiation (APBI) [6, 7]. Conceptually, during APBI only the tumor bed is treated with confined and high amounts of radiation. The prescribed dose is delivered only to the lumpectomy cavity and its vicinity. Since the tumor mass is removed with surgery, the target volume during radiotherapy is much smaller so the treatment can be 'accelerated' by decreasing the number of fractions while increasing the radiation dose [8]. This makes APBI particularly attractive to patients for both time and delivery convenience. Traditional radiotherapy takes about 6–8 weeks [9], while APBI can be delivered within 5 days, BID (twice a day treatment delivery) [10]. Following the BCS, APBI treatment may begin anywhere from 2–21 days post BCS [11].

Aside from the rapid treatment delivery, APBI can also be delivered with either external beam irradiation or brachytherapy [12]. The most common practice of brachytherapy APBI is typically applied with the use of a balloon applicator.

doi:10.1088/978-0-7503-2396-3ch18

MammoSite is the most well-known and historically performed applicator. That being said, recent studies comparing EBRT and BT conveyed controversy to APBI outcomes. As an example, some studies showed cosmesis problems and higher long-term toxicity compared to WBI [13]. This proves the need for development of APBI applications, potentially improving the results while addressing the limitations. To this end, the use of nanoparticles in conjunction with radiotherapy helps advance the use of APBI. It is already proven that the presence of nanoparticles of high-Z materials during radiotherapy can increase the local dose deposition [14] in the tumor volume. As explained in the introduction, when low energy photons interact with high-Z material, it results in emitting electrons from various orbits of the high-Z atoms. This concept is known as the photoelectric effect. These electrons will have low energy hence short range to travel. Thus, this additional dose, which is defined as the amount of energy deposited in mass of tissue, will be deposited in the near vicinity of where the photon/electron interaction occurred. While a large number of high-Z materials have been under focus for nanoparticle-aided radiotherapy, many researchers focused on gold nanoparticles. Gold is relatively more attractive for a couple reasons; its biocompatibility [15] and non-toxicity [16] has been proven by several researchers. Because of its known characteristics, investigation of its radiosensitization effects is well understood [14, 17].

This work particularly investigates the dosimetric feasibility of gold nanoparticles (GNPs) during delivery of APBI. The quantitative radiosensitivity of GNPs during radiotherapy using both external beam radiotherapy and brachytherapy is taken into account. By virtue of the concept of dose enhancement due to nanoparticle-aided radiotherapy, dose to healthy tissue could potentially be decreased. This could result in better treatment outcomes, reducing long-term toxicity and cosmesis problems, potentially.

18.1 Methods

After the BCS, the tissue around the lumpectomy cavity (from where the primary tumor has been surgically removed) is irradiated via either brachytherapy or external beam therapy. During brachytherapy, a balloon applicator is inserted into the lumpectomy cavity and the irradiation can be performed using the 50 kVp Xoft electronic brachytherapy source [18–20]. In the case of external beam irradiation, the lumpectomy cavity site is irradiated by a 6 MV linac source. For the electronic brachytherapy case, our proposed method is to deliver GNPs via *in situ* release from a GNP-loaded polymer film that is coated on the surface of the balloon applicator (figure 18.1(a)). For the external beam irradiation, our proposed method of administration of the GNPs is administering the NPs within the saline solution, which will be used to expand the lumpectomy cavity (figure 18.1(b)). The spectra for the 50 kVp Xoft electronic brachytherapy device was generated using the Spekcalc program [21, 22]. Monte Carlo generated 6 MV spectra for 4 cm × 4 cm field size at 1.5 cm depth [23] was also used.

Two different GNP sizes, 10 nm and 2 nm, were investigated in this work in order to understand the diffusion characteristics of GNPs. The impact of of size on GNP

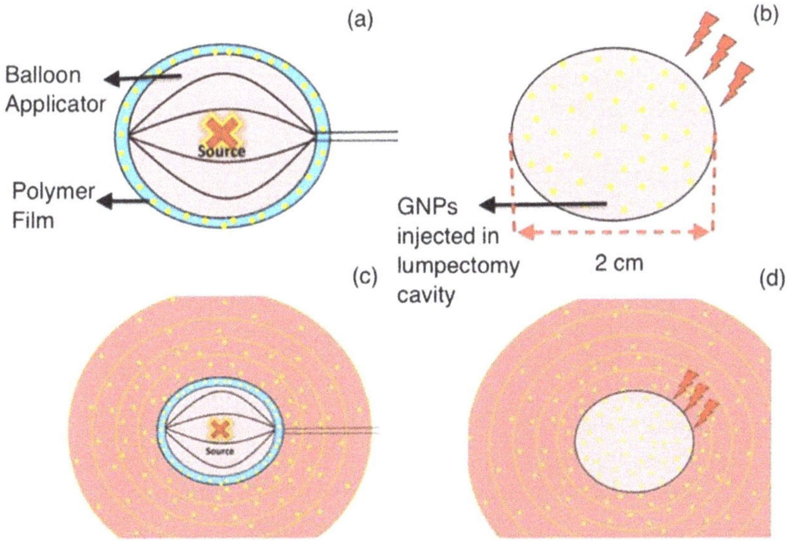

Figure 18.1. A schematic diagram of the distribution of GNPs in lumpectomy cavity for; (a) case I, (b) case II. Case I represents GNPs incorporated in polymer film on the surface of the Xoft balloon applicator. Case II shows GNPs injected inside lumpectomy cavity via syringe-like tool. (c) Diffusion of NP for case I and (d) diffusion of NP for case II.

diffusion could potentially be significant, resulting in important changes during the time of irradiation. Hence, in order to calculate the dose enhancement to the target volume, which was defined as the volume that is 1 cm away from the surface of the lumpectomy cavity, the diffusion profiles of 2 and 10 nm GNPs were acquired. These profiles were associated with time of GNP delivery and only then the dose enhancement ratios with respect to radiotherapy delivery were calculated. In order to generate the diffusion profiles, we first used an experimentally determined diffusion coefficient for 10 nm particles [24] $D = 2.2 \times 10^{-8}$ cm^2 s^{-1}, and then extrapolated it to 2 nm GNPs by using the Stokes–Einstein equation (equation (18.1)):

$$D = \frac{k_B T}{6\pi\eta r}, \tag{18.1}$$

where, k_B is Boltzmann's constant, T is the absolute temperature, η is the dynamic viscosity of the medium and r is the radius of the nanoparticles. The diffusion coefficient for 2 nm particles was found $D = 11 \times 10^{-8}$ cm^2 s^{-1}. We assumed that the Stokes–Einstein relation for the diffusion coefficient of nanoparticles is valid in tissue media, and that the mean viscosity is constant in the particle size and concentration ranges considered in this paper. Since the motion of nanoparticles is assumed to be only in radial direction, 1D Stokes–Einstein approximation is assumed to be appropriate.

We used Fick's second law to determine the GNP concentration at any time/point in time inside the target volume. For given boundary conditions, such as initial concentration, concentration of GNPs inside the source (lumpectomy cavity surface in our case), time-controlled release profiles can be generated by Fick's second law:

$$\frac{C(x, t) - C_0}{C_s - C_0} = 1 - erf\left(\frac{x}{2\sqrt{Dt}}\right). \tag{18.2}$$

As provided by Fick's second law, it is important to define the initial conditions. For that reason, it is necessary to know the number of gold nanoparticles present inside the lumpectomy cavity, whether on the applicator surface or inside the lumpectomy cavity. The number of GNPs interacting with photons in the target area depends on the initial concentration as well as the diffusion rate of the nanoparticles. Although the characteristics of GNPs are well understood and gold is considered to be inert, two different concentrations of GNPs was investigated in order to determine the dose enhancement impact under conditions in which administration of high concentrations are not feasible. The two initial GNP concentrations (C_0) were used in this work are; 7 mg g^{-1} and 43 mg g^{-1} for a lumpectomy cavity size of 2 cm in diameter. An *in vivo* animal study showed that there are no toxic side effects of GNPs when used with a 7 mg g^{-1} concentration [25, 26]. We took that as our base low concentration to be used under conditions where higher concentrations are not feasible. In addition, we used 43 mg g^{-1} GNP concentration since it is the FDA approved concentration of cisplatin, which is relatively more toxic than gold [27].

The hypothesis behind the dose enhancement due to interactions of radiation with GNPs is based on the photoelectric effect. The localized dose boost to tumor cells will result from micrometer ranged photo-/Auger electrons emitted from the high-*Z* GNPs due to the interactions with low energy photons during APBI. In order to understand the true 'enhancement' in dose delivery, we performed analytical calculations, which allowed us to eliminate dependence of initial/prescribed dose. The dose enhancement factor, DEF, is defined as the ratio of dose to each tumor voxel with and without GNPs. Physically, for example, if the DEF is 2, it means the delivered dose in the presence of GNPs is doubled (or 100% higher) compared to dose without nanoparticles.

The analytical calculation method is explained further in previous publications by Ngwa [28] and Sinha [29] and by previous chapters in this book. Briefly, in this approach a tumor voxel is modeled as a slab of 10 μm × 10 μm × 10 μm, representing a sub-volume containing a tumor cell of diameter 10 μm. The energy deposited by an emitted electron, *E*, is calculated by Cole's electron energy loss formula [30] (equation (18.3)):

$$\frac{dE}{dR} = 3.316(R + 0.007)^{0.435} + 0.0055R^{0.33}. \tag{18.3}$$

Here $R = R_{\text{tot}} - r$, where r is the distance from the photoelectron emission site and R_{tot} is the total range of the photoelectron (equation (18.4)).

$$R_{tot} = 0.431(E + 0.367)^{1.77}0.007 \quad (18.4)$$

By integrating equation (18.4) over the range of emitted electron energies, the total energy deposited in a tumor sub-volume was calculated.

There are, however, some underlying assumptions to this model. For example, the GNPs are assumed to be distributed homogeneously within the source, inside the lumpectomy cavity and/or on or within the polymer film on the balloon applicator. The analytical calculation does *not* depend on the uniformity of GNP distribution, hence it would not alter the DEF result. Moreover, the behavior of GNPs within a human/animal system is unpredictable. Past studies showed that NPs tend to accumulate near tumor vasculature and the direction through which they will diffuse could vary depending on multiple reasons. In the grand scheme of things, however, we considered a uniform and homogenous diffusion of GNPs within the tumor volume and did not alter the Fick's second law. Furthermore, upon insertion of GNPs inside the lumpectomy cavity, it is also reasonable to expect a burst release initially. This could result in a shift in GNP release and diffusion profiles that are acquired by the diffusion model.

The consequence of these assumptions and that of the burst release will be addressed in the discussion section.

Due to the short range of photo/Auger electrons emitted by GNPs, the dose enhancement is expected to be localized almost entirely within the planning target volume (PTV) containing any residual tumor cells. This is one of the strengths of nanoparticle-aided radiotherapy as long as the location of nanoparticles is well known and can be controlled. This makes our proposed method of delivering GNPs during ABPI particularly of interest. Successive delivery of GNPs within the lumpectomy cavity and time-controlled release and delivery of radiation could allow for sub-volume dose boosting while sparing the dose to surrounding healthy tissue.

18.2 Results

The first results shown in figures 18.2(a) and (b) are illustrations of diffusion profiles of 2 and 10 nm GNPs, respectively. The diffusion profiles were analyzed for 1, 3, 5 and 7 days, denoted as blue, green, red and cyan colors, with respect to distance from the lumpectomy cavity. For therapeutic purposes, distance diffusion profiles were only analyzed up to 1 cm away from the lumpectomy cavity. The first take away from these results is the dependency of diffusion on the size of the nanoparticle. As previous diffusion models also suggest, smaller NPs travel faster compared to bigger NPs. It is evident that 2 nm GNPs diffuse faster compared to 10 nm GNPs. This analysis was performed only up to 7 days following injection of GNPs since 7 days is the typical time required for APBI treatment delivery [6]. It is evident that the size and concentration of GNPs would allow acquiring different diffusion models, potentially permitting the customization of treatment for individuals.

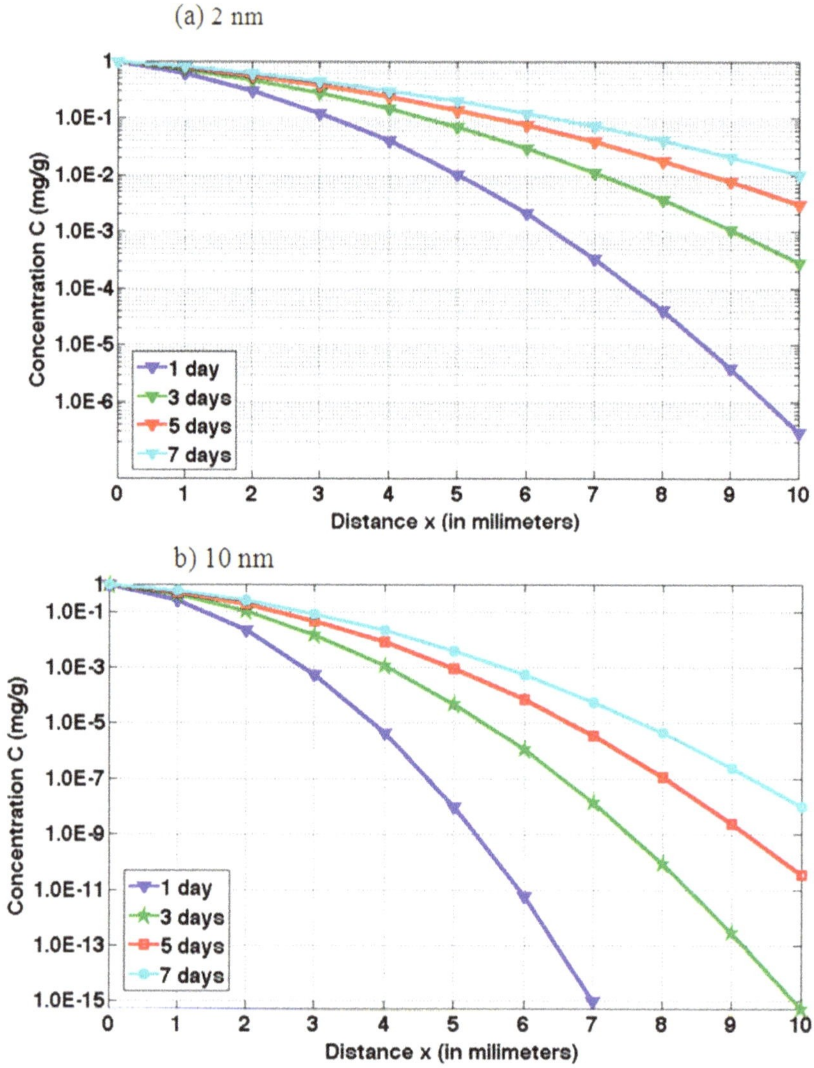

Figure 18.2. Diffusion profiles for 2 and 10 nm GNPs, up to 1 cm at different times and positions.

Following the analysis of GNP diffusion profiles, DEF with respect to distance was performed. The results presented in figures 18.3 and 18.4 show DEF values 7 days post administration of GNPs, that are exposed to irradiation with 50-kVp electronic brachytherapy and 6 MV linac sources, respectively. Since variety concentrations of GNPs can be delivered to lumpectomy cavity, concentration range from 7 mg g^{-1} to 43-mg g^{-1} was chosen in order to identify DEF variation. Figure 18.3 presents DEF versus distance for 50 kVp electronic source for 2 and 10 nm GNPs up to 1 cm away from lumpectomy cavity surface. DEF is higher for 2 nm GNPs compared to 10 nm GNPs as expected, supporting our earlier results. DEF values were also found to be higher in areas of near proximity to lumpectomy cavity compared to distal sites, due

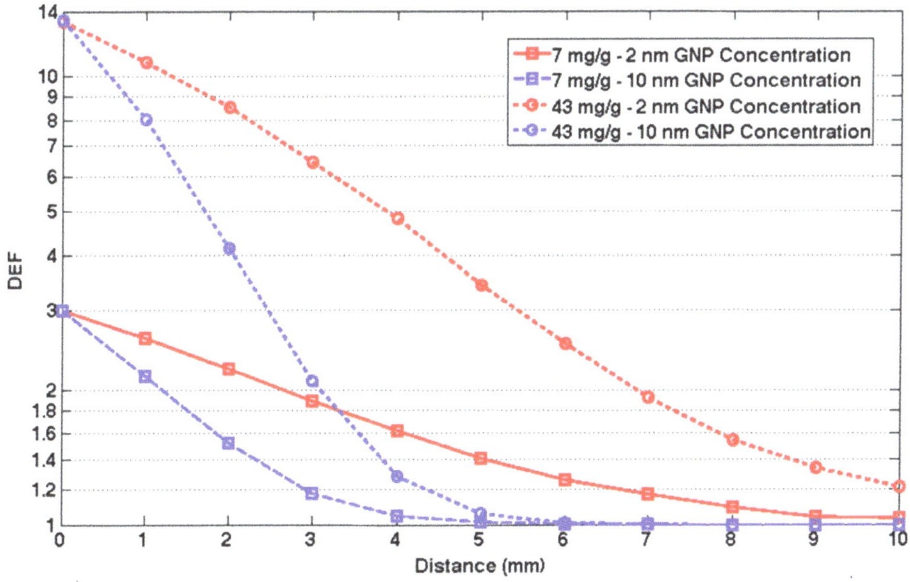

Figure 18.3. DEF versus distance for 2 and 10 nm GNPs, with irradiation performed 7 days post injection using a 50 kVp x-ray source with 7 mg g^{-1} and 43 mg g^{-1} GNP concentrations.

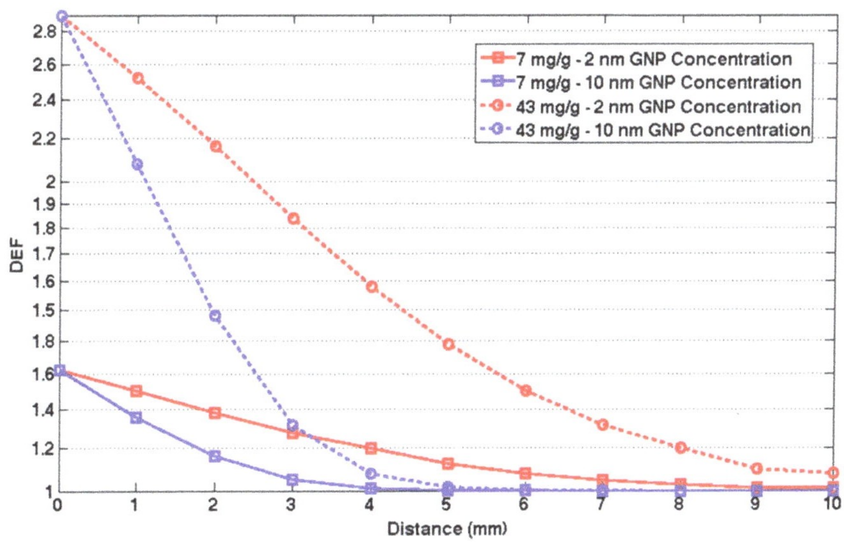

Figure 18.4. DEF versus distance for 2 and 10 nm GNPs, with irradiation performed 7 days post injection with 6 MV linac source 4 cm × 4 cm field size at 1.5 cm depth with 7 mg g^{-1} and 43 mg g^{-1} concentrations.

to higher GNP concentration. DEF values indicating 20% higher dose overall in the presence of GNPs (DEF > 1.2) were achievable using both 2 nm and 10 nm GNPs with 43 mg g^{-1} concentrations. These were found at 10 mm and 4 mm distance, respectively. This result also implies that DEF is much higher up to these distances.

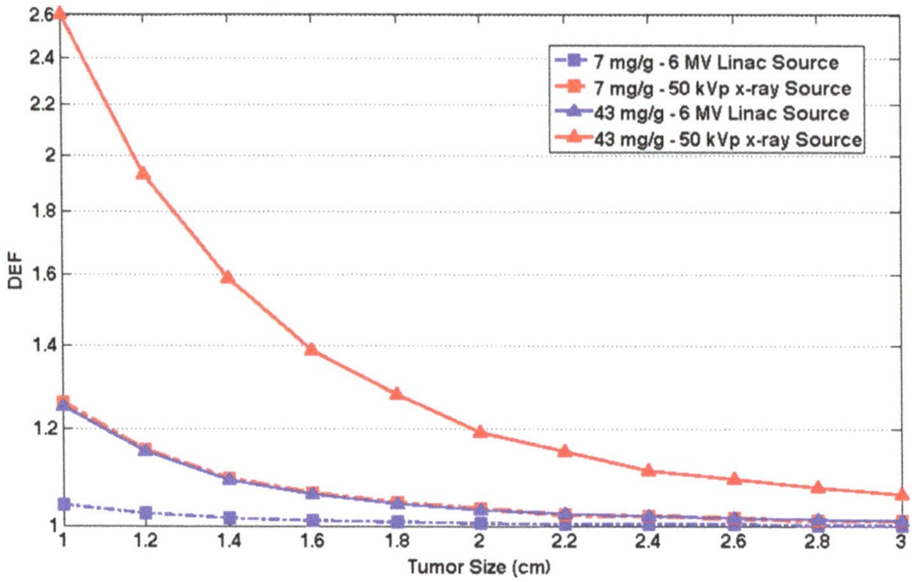

Figure 18.5. DEF values with respect to different tumor sizes for 7 mg g^{-1} and 43 mg g^{-1} concentrations of 2 nm GNPs irradiated with 50 kVp x-ray source and 6 MV linac source.

Figure 18.4 shows results in a similar way for a 6 MV linac source. As expected, DEF values are lower for the 6 MV linac source, compared to 50 kVp electronic brachytherapy source. The parameters for the simulated 6 MV linac source is 4 cm × 4 cm field size at 1.5 cm depth. Depth of 1.5 cm was chosen since it is the appropriate depth for target during breast irradiation. Similar to results on figure 18.3, DEF values of (DEF > 1.2) with 43 mg g^{-1} concentration of 2 and 10 nm GNPs were found at 6 mm and 2 mm away from the lumpectomy cavity, respectively.

Lastly, the DEF analysis for various tumor sizes was performed in order to account for customization for individuals. Keeping the concentration interval the same as with other analysis, the DEF was calculated for tumor volume sizes ranging from 1 cm to 3 cm. Deservedly, figure 18.5 shows lower DEF values for larger tumor volumes. This can be solely explained for the decrease of the GNP concentration over the larger target volume, referencing our earlier results above.

18.3 Discussion

This chapter is focused on the dose enhancement in the presence of GNPs to an APBI PTV following BCS. The PTV is expected to contain remaining tumor cells after BCS and two types of treatment approaches were considered; 6 MV linac and 50 kVp electronic brachytherapy sources. The analysis of dose enhancement with respect to two initial GNP concentrations and their corresponding diffusion profiles, along with two different GNP sizes shows that significant DEF can be achieved. Moreover, our results prove that this approach could be customized and various DEFs could be achievable, which would allow customized treatment delivery for individuals.

The motivation behind nanoparticle-aided therapy arises from previous clinical studies proving that radiation dose boost can help prevent cancer recurrence [1, 30, 31]. While in theory GNPs could help boost dose to tumor sub-volumes, it is imperative to point out the clinical applicability of delivery method. Since, APBI is usually delivered soon after BCS, it is important to determine the release and diffusion profiles of GNPs from lumpectomy cavity to tumor sub-volumes. Our results indicate that, when sufficient concentrations are used, even after 7 days following insertion of GNPs, substantial dose boost would be attained. APBI delivered by brachytherapy is usually delivered within a week, which would allow the GNPs to diffuse far enough to reach remaining cancerous cells, while still remaining in the shallow distances away from the lumpectomy cavity, eliminating boosting dose to healthy tissue. This is true since the dose boost comes from the photo and Auger electrons which are emitted by the nanoparticles. The energy and the range of these nanoparticles are considerably small hence the dose boost would only occur in the near vicinity of the nanoparticle. Therefore, the biodistribution of GNPs from the lumpectomy cavity to distal areas is an important parameter in the efficacy of such nanoparticle-aided APBI.

The analytical approach used here was published in previous work and the results have been parallel to those of experimental and Monte Carlo results, which have also shown significant dose enhancement [32, 33]. One other theoretical study by Sinha *et al* [29] considered the release of GNPs from the surface of a brachytherapy spacer using the same analytical approach, and also showed significant DEF values similar to the ones presented here. In both the incidences, a burst release form was observed, resulting in diffusion through the lumpectomy cavity surface, immediately. However, for case 1, in practice, GNPs will be incorporated into a polymer film, and their release rate from such films must be accounted for. That being said, the release can potentially be controlled, and customized for particular cases, by modifying the polymer film parameters, such as polymer weight or type [34]. Specific locations of GNPs were not considered in the tumor sub-volume or the cell in our analytical calculations. Therefore, the actual DEF could vary a small amount in reality. Furthermore, since the actual DNA damage occurs in the sub-atomical level, meaning the DNA damage emanates when the emitted electrons are close enough to reach the cell's nucleus, the DEF is expected to be higher. However, our analytical approach disregards the location of nanoparticles. A recent study [35] shows that nuclear targeting with nanoparticles is achievable and could, thus, be employed here to maximize damage to the tumor cells' DNA.

Further investigation regarding targeting cell nucleus/DNA would improve the dosimetric feasibility of GNPs [35–37]. Such methods could include functionalizing GNPs via binding agents to cancerous cells. This would also result in potentially sparing healthy tissue since dose boost to tumor cells would permit the decrease of the prescribed dose, resulting in lower exposure to normal tissue. This would potentially help overcome long-term toxicity side effects and cosmesis problems currently associated with APBI.

We could also argue that the same concentrations of GNPs within lumpectomy cavity could result in higher dose enhancement via coating the balloon applicator method since higher number of GNPs would in fact be diffusing through the lumpectomy surface. Consequently, this delivery of GNPs to tumor sub-volumes would result in higher DEF values.

Furthermore, the choice of RT delivery could play a vital role in terms of GNP release of diffusion control. As mentioned previously, APBI may begin anywhere from 2–21 days after BCS [11]. In this work, we followed a conservative approach and assumed APBI to be delivered immediately after BCS. If GNPs were administrated inside the lumpectomy cavity at the end of the surgery, and APBI delivery was delayed for any possible reason, GNPs could reach distal volumes. This could result in successive targeting of cancerous cells that are father away or unintentionally harming healthy tissue. On the other hand, this concept could also allow the customization of the treatment delivery and boost for individuals. Earlier release of GNPs would result in higher number of GNPs released from the lumpectomy cavity surface, resulting in higher DEF values.

As mentioned above, two different concentrations of GNPs were considered in this work both for justifiable reasons. However, the maximum amount of GNPs that can be incorporated with polymer films is yet to be determined experimentally. Experimental study, could potentially yield more information regarding the GNP capacity of polymer film, depending on its size and thickness. As a result, GNP concentrations that are in fact feasible could be different than what is demonstrated here. That being said, our results demonstrate feasibility providing valuable insight for planning experimental investigations.

18.4 Conclusion

APBI has been growing in popularity over recent years and it is the preferred method of treatment amongst early stage breast cancer patients. Most of the time, radiation boost follows BCS and it has been shown that boosting dose to tumor sub-volumes helps prevent cancer recurrence. Our suggested method offers such delivery with no additional inconvenience or harm to patients, and in fact, it could potentially help eliminate dose to healthy tissue. Our preliminary results suggest that significant dose enhancement can be achieved to residual tumor cells by administering GNPs to tumor cells. During APBI treatment delivery, the interaction of radiation with nanoparticles of high-Z nanoparticles would result in dose boost due to emission of secondary electrons. Our findings motivate further studies, particularly experimental work towards development of such novel work to understand the characteristics of nanoparticles in the human system as well as the functionalization of nanoparticles. This method could potentially address the current limitations of APBI and toxicity related skin problems.

References

[1] https://nationalbreastcancer.org/

[2] Fisher B *et al* 2002 Twenty-year follow-up of a randomized trial comparing total mastectomy, lumpectomy, and lumpectomy plus irradiation for the treatment of invasive breast cancer *N. Engl. J. Med.* **347** 1233–41

[3] Jagsi R and Haffty B G 2013 External-beam accelerated partial-breast irradiation: exploring the limits of tolerability *J. Clin. Oncol.* **31** 4029–31
[4] Arthur D W *et al* 2003 Partial breast brachytherapy after lumpectomy: low-dose-rate and high-dose-rate experience *Int. J. Radiat. Oncol. Biol. Phys.* **56** 681–9
[5] Veronesi U *et al* 2002 Twenty-year follow-up of a randomized study comparing breast-conserving surgery with radical mastectomy for early breast cancer *N. Engl. J. Med.* **347** 1227–32
[6] Sanders M E *et al* 2007 Accelerated partial breast irradiation in early-stage breast cancer *J. Clin. Oncol.* **25** 996–1002
[7] Benitez P R *et al* 2004 Partial breast irradiation in breast conserving therapy by way of intersitial brachytherapy *Am. J. Surg.* **188** 355–64
[8] Lewin A A *et al* 2012 Accelerated partial breast irradiation is safe and effective using intensity-modulated radiation therapy in selected early-stage breast cancer *Int. J. Radiat. Oncol. Biol. Phys.* **82** 2104–10
[9] Froud P J *et al* 2000 Effect of time interval between breast-conserving surgery and radiation therapy on ipsilateral breast recurrence *Int. J. Radiat. Oncol. Biol. Phys.* **46** 363–72
[10] Tsai P I *et al* 2006 Accelerated partial breast irradiation using the mammosite device: early technical experience and short-term clinical follow-up *Am. Surg.* **72** 929–34
[11] Lori L and Vanyo M D 2009 *Accelerated Partial Breast Irradiation (APBI)* (Pomona, CA: The Robert and Beverly Lewis Family Cancer Care Center)
[12] Njeh C F, Saunders M W and Langton C M 2010 Accelerated Partial Breast Irradiation (APBI): a review of available techniques *Radiat. Oncol.* **5** 90
[13] Piroth M D 2013 [Risks of unfavorable cosmetic and toxicity after percutaneous accelerated partial breast irradiation (APBI). Interim analysis from the Canadian RAPID trial] *Strahlenther. Onkol.* **189** 1054–5
[14] Ngwa W *et al* 2014 Targeted radiotherapy with gold nanoparticles: current status and future perspectives *Nanomedicine* **9** 1063–82
[15] Grant S A *et al* 2014 Assessment of the biocompatibility and stability of a gold nanoparticle collagen bioscaffold *J. Biomed. Mater. Res.* A **102** 332–9
[16] Alkilany A M and Murphy C J 2010 Toxicity and cellular uptake of gold nanoparticles: what we have learned so far? *J. Nanopart. Res.* **12** 2313–33
[17] Hainfeld J F, Slatkin D N and Smilowitz H M 2004 The use of gold nanoparticles to enhance radiotherapy in mice *Phys. Med. Biol.* **49** N309–15
[18] Park C C *et al* 2010 American Society for Therapeutic Radiology and Oncology (ASTRO) Emerging Technology Committee report on electronic brachytherapy *Int. J. Radiat. Oncol. Biol. Phys.* **76** 963–72
[19] Shaikh T *et al* 2010 Improvement in interobserver accuracy in delineation of the lumpectomy cavity using fiducial markers *Int. J. Radiat. Oncol. Biol. Phys.* **78** 1127–34
[20] Park C K *et al* 2012 Validating fiducial markers for image-guided radiation therapy for accelerated partial breast irradiation in early-stage breast cancer *Int. J. Radiat. Oncol. Biol. Phys.* **82** e425–31
[21] Poludniowski G *et al* 2009 SpekCalc: a program to calculate photon spectra from tungsten anode x-ray tubes *Phys. Med. Biol.* **54** N433–8
[22] Spekcalc_Program_http://spekcalc.weebly.com.

[23] Liu H H and Verhaegen F 2002 An investigation of energy spectrum and lineal energy variations in mega-voltage photon beams used for radiotherapy *Radiat. Prot. Dosimetry* **99** 425–7

[24] Wong C *et al* 2011 Multistage nanoparticle delivery system for deep penetration into tumor tissue *Proc. Natl Acad. Sci. USA* **108** 2426–31

[25] Cho S H, Jones B L and Krishnan S 2009 The dosimetric feasibility of gold nanoparticle-aided radiation therapy (GNRT) via brachytherapy using low-energy gamma-/x-ray sources *Phys. Med. Biol.* **54** 4889–905

[26] Hainfeld J F *et al* 2006 Gold nanoparticles: a new X-ray contrast agent *Br. J. Radiol.* **79** 248–53

[27] FDA-Database.http://accessdata.fda.gov/drugsatfda_docs/label/2011/018057s080lbl.pdf.

[28] Ngwa W, Makrigiorgos G M and Berbeco R I 2012 Gold nanoparticle-aided brachytherapy with vascular dose painting: estimation of dose enhancement to the tumor endothelial cell nucleus *Med. Phys.* **39** 392–8

[29] Sinha N *et al* 2014 Brachytherapy application with *in situ* dose painting administered by gold nanoparticle eluters *Int. J. Radiat. Oncol. Biol. Phys.* **91** 385–92

[30] Cole A 1969 Absorption of 20-eV to 50,000-eV electron beams in air and plastic *Radiat. Res.* **38** 7–33

[31] Bartelink H *et al* 2007 Impact of a higher radiation dose on local control and survival in breast-conserving therapy of early breast cancer: 10-year results of the randomized boost versus no boost EORTC 22881-10882 trial *J. Clin. Oncol.* **25** 3259–65

[32] Ngwa W, Makrigiorgos G M and Berbeco R I 2010 Applying gold nanoparticles as tumor-vascular disrupting agents during brachytherapy: Estimation of endothelial dose enhancement *Phys. Med. Biol.* **55** 6533–48

[33] Berbeco R I, Ngwa W and Makrigiorgos G M 2011 Localised dose enhancement to tumor blood vessel endothelial cells via megavoltage x-rays and targeted gold nanoparticles: New potential for external beam radiotherapy *Int. J. Radiat. Oncol. Biol.Phys.* **81** 270–6

[34] Nagesha D K *et al* 2010 Radiosensitizer-eluting nanocoatings on gold fiducials for biological *in situ* image-guided radio therapy (BIS-IGRT) *Phys. Med. Biol.* **55** 6039–52

[35] Yang C *et al* 2014 Peptide modified gold nanoparticles for improved cellular uptake, nuclear transport, and intracellular retention *Nanoscale* **6** 12026–33.

[36] Chithrani B D, Ghazani A A and Chan W C 2006 Determining the size and shape dependence of gold nanoparticle uptake into mammalian cells *Nano Lett.* **6** 662–8

[37] Perrault S D *et al* 2009 Mediating tumor targeting efficiency of nanoparticles through design *Nano Lett.* **9** 1909–15

www.ingramcontent.com/pod-product-compliance
Ingram Content Group UK Ltd.
Pitfield, Milton Keynes, MK11 3LW, UK
UKHW051903100926
8556IPUK00005B/740

9 780750 323949